T0198202

Advances in Clinical Cytometry

Editor

CHRISTOPHER B. HERGOTT

CLINICS IN LABORATORY MEDICINE

www.labmed.theclinics.com

Consulting Editor
MILENKO JOVAN TANASIJEVIC

September 2023 • Volume 43 • Number 3

ELSEVIER

1600 John F. Kennedy Boulevard ● Suite 1800 ● Philadelphia, Pennsylvania, 19103-2899

http://www.theclinics.com

CLINICS IN LABORATORY MEDICINE Volume 43, Number 3
September 2023 ISSN 0272-2712, ISBN-13: 978-0-443-18284-6

Editor: Taylor Hayes
Developmental Editor: Akshay Samson

© **2023 Elsevier Inc. All rights reserved.**

This periodical and the individual contributions contained in it are protected under copyright by Elsevier, and the following terms and conditions apply to their use:

Photocopying
Single photocopies of single articles may be made for personal use as allowed by national copyright laws. Permission of the Publisher and payment of a fee is required for all other photocopying, including multiple or systematic copying, copying for advertising or promotional purposes, resale, and all forms of document delivery. Special rates are available for educational institutions that wish to make photocopies for non-profit educational classroom use. For information on how to seek permission visit www.elsevier.com/permissions or call: (+44) 1865 843830 (UK)/(+1) 215 239 3804 (USA).

Derivative Works
Subscribers may reproduce tables of contents or prepare lists of articles including abstracts for internal circulation within their institutions. Permission of the Publisher is required for resale or distribution outside the institution. Permission of the Publisher is required for all other derivative works, including compilations and translations (please consult www.elsevier.com/permissions).

Electronic Storage or Usage
Permission of the Publisher is required to store or use electronically any material contained in this periodical, including any article or part of an article (please consult www.elsevier.com/permissions). Except as outlined above, no part of this publication may be reproduced, stored in a retrieval system or transmitted in any form or by any means, electronic, mechanical, photocopying, recording or otherwise, without prior written permission of the Publisher.

Notice
No responsibility is assumed by the Publisher for any injury and/or damage to persons or property as a matter of products liability, negligence or otherwise, or from any use or operation of any methods, products, instructions or ideas contained in the material herein. Because of rapid advances in the medical sciences, in particular, independent verification of diagnoses and drug dosages should be made.

Although all advertising material is expected to conform to ethical (medical) standards, inclusion in this publication does not constitute a guarantee or endorsement of the quality or value of such product or of the claims made of it by its manufacturer.

Reprints. For copies of 100 or more, of articles in this publication, please contact the Commercial Reprints Department, Elsevier Inc., 360 Park Avenue South, New York, New York 10010-1710. Tel. 212-633-3874, Fax: 212-633-3820, E-mail: reprints@elsevier.com.

Clinics in Laboratory Medicine (ISSN 0272-2712) is published quarterly by Elsevier Inc., 360 Park Avenue South, New York, NY 10010-1710. Months of issue are March, June, September, and December. Business and Editorial offices: 1600 John F. Kennedy Blvd., Suite 1800, Philadelphia, PA 19103-2899. Periodicals postage paid at New York, NY and additional mailing offices. Subscription prices are $291.00 per year (US individuals), $657.00 per year (US institutions), $100.00 per year (US students), $374.00 per year (Canadian individuals), $798.00 per year (Canadian institutions), $100.00 per year (Canadian students), $416.00 per year (international individuals), $798.00 per year (international institutions), $185.00 (international students). Foreign air speed delivery is included in all Clinics subscription prices. All prices are subject to change without notice. POSTMASTER: Send address changes to *Clinics in Laboratory Medicine*, Elsevier Health Sciences Division, Subscription Customer Service, 3251 Riverport Lane, Maryland Heights, MO 63043. **Customer Service: 1-800-654-2452 (US). From outside of the US and Canada, call 1-314-447-8871. Fax: 1-314-447-8029. E-mail: journalscustomerservice-usa@elsevier.com (for print support) or journalsonlinesupport-usa@elsevier.com (for online support).**

Clinics in Laboratory Medicine is covered in *EMBASE/Exerpta Medica, MEDLINE/PubMed (Index Medicus), Cinahl, Current Contents/Clinical Medicine, BIOSIS and ISI/BIOMED.*

Contributors

EDITOR-IN-CHIEF

MILENKO JOVAN TANASIJEVIC, MD, MBA
Vice Chair for Clinical Pathology and Quality, Department of Pathology, Director of Clinical Laboratories, Brigham and Women's Hospital, Dana-Farber Cancer Institute, Associate Professor of Pathology, Harvard Medical School, Boston, Massachusetts

EDITOR

CHRISTOPHER B. HERGOTT, MD, PhD
Associate Pathologist, Department of Pathology, Brigham and Women's Hospital, Harvard Medical School, Boston, Massachusetts

AUTHORS

FERAS ALLY, MD
Department of Laboratory Medicine and Pathology, Seattle, WA

BACHIR ALOBEID, MD
Professor, Department of Pathology and Cell Biology, Columbia University Irving Medical Center, New York, New York

ANDREW A. BORKOWSKI, MD
AI Facility Lead, National Artificial Intelligence Institute, Washington, DC; Chief, Artificial Intelligence Service, James A. Haley Veterans' Hospital, Professor of Pathology and Cell Biology, University of South Florida Morsani School of Medicine, Tampa, Florida

ELIZABETH L. COURVILLE, MD
Department of Pathology, University of Virginia Health, Charlottesville, Virginia

KRISZTIÁN CSOMÓS, PhD
Division of Pediatric Allergy/Immunology, University of South Florida, Johns Hopkins All Children's Hospital, St Petersburg, Florida

KARA L. DAVIS, DO
Assistant Professor, Department of Pediatrics, Stanford University School of Medicine, Center for Cancer Cell Therapy, Stanford University, Stanford, California

SIBA EL HUSSEIN, MD
Department of Pathology, University of Rochester Medical Center, Rochester, New York

ANDREW L. FRELINGER III, PhD
Center for Platelet Research Studies, Dana-Farber/Boston Children's Cancer and Blood Disorders Center, Harvard Medical School, Boston, Massachusetts

JONATHAN R. FROMM, MD, PhD
Department of Laboratory Medicine and Pathology, University of Washington, Seattle, WA

DAVID GAJZER, MD
Department of Laboratory Medicine and Pathology, University of Washington, Seattle, WA

QI GAO, DCLS, MLS ASCP(CM)
Department of Pathology and Laboratory Medicine, Memorial Sloan Kettering Cancer Center, New York, New York

DAVID A. GORLIN, MS
Medical Doctoral Candidate, University of Florida, College of Medicine, Gainesville, Florida

CHRISTOPHER B. HERGOTT, MD, PhD
Associate Pathologist, Department of Pathology, Brigham and Women's Hospital, Harvard Medical School, Boston, Massachusetts

ABHISHEK KOLADIYA, PhD
Post-doctoral fellow, Department of Pediatrics, Stanford University School of Medicine, Stanford, California

ATTILA KUMÁNOVICS, MD
Department of Laboratory Medicine and Pathology, Mayo Clinic, Rochester, Minnesota

JASON H. KURZER, MD, PhD
Clinical Assistant Professor, Department of Pathology, Stanford University School of Medicine, Stanford, California

ANAND SHREERAM LAGOO, MD, PhD, FCAP
Professor of Pathology, Director, Clinical Flow Cytometry Laboratory, Duke University Health System, Duke University School of Medicine, Durham, North Carolina

JOSHUA E. LEWIS, MD, PhD
Resident, Department of Pathology, Brigham and Women's Hospital, Harvard Medical School, Boston, Massachusetts

SANAM LOGHAVI, MD
Department of Hematopathology, The University of Texas MD Anderson Cancer Center, Houston, Texas

FABIENNE LUCAS, MD, PhD
Senior Clinical Pathology Resident, Department of Pathology, Brigham and Women's Hospital, Boston, Massachusetts

HIBBAH NABEEL, MD
Clinical Fellow, Department of Pathology and Cell Biology, Columbia University Irving Medical Center, New York, New York

MIKHAIL ROSHAL, MD, PhD
Department of Pathology and Laboratory Medicine, Memorial Sloan Kettering Cancer Center, New York, New York

AMIR A. SADIGHI AKHA, MD, DPhil
Department of Laboratory Medicine and Pathology, Mayo Clinic, Rochester, Minnesota

ROBERT P. SEIFERT, MD
Associate Professor, Department of Pathology, Immunology and Laboratory Medicine, University of Florida, College of Medicine, Gainesville, Florida

AMRIT P. SINGH, MD
Department of Pathology, University of Virginia Health, Charlottesville, Virginia

BENJAMIN E.J. SPURGEON, PhD
Center for Platelet Research Studies, Dana-Farber/Boston Children's Cancer and Blood Disorders Center, Harvard Medical School, Boston, Massachusetts

BOGLÁRKA UJHÁZI, MSc
Division of Pediatric Allergy/Immunology, University of South Florida, Johns Hopkins All Children's Hospital, St Petersburg, Florida

JOLÁN E. WALTER, MD, PhD
Division of Pediatric Allergy/Immunology, University of South Florida, Johns Hopkins All Children's Hospital, St Petersburg, Florida

OLGA K. WEINBERG, MD
Department of Pathology, The University of Texas Southwestern Medical Center, Dallas, Texas

Contents

Flow cytometry enables multiparametric characterization of hematopoietic cell immunophenotype. Deviations from normal immunophenotypic patterns comprise a cardinal feature of many hematopoietic neoplasms, underscoring the ongoing essentiality of flow cytometry as a diagnostic tool. However, understanding of aberrant hematopoiesis requires an equal understanding of normal hematopoiesis as a comparator. In this review, we outline key features of healthy adult hematopoiesis and lineage specification as illuminated by flow cytometry and provide diagrams illustrating what a diagnostician may observe in flow cytometric plots. These features provide a profile of baseline hematopoiesis, to which clinical samples with suspected neoplasia may be compared.

Multiparametric flow cytometry assays are long recognized as an essential diagnostic test for leukemias and lymphomas. Lacking Food and Drug Administration–approved standardized tests, these assays remain laboratory developed tests. The recently published guidelines, CLSI H62, are the most detailed and up-to-date instructions for designing and validating clinical flow cytometry assays. This review provides a historical background for the current situation, summarizes key points from the CLSI guidelines, and lists practical points for assay development gained from personal experience.

Flow cytometry (FC) is a well-established method important in the diagnosis and subclassification of lymphoma. In this article, the role of FC in lymphoma prognostication will be explored, and the clinical role for FC minimal/measurable residual disease testing as a monitoring tool for mature lymphoma will be introduced. Potential pitfalls of monitoring for residual/recurrent disease following immunotherapy will be presented.

Flow cytometry plays a critical role in the diagnosis, prognostication, therapy response evaluation, and clinical management of plasma cell neoplasms. The review summarizes how flow cytometry is used in the initial evaluation to distinguish primary and secondary clonal plasma cell populations from each other and from reactive plasma cells. We further illustrate the kinds of prognostic information the assessment can provide at diagnosis and disease follow-up of primary plasma cell neoplasms. Technical requirements for MRD assays and their use in therapy efficacy assessment and clinical decision-making in multi-myeloma are discussed.

Although final classification of acute myeloid leukemia (AML) integrates morphologic, cytogenetic, and molecular data, flow cytometry remains an essential component of modern AML diagnostics. Here, we review the current role of flow cytometry in the classification, prognostication, and monitoring of AML. We cover immunophenotypic features of key genetically defined AML subtypes and their effects on biological and clinical behaviors, review clinically tractable strategies to differentiate leukemias with ambiguous immunophenotypes more accurately, and discuss key principles of standardization for measurable residual disease monitoring. These advances underscore flow cytometry's continued growth as a powerful diagnostic, management, and discovery tool.

This review discusses recent updates in the diagnosis of acute leukemias of ambiguous lineage and emphasizes the necessary elements for proper flow cytometric evaluation of these cases. The current emphasis of the classification system is toward interpreting the marker expression in light of the intensity of lineage markers and avoiding a diagnosis of mixed phenotype acute leukemia based solely on immunophenotyping without considering underlying genetic findings. Novel entities including mixed phenotype acute leukemia with ZNF384 rearrangements and acute leukemias of ambiguous lineage with BCL11B rearrangements seem to show characteristic flow cytometric immunophenotypes discussed here.

The utility of flow cytometry analysis in the evaluation of chronic myeloid neoplasms, such as myelodysplastic neoplasms and chronic myeloproliferative neoplasms, continues to be emphasized and explored. Recently flow cytometry analysis has been also proven to be able to distinguish persistent clonal hematopoiesis from measurable residual disease in patients with acute myeloid leukemia (AML), a finding with potential critical treatment impact in the management of patients with AML.

Classic Hodgkin lymphoma, nodular lymphocyte predominant Hodgkin lymphoma, and T cell/histiocyte-rich large B cell lymphoma form a unique set of lymphomas with similar morphologic growth patterns (occasional neoplastic cells within a prominent cellular cell background) that are pathobiologically related. Distinguishing these entities has been historically difficult by flow cytometry; however, our laboratory has developed antibody-fluorochrome combinations capable of immunophenotyping these lymphomas. Additionally, characterization of the background reactive lymphocytes can aid in narrowing the differential diagnosis. This review summarizes the immunophenotypic features and insights of the neoplastic and reactive populations found in this unique group of lymphomas.

Clinical flow cytometry tests for inherited and acquired platelet disorders are useful diagnostic tools but are not widely available. Flow cytometric methods are available to detect inherited glycoprotein deficiencies, granule release (secretion defects), drug-induced thrombocytopenias, presence of antiplatelet antibodies, and pharmacodynamic inhibition by antiplatelet agents. New tests take advantage of advanced multicolor cytometers and allow identification of novel platelet subsets by high-dimensional immunophenotyping. Studies are needed to evaluate the value of these new tests for diagnosis and monitoring of therapy in patients with platelet disorders.

Flow cytometry analysis has stood the test of time as a powerful tool in the assessment of hematologic neoplasms. The role of flow cytometry has expanded to evaluate various nonhematologic neoplasms encountered in body cavity malignant effusions, lymph nodes, and other body sites. This review explores the use of routine antibody panels as well as specially designed multicolor antibody panels that have been investigated by different groups and reported in the literature for evaluating nonhematologic neoplasms. In this context, the limitations, pitfalls, future directions, and promising applications of flow cytometry analysis are also discussed.

Primary immunodeficiencies were initially identified on the basis of recurrent, severe or unusual infections. Subsequently, it was noted that these diseases can also manifest with autoimmunity, autoinflammation, allergy,

CLINICS IN LABORATORY MEDICINE

SERIES OF RELATED INTEREST

Advances in Molecular Pathology
Available at: https://www.journals.elsevier.com/advances-in-molecular-pathology

---

THE CLINICS ARE NOW AVAILABLE ONLINE!
Access your subscription at:
www.theclinics.com

Preface

The Enduring and Expanding Importance of Clinical Cytometry

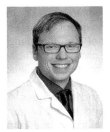

Christopher B. Hergott, MD, PhD
Editor

Clinical cytometry is changing. Building upon decades of proven utility in diagnostic medicine, the field is now expanding to provide actionable clinical information beyond the initial diagnosis for an ever-expanding number of diseases. This advancement is driven in part by new technologies that make cytometry more sensitive, more precise, and easier to use for a wider population of providers. However, as the issue shows, the progress is equally due to the enduring ingenuity of physicians and scientists who push the boundaries of cytometry's capability, looking deeply into available data to unearth new clinical applications. This 2023 issue of *Clinics in Laboratory Medicine* gathers many of these leading experts to update us on the current state of the field and to illuminate the most exciting advances that will define it in the years to come.

First, Dr Joshua Lewis reviews the key immunophenotypic features of healthy human hematopoiesis, providing an important foundation for understanding the aberrancies associated with hematopoietic disease. Dr Anand Lagoo then provides a practical, stepwise guide for designing and validating new clinical flow cytometry assays in accordance with current guidelines. We then explore new applications for flow cytometry in diseases long associated with the technique for initial diagnosis. Drs Singh and Courville focus on non-Hodgkin lymphomas, highlighting the prognostic implications of key immunophenotypic aberrancies, robust assays for measurable residual disease (MRD) in chronic lymphocytic leukemia/small lymphocytic lymphoma, and new cytometric approaches for diagnosing and monitoring T-cell lymphomas. Dr Roshal and Qi Gao discuss the principles of plasma cell cytometry and provide guidance for establishing cytometric MRD assays that predict therapy outcomes in multiple myeloma. Dr Fabienne Lucas then reviews acute myeloid leukemia cytometry and details how our deepening knowledge of genotype-immunophenotype correlations enhances disease classification and monitoring. Finally, Drs Kurzer and Weinberg highlight refinements in

Clin Lab Med 43 (2023) xiii–xiv
https://doi.org/10.1016/j.cll.2023.04.002
0272-2712/23/© 2023 Published by Elsevier Inc.

flow cytometry techniques that can clarify immunophenotypically ambiguous, diagnostically challenging leukemias.

This issue also reflects recent advances that expand the list of diseases for which clinical cytometry is likely to be used widely in the future. Drs Hussein and Loghavi discuss developments in flow cytometry in the evaluation of myelodysplastic syndrome and other chronic myeloid neoplasms, including an especially exciting role for cytometry in distinguishing residual clonal hematopoiesis from residual acute myeloid leukemia after treatment. Dr Jonathan Fromm and colleagues review groundbreaking work that allows Hodgkin lymphoma and related entities to be evaluated with cytometry, detecting both microenvironmental changes and the neoplastic cells themselves. Drs Frelinger and Spurgeon highlight high-dimensional immunophenotyping for platelet disorders and its emerging applications in the clinic. Drs Nabeel and Alobeid evaluate the utility of flow cytometry to evaluate nonhematopoietic neoplasms, a long-underrecognized capability now bolstered by several recent technical advances. Rounding out this section, Dr Attila Kumanovics and colleagues discuss clinical cytometry's role in evaluating immunodeficiencies and errors of immunity, with particular focus on a recently discovered subset of B cells implicated in multiple realms of immune dysregulation.

Finally, the issue discusses new technical advances that may change the very foundation of how clinical cytometry is performed and analyzed. Drs Seifert, Gorlin, and Borkowski provide a landmark overview of machine learning and artificial intelligence in clinical cytometry, notable for both its comprehensiveness and its accessibility to diagnosticians less familiar with these techniques. Abhishek Koladiya and Dr Kara Davis then highlight mass cytometry as a rapidly advancing, data-rich alternative to traditional flow cytometry and discuss the myriad potential clinical applications for this technology. This issue is named "Advances in Clinical Cytometry" (as opposed to "Clinical Flow Cytometry") to reflect the growing promise of these new platforms.

I would like to express my deepest gratitude to all the authors of this series for contributing articles of exemplary insight and clarity. I believe that readers will share my conclusion, upon reading these works, that the future of clinical cytometry will be one of striking innovation and enduring clinical relevance.

Christopher B. Hergott, MD, PhD
Department of Pathology
Brigham and Women's Hospital and Harvard Medical School
75 Francis Street
Boston, MA 02115, USA

E-mail address:
christopher_hergott@dfci.harvard.edu

The Immunophenotypic Profile of Healthy Human Bone Marrow

Joshua E. Lewis, MD, PhD[a,b], Christopher B. Hergott, MD, PhD[a,b],*

KEYWORDS

- Hematopoiesis • Bone marrow • Flow cytometry • Myeloid • Monocytic • Erythroid
- Megakaryocytic • Lymphoid

KEY POINTS

- Flow cytometry provides multiparametric, single-cell immunophenotypic profiles of hematopoietic cells.
- Familiarity with the immunophenotypic profile of healthy bone marrow is essential for understanding aberrancies that arise with hematologic malignancies.
- Flow cytometry correlates well with the molecular features of human hematopoiesis and can provide clinically tractable markers for lineage and differentiation state.

INTRODUCTION

After birth, nearly all hematopoietic cells in humans are produced within the bone marrow.[1] Detailed characterization of bone marrow hematopoiesis can therefore provide significant insight into the function (or dysfunction) of a patient's blood-forming system. Flow cytometry provides a clinically tractable, multiparametric approach to determine the immunophenotypic characteristics of hematopoietic cells. The resulting profile can highlight abnormalities in the differentiation or maturation of bone marrow elements, which has proven particularly useful in the diagnosis of hematologic malignancies.[2] Despite the advent of transcriptional and proteomic technologies providing ever-deeper characterization of the biology of hematopoiesis, flow cytometry remains the clinical standard for immunophenotypic diagnosis. However, any actionable understanding of hematopoietic dysfunction requires an equal understanding of healthy hematopoiesis, providing a baseline from which the diseased marrow diverges.

Here, we provide a brief review of the current understanding of normal hematopoiesis in the healthy human bone marrow as characterized by flow cytometry. We also

a Department of Pathology, Brigham and Women's Hospital, 75 Francis Street, Boston, MA 02115, USA; b Harvard Medical School, 25 Shattuck St, Boston, MA 02115, USA
* Corresponding author.
E-mail address: Christopher_Hergott@DFCI.HARVARD.EDU

Clin Lab Med 43 (2023) 323–332
https://doi.org/10.1016/j.cll.2023.04.003   labmed.theclinics.com
0272-2712/23/© 2023 Elsevier Inc. All rights reserved.

explore the immunophenotypic changes associated with lineage specification and differentiation in humans, which can differ significantly from well-studied murine models.[3] We use illustrative diagrams modeling normal patterns of maturation to illustrate concisely the patterns a diagnostician may see in flow cytometry plots. These examples should provide a guide for the phenotypic assessment of hematopoietic stem cells, lineage precursors, and maturing lineage-defined cells. From a clear picture of healthy hematopoiesis, diagnosticians may more easily make comparisons with clinical samples and render accurate flow cytometric diagnoses for hematologic disorders.

HEMATOPOIETIC STEM CELLS AND PROGENITORS

Multipotent long-term hematopoietic stem cells (LT-HSCs), which are capable of durable self-renewal, are characterized by surface expression of CD34, CD49c (integrin α3), CD49f (integrin α6), CD90 (Thy-1), and CD135 (FLT3) (**Fig. 1**A).[4–7] Differentiation into short-term HSCs is associated with loss of CD49c, the function of which was shown to be important for long-term engraftment of LT-HSCs.[6] Differentiation into multipotent progenitors (MPPs) is associated with loss of CD49f,[8] highlighting this surface integrin as a potentially specific marker for HSCs. Sources also report downregulation of CD90 expression during LT-HSC differentiation, although debate remains

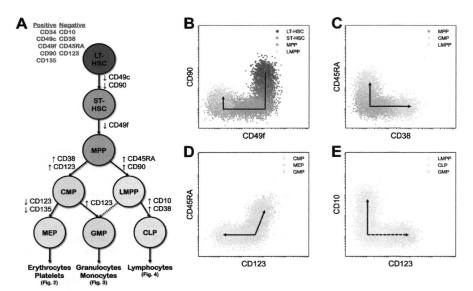

Fig. 1. Flow cytometry immunophenotype of hematopoietic stem cells and lineage precursor cells. (A) Differentiation pathway of hematopoietic stem and progenitor cells. The immunophenotype of LT-HSCs, and the flow cytometry markers gained or lost along the differentiation pathway, are shown. Illustrative recreation of typical flow cytometry plots for (B) CD90 versus CD49f expression along differentiation from LT-HSCs to LMPPs, (C) CD45RA versus CD38 expression at the split of MPPs to either CMPs or LMPPs, (D) CD45RA versus CD123 expression at the split of CMPs to either MEPs or GMPs, and (E) CD10 versus CD123 expression at the split of LMPPs to either GMPs or CLPs. CLP, common lymphoid progenitors; CMP, common myeloid progenitors; GMP, granulocyte-monocyte progenitors; LMPP, lymphoid-primed multipotent progenitors; MEP, megakaryocyte-erythroid progenitors; MPP, multipotent progenitors; ST-HSC, short-term hematopoietic stem cells.

regarding the precise stage when loss of CD90 surface expression is observed (**Fig. 1B**; **Box 1** for details regarding illustrative plot generation).[5,6]

MPPs are capable of differentiating into common myeloid progenitors (CMPs) and lymphoid-primed MPP (LMPPs).[4,9] The transition to CMP is characterized by gain of CD38 (cyclic ADP ribose hydrolase),[4] which is lost early in the differentiation of myeloid and erythroid cells[10] and is gained soon after the LMPP stage in lymphoid progenitor differentiation (**Fig. 1C**).[9] Dim expression of CD123 (IL3 receptor α) is also seen in CMPs and further increased in granulocyte-monocyte progenitors (GMPs) (**Fig. 1D**).[11] Variable CD123 expression on megakaryocyte-erythroid progenitors is reported among sources, with some reporting loss of expression[4] and others demonstrating continued expression.[11] Transition from MPPs to LMPPs is characterized by gain of CD45RA (RA isoform of protein tyrosine phosphatase, receptor type, C).[12] Additionally, some sources report dim CD90 expression in LMPPs.[13] Although most LMPPs are presumed to transition to common lymphoid progenitors with associated increases in CD10 (neprilysin) and CD38 expression, a subset can transition into GMPs and gain CD123 expression (**Fig. 1E**).[9,11]

ERYTHROID AND MEGAKARYOCYTIC LINEAGES

Megakaryocyte-erythroid progenitors are capable of differentiating into burst-forming unit-megakaryocyte and burst-forming unit-erythroid. Both are characterized by loss of CD38[10] and the latter is associated with acquisition of dim CD71 (transferrin receptor 1) expression (**Fig. 2A, B**).[14,15] The transitions from burst-forming unit-megakaryocyte to colony-forming unit-megakaryocytes, megakaryoblasts, and megakaryocytes are associated with gains of megakaryocyte markers CD41a (integrin α2b), CD61 (integrin β3), and CD42b (glycoprotein 1b), respectively, all proteins that ultimately are necessary for platelet function (**Fig. 2C, D**).[16–18] Loss of CD34 expression is believed to occur following gain of CD41 expression and near the point of CD61 upregulation, although the exact megakaryocytic precursor stage at which this occurs is not entirely clear.[16,17]

Box 1
Method for generating illustrative flow cytometry diagrams

Per the references cited in this article, the expression levels of flow cytometry markers for various cell stages were assigned one of the following values: bright, positive, dim-positive, dim, dim-negative, negative, variable. Each value is assigned an associated mean and variance value.
- Bright: mean = 3, var = 0.25
- Positive: mean = 2, var = 0.25
- Dim-positive: mean = 1.5, var = 0.25
- Dim: mean = 1, var = 0.25
- Dim-negative: mean = 0.5, var = 0.25
- Negative: mean = 0, var = 0.25
- Variable: mean = 1.5, var = 0.5

To visualize on a two-dimensional (2D) plot the change in expression of two flow cytometry markers along a cell stage transition, a line is drawn between the mean values of the two expression values represented by the two cell states. Around this line, a 2D Gaussian distribution was drawn, with the variance of each dimension equal to the average of the two variance values of the associated marker expression values. For each cell stage transition, 3000 random points were drawn from the 2D Gaussian distribution. The color of each point is determined based on how far along the cell stage transition it is placed. A custom Python script was written to create these 2D flow cytometry plots.

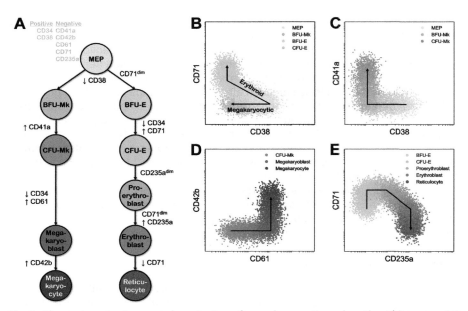

Fig. 2. Flow cytometry immunophenotyping of megakaryocytic and erythroid lineages. (*A*) Differentiation pathway of megakaryocytic and erythroid lineages. The immunophenotype of MEPs, and the flow cytometry markers gained or lost along the differentiation pathway, are shown. Illustrative recreation of typical flow cytometry plots for (*B*) CD71 versus CD38 expression at the split of MEPs into the megakaryocytic (BFU-Mk) and erythroid (BFU-E and CFU-E) lineages, (*C*) CD41a versus CD38 expression along megakaryocytic differentiation from MEPs to CFU-Mks, (*D*) CD42b versus CD61 along megakaryocytic differentiation from CFU-Mks to megakaryocytes, and (*E*) CD71 versus CD235a expression along erythroid differentiation from BFU-Es to reticulocytes. BFU-E, burst-forming unit-erythroid; BFU-Mk, burst-forming unit-megakaryocyte; CFU-E, colony-forming unit-erythroid; CFU-Mk, colony-forming unit-megakaryocyte.

Differentiation from burst-forming unit-erythroid to colony-forming unit-erythroid is characterized by continued gain of CD71 expression, a change necessary for optimal iron sensing in erythroid precursors.[14,15,19] Loss of CD34 expression is reported by some sources to take place at this transition,[14] whereas others report CD34 loss occurs later during differentiation into proerythroblasts.[15,19] Continuing differentiation from colony-forming unit-erythroid, proerythroblast, and erythroblast is associated with continually increased expression of CD235a (glycophorin A), which shares a role with glycophorin B (CD235b) in the MNS antigen system (**Fig. 2**E).[19] Loss of CD71 expression (absent by the reticulocyte stage) is also observed during the differentiation pathway.[15,19,20]

GRANULOCYTIC AND MONOCYTIC LINEAGES

Differentiation of GMPs into forms with myeloblastic or monoblastic morphology is associated with gain of CD13 (alanyl aminopeptidase) and CD33 (Siglec-3) expression,[21,22] with CD33 expression possibly being acquired earlier than CD13 (**Fig. 3**A).[23] This transition is also characterized by dim CD45 expression.[24] Further differentiation to the promonocyte/myelocyte and monocyte/myelocyte stages in both

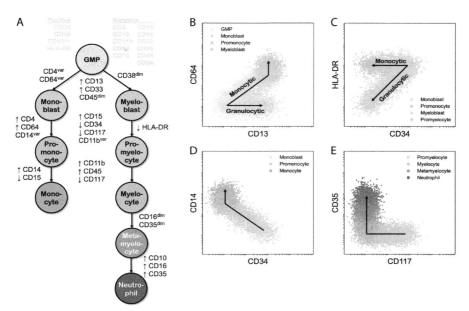

Fig. 3. Flow cytometry immunophenotyping of monocytic and granulocytic lineages. (*A*) Differentiation pathway of monocytic and granulocytic lineages. The immunophenotype of GMPs, and the flow cytometry markers gained or lost along the differentiation pathway, are shown. Marker expression changes shown in the middle of the monocytic and granulocytic lineages reflect changes observed in both lineages. Illustrative recreation of typical flow cytometry plots for (*B*) CD64 versus CD13 expression at the split of GMPs into the monocytic (monoblast and promonocyte) and granulocytic (myeloblast) linages, (*C*) HLA-DR versus CD34 expression along the monocytic (monoblast and promonocyte) and granulocytic (myeloblast and promyelocyte) linages, (*D*) CD14 versus CD34 expression along monocytic differentiation from monoblasts to monocytes, and (*E*) CD35 versus CD117 expression along granulocytic differentiation from promyelocytes to neutrophils.

lineages is associated with loss of CD34 and CD117 (KIT), and gradual gain of CD11b (integrin αM).[21,22] Thus, CD11b is not valuable in differentiating between granulocytic versus monocytic lineages. CD15 (Sialyl-Lewis X) is also upregulated at the promonocyte and promyelocyte stage. However, maturing granulocytes maintain CD15 expression at high levels, whereas maturing monocytes exhibit lower CD15 levels.

Transition to the monocytic lineage is associated with gain of CD4 and CD64 (FcγRI) expression at variable levels, which are increased further during differentiation to promonocytes (**Fig. 3**B).[25] In contrast, transition to the granulocytic lineage is mainly categorized by downregulation of HLA-DR, which begins during differentiation from myeloblast to promyelocyte (**Fig. 3**C).[26,27] Myeloblasts may also demonstrate dimmer CD38 expression compared with monoblasts.[28] Of note, exposure of neutrophils to cytokine/growth factor treatment (including interferon-γ and granulocyte colony–stimulating factor) can induce expression of CD64 as an activation marker[29,30]; nonetheless, expression of other key markers at the neutrophil stage should aid in differentiating these from monocytic cells (eg, CD15[hi], CD66b, CD10).

Downstream monocyte differentiation is characterized by gradually increased CD14 expression between monoblasts, promonocytes, and monocytes, allowing monocytes/macrophages to bind to bacterial lipopolysaccharides and exert innate immune function (**Fig. 3**D).[21,31] Circulating monocytes further evolve from a classical/inflammatory phenotype (CD14[hi], CD16[low]) to a nonclassical/patrolling phenotype (CD14[low], CD16[hi]). Overrepresentation of the classical/inflammatory phenotype may represent a diagnostic signature distinguishing chronic myelomonocytic leukemia from reactive monocytosis.[32] Granulocyte differentiation is associated with gradual gain of CD16 (FcγRIII) and CD66b,[21] gain of CD35 (complement receptor 1) either at the metamyelocyte or band stage,[33,34] and gain of CD10 at the final transition from metamyelocyte to neutrophil (**Fig. 3**E).[35]

LYMPHOID LINEAGES

Common lymphoid progenitors differentiate into T-cell precursors, which mature in the thymus, and B-cell precursors (hematogones), which continue to mature in the bone marrow (**Fig. 4**A). Evidence from mouse models suggests that early thymic hematopoietic precursors are uncommitted to the T lineage and commit to the T lineage through Notch signaling in the thymus.[36] Early hematogone differentiation begins with acquisition of dim CD19 and CD22 (Siglec-2) expression and bright CD38 expression (**Fig. 4**B).[37–39] CD19 intensity continues to increase between stage 1 and 2 hematogones, whereas bright levels of CD22 are generally not reached until the mature B-cell stage.[40]

Maturation from stage 1 to 2 hematogones is additionally characterized by loss of CD34 and TdT, decreased intensity of CD10 expression, and gain of dim CD20 and immunoglobulin heavy and light chain surface expression (**Fig. 4**C).[40–42] CD20 levels continue to increase between stage 2 and 3 hematogones (**Fig. 4**D)[40]; surface immunoglobulin expression is also gained during this transition.[40–42] Finally, differentiation to mature B cell is associated with further decrease in CD10 expression, and increased CD22 and CD45 expression (**Fig. 4**E, F).[40,43] Mature B cells undergo additional immunophenotypic changes outside of the bone marrow, including gain of

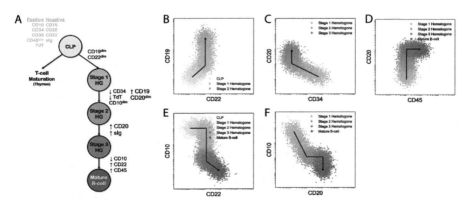

Fig. 4. Flow cytometry immunophenotyping of lymphocytic lineages. (*A*) Differentiation pathway of lymphocytes. The immunophenotype of CLPs, and the flow cytometry markers gained or lost along the differentiation pathway, are shown. Illustrative recreation of typical flow cytometry plots for (*B*) CD19 versus CD22 expression along differentiation from CLPs to stage 2 hematogones, (*C*) CD20 versus CD34 expression along differentiation from stage 1 to stage 3 hematogones, (*D*) CD20 versus CD45 expression along differentiation from stage 1 hematogones to mature B cells, (*E*) CD10 versus CD22 expression along differentiation from CLPs to mature B cells, and (*F*) CD10 versus CD20 expression along differentiation from stage 1 hematogones to mature B cells. HG, hematogones.

CD10 and CD38 within lymph node germinal centers, and gain of CD38 and CD138 during differentiation into plasma cells.[38]

CORRELATION OF FLOW CYTOMETRY WITH MOLECULAR PHENOTYPES

Newer methodologies for cellular characterization including mass cytometry (cyTOF), single-cell RNA sequencing (scRNA-seq), and cellular indexing of transcriptomes and epitopes by sequencing (CITE-seq), have been shown to provide additional layers of information regarding hematopoiesis, and molecular correlates to flow cytometry markers. Oetjen and colleagues[44] demonstrated that flow cytometry, cyTOF, and scRNA-seq report well-matched quantification abilities for hematopoietic stem and precursor cells and most fully differentiated hematopoietic cells (excepting T cells and natural killer cells), suggesting that correlations between flow cytometry and molecular profiling are tractable. Lee and colleagues[45] showed that CITE-seq analysis could recapitulate B-cell differentiation as previously defined by flow cytometry and identify new markers for B-cell differentiation when combined with gene expression analysis. Similarly, Huang and colleagues[46] evaluated the roles of novel signaling proteins on erythroid differentiation by performing knockdown experiments and correlating with flow cytometry findings. Finally, Li and colleagues[47] used scRNA-seq data and lists of available antibodies to identify cell type–specific surface markers that could be used as novel flow cytometry markers for peripheral blood and bone marrow samples. These studies demonstrate that these newer technologies correlate directly with flow cytometric analysis of surface phenotypes and can be used to expand the biologic mechanisms and novel markers associated with hematopoietic cell differentiation in the bone marrow.

SUMMARY

In this review, we provide an overview of the immunophenotypic profile of the human bone marrow, with particular emphasis on changes in flow cytometry marker expression associated with differentiation of hematopoietic stem cells, lineage precursors, and maturing lineage-defined cell types. This overview provides a baseline for flow cytometric characterization of healthy bone marrow, to which clinical samples can be compared for diagnosis of hematologic disorders. Additionally, the changes in surface marker expression outlined here provide insight into the biologic changes associated with differentiating hematopoietic elements, and how aberrant marker expression in hematologic neoplasms may alter the function and therapeutic susceptibility of malignant cells. Finally, we have highlighted recent progress in using newer cell characterization technologies including cyTOF, scRNA-seq, and CITE-seq, for identifying novel biomarkers with greater specificity for hematopoietic cell characterization and assessment of cell differentiation. We hope that this review can serve as a reference for current and future investigations into the flow cytometric evaluation of the human bone marrow.

CLINICS CARE POINTS

- Flow cytometry can capture essential transitions in hematopoietic cell differentiation through evaluation of cell surface marker expression.
- Differentiation of hematopoietic stem cells and lineage precursors is characterized by sequential branching events, leading to different pathways for myeloid/granulocytic, monocytic, erythroid, megakaryocytic, and lymphoid cell progression.

- Newer technologies including cyTOF, scRNA-seq, and CITE-seq are identifying novel cell surface markers with greater cell type specificity, which could be used for patient-level flow cytometry assessment of hematopoiesis.

DISCLOSURE

The authors have no financial interests or relationships to disclose.

FUNDING

CBH is funded by a Society of '67 Scholar Award from the Association of Pathology Chairs, a Young Investigator Grant from the Academy of Clinical Laboratory Physicians and Scientists, and by NIH 5T32CA251062.

REFERENCES

1. Keohane E, Otto CN, Walenga J. Rodak's hematology-e-book: clinical principles and applications. Amsterdam, The Netherlands: Elsevier Health Sciences; 2019.
2. Craig FE, Foon KA. Flow cytometric immunophenotyping for hematologic neoplasms. Blood 2008;111(8):3941–67.
3. Rieger MA, Schroeder T. Hematopoiesis. Cold Spring Harb Perspect Biol 2012;4(12).
4. Seita J, Weissman IL. Hematopoietic stem cell: self-renewal versus differentiation. Wiley Interdisciplinary Reviews 2010;2(6):640–53.
5. Challen GA, Goodell MA. Bridge over troubled stem cells. Mol Ther 2011;19(10): 1756–8.
6. Tomellini E, Fares I, Lehnertz B, et al. Integrin-α3 is a functional marker of ex vivo expanded human long-term hematopoietic stem cells. Cell Rep 2019;28(4): 1063–73.e5.
7. Kikushige Y, Yoshimoto G, Miyamoto T, et al. Human Flt3 is expressed at the hematopoietic stem cell and the granulocyte/macrophage progenitor stages to maintain cell survival. J Immunol 2008;180(11):7358–67.
8. Notta F, Doulatov S, Laurenti E, et al. Isolation of single human hematopoietic stem cells capable of long-term multilineage engraftment. Science 2011; 333(6039):218–21.
9. Ostendorf BN, Flenner E, Flörcken A, et al. Phenotypic characterization of aberrant stem and progenitor cell populations in myelodysplastic syndromes. PLoS One 2018;13(5):e0197823.
10. Belay E, Miller CP, Kortum AN, et al. A hyperactive Mpl-based cell growth switch drives macrophage-associated erythropoiesis through an erythroid-megakaryocytic precursor. Blood 2015;125(6):1025–33.
11. Gill S, Tasian SK, Ruella M, et al. Preclinical targeting of human acute myeloid leukemia and myeloablation using chimeric antigen receptor-modified T cells. Blood 2014;123(15):2343–54.
12. Görgens A, Ludwig A-K, Möllmann M, et al. Multipotent hematopoietic progenitors divide asymmetrically to create progenitors of the lymphomyeloid and erythromyeloid lineages. Stem Cell Rep 2014;3(6):1058–72.
13. Doulatov S, Notta F, Eppert K, et al. Revised map of the human progenitor hierarchy shows the origin of macrophages and dendritic cells in early lymphoid development. Nat Immunol 2010;11(7):585–93.

14. Nandakumar SK, Ulirsch JC, Sankaran VG. Advances in understanding erythro-poiesis: evolving perspectives. Br J Haematol 2016;173(2):206–18.
15. Yang L, Lewis K. Erythroid lineage cells in the liver: novel immune regulators and beyond. J Clin Transl Hepatol 2020;8(2):177.
16. Pineault N, Boisjoli G. Megakaryopoiesis and ex vivo differentiation of stem cells into megakaryocytes and platelets. ISBT Sci Ser 2015;10(S1):154–62.
17. Lee E-j, Godara P, Haylock D. Biomanufacture of human platelets for transfusion: rationale and approaches. Expl Hematol 2014;42(5):332–46.
18. Cortin V, Pineault N, Garnier A. Ex vivo megakaryocyte expansion and platelet production from human cord blood stem cells. In: Audet J, Stanford WL, editors. Stem cells in regenerative medicine. New York, NY, USA: Springer; 2009. p. 109–26.
19. Macrì S, Pavesi E, Crescitelli R, et al. Immunophenotypic profiling of erythroid progenitor-derived extracellular vesicles in diamond-blackfan anaemia: a new diagnostic strategy. PLoS One 2015;10(9):e0138200.
20. Lim ZR, Vassilev S, Leong YW, et al. Industrially compatible transfusable iPSC-derived RBCs: progress, challenges and prospective solutions. Int J Mol Sci 2021;22(18):9808.
21. Van Lochem E, Van der Velden V, Wind H, et al. Immunophenotypic differentiation patterns of normal hematopoiesis in human bone marrow: reference patterns for age-related changes and disease-induced shifts. Cytometry Part B: Clinical Cytometry: The Journal of the International Society for Analytical Cytology 2004; 60(1):1–13.
22. Marti LC, Bacal NS, Bento LC, et al. Phenotypic markers and functional regulators of myelomonocytic cells. In: Ghosh A, editor. Biology of myelomonocytic cells. London, UK: IntechOpen; 2017.
23. Plesa A, Ciuperca G, Genieys S, et al. A biomathematical analysis of immunophe-notypic characteristics in patients with acute myeloblastic leukemia. Washington, DC, USA: American Society of Hematology; 2006.
24. Lacombe F, Durrieu F, Briais A, et al. Flow cytometry CD45 gating for immunophe-notyping of acute myeloid leukemia. Leukemia 1997;11(11):1878–86.
25. Naeim F. Atlas of hematopathology: morphology, immunophenotype, cytoge-netics, and molecular approaches. Cambridge, MA, USA: Academic Press; 2012.
26. Czader M. Clinical flow cytometry. In: Cheng L, Zhang DY, Eble JN, editors. Molecular genetic pathology. New York, NY, USA: Springer; 2008. p. 155–83.
27. Leach M, Drummnond M, Doig A. Practical flow cytometry in haematology diagnosis. Hoboken, NJ: Wiley-Blackwell; 2013.
28. Roshal M, Chien S, Othus M, et al. The proportion of CD34+ CD38low or neg my-eloblasts, but not side population frequency, predicts initial response to induction therapy in patients with newly diagnosed acute myeloid leukemia. Leukemia 2013;27(3):728–31.
29. Perussia B, Dayton ET, Lazarus R, et al. Immune interferon induces the receptor for monomeric IgG1 on human monocytic and myeloid cells. J Exp Med 1983; 158(4):1092–113.
30. Repp R, Valerius T, Sendler A, et al. Neutrophils express the high affinity receptor for IgG (Fc gamma RI, CD64) after in vivo application of recombinant human granulocyte colony-stimulating factor. 1991.
31. Matarraz S, Almeida J, Flores-Montero J, et al. Introduction to the diagnosis and classification of monocytic-lineage leukemias by flow cytometry. Cytometry B Clin Cytometry 2017;92(3):218–27.

32. Selimoglu-Buet D, Wagner-Ballon O, Saada V, et al. Characteristic repartition of monocyte subsets as a diagnostic signature of chronic myelomonocytic leukemia. Blood 2015;125(23):3618–26.
33. McKenna E, Mhaonaigh AU, Wubben R, et al. Neutrophils: need for standardized nomenclature. Front Immunol 2021;12:602963.
34. Elghetany MT, Patel J, Martinez J, et al. CD87 as a marker for terminal granulocytic maturation: assessment of its expression during granulopoiesis. Cytometry Part B: Clinical Cytometry: The Journal of the International Society for Analytical Cytology 2003;51(1):9–13.
35. Marini O, Costa S, Bevilacqua D, et al. Mature CD10+ and immature CD10− neutrophils present in G-CSF–treated donors display opposite effects on T cells. Blood 2017;129(10):1343–56.
36. Heinzel K, Benz C, Martins VC, et al. Bone marrow-derived hemopoietic precursors commit to the T cell lineage only after arrival in the thymic microenvironment. J Immunol 2007;178(2):858–68.
37. Marti LC, Bacal NS, Bento LC, et al. In: Lymphoid hematopoiesis and lymphocytes differentiation and maturation, In: Isvoranu G., Lymphocyte updates-cancer, autoimmunity and infection. London, UK: IntechOpen; 2017.
38. Perez-Andres M, Paiva B, Nieto WG, et al. Human peripheral blood B-cell compartments: a crossroad in B-cell traffic. Cytometry B Clin Cytometry 2010; 78(S1):S47–60.
39. Qin H, Ramakrishna S, Nguyen S, et al. Preclinical development of bivalent chimeric antigen receptors targeting both CD19 and CD22. Molecular Therapy-Oncolytics 2018;11:127–37.
40. Chantepie S, Cornet E, Salaün V, et al. Hematogones: an overview. Leuk Res 2013;37(11):1404–11.
41. McKenna RW, Washington LT, Aquino DB, et al. Immunophenotypic analysis of hematogones (B-lymphocyte precursors) in 662 consecutive bone marrow specimens by 4-color flow cytometry. Blood, The Journal of the American Society of Hematology 2001;98(8):2498–507.
42. Babusikova O, Zeleznikova T. Normal maturation sequence of immunoglobulin light and heavy chains in hematogone stages 1, 2 and 3 in acute leukemia after treatment. Neoplasma 2008;55(6):501–6.
43. Morgan D, Tergaonkar V. Unraveling B cell trajectories at single cell resolution. Trends Immunol 2022;43(3):210–29.
44. Oetjen KA, Lindblad KE, Goswami M, et al. Human bone marrow assessment by single-cell RNA sequencing, mass cytometry, and flow cytometry. JCI insight 2018;3(23).
45. Lee RD, Munro SA, Knutson TP, et al. Single-cell analysis identifies dynamic gene expression networks that govern B cell development and transformation. Nat Commun 2021;12(1):1–16.
46. Huang P, Zhao Y, Zhong J, et al. Putative regulators for the continuum of erythroid differentiation revealed by single-cell transcriptome of human BM and UCB cells. Proc Natl Acad Sci USA 2020;117(23):12868–76.
47. Li R, Banjanin B, Schneider RK, et al. Detection of cell markers from single cell RNA-seq with sc2marker. BMC Bioinf 2022;23(1):1–19.

How to Design and Validate a Clinical Flow Cytometry Assay

Anand Shreeram Lagoo, MD, PhD

KEYWORDS

- Laboratory developed tests (LDTs)
- Clinical and Laboratory Standards Institute (CLSI) • Spillover • Compensation
- Spread • Quasi-quantitative assay • Limit of blank (LoB)

KEY POINTS

- Panel design for multiparametric flow cytometry assays is initiated using accepted principles but often requires one or more changes based on practical performance of the panel.
- Ideally, assay design should be completed before beginning the steps for assay validation.
- Assay validation steps are more or less rigorous depending on the nature of the assay (qualitative vs quasi-quantitative) and its intended purpose.

INTRODUCTION

The immunologic classification of leukemias and lymphomas was initially proposed in the mid-1980s.[1] Since the Revised European-American Classification of Lymphomas[2] and subsequent World Health Organization classifications,[3–5] immunophenotyping is accepted as a key required feature in accurate classification of lymphomas and is now routinely performed by multiparameter flow cytometry. However, a standardized clinical flow cytometry assay approved by the Food and Drug Administration (FDA) is not available for leukemia/lymphoma diagnosis. Most clinical flow cytometry assays are laboratory developed tests (LDTs), and the medical director of a clinical flow cytometry laboratory is responsible for their development and validation.[6] These assays are "high complexity tests" and are subject to regulation by Centers for Medicare and Medicaid Services, usually enforced by deemed entities such as the College of American Pathologists (CAP). The guidance provided in the current CAP laboratory general checklist COM.40350 for LDTs requires that for each LDT assay the laboratory must determine and document the analytical accuracy, precision, sensitivity, specificity, reportable range, and any other performance characteristic required to ensure analytical test performance, before clinical use of each LDT. The actual steps for development and validation of flow cytometry tests have been recently published by the

Department of Pathology, Duke University School of Medicine, Box 3712 DUMC, NC 27710, USA
E-mail address: anand.lagoo@duke.edu

Clin Lab Med 43 (2023) 333–349
https://doi.org/10.1016/j.cll.2023.04.004
0272-2712/23/© 2023 Elsevier Inc. All rights reserved.

labmed.theclinics.com

Clinical and Laboratory Standards Institute (CLSI, formerly National Committee for Clinical Laboratory Standards [NCCLS]) as Guidance H62.[7] These guidelines will likely form the basis for detailed checklist items for accreditation of clinical flow cytometry laboratories, and this review is primarily based on them.

HISTORY

Accurate enumeration of various peripheral blood cells by flow cytometry predates the use of this technique for diagnosis of leukemia and lymphoma by more than 3 decades. The ability to interrogate subset-defining properties of viable white blood cells in suspension using a laser beam was described in 1965.[8] These early flow cytometers used forward scatter and side scatter to identify the major subsets of unstained white blood cells. After the introduction of monoclonal antibodies (MoAbs) in 1976, flow cytometry was used to determine the reactivity of newly developed monoclonal antibodies to lymphocyte subsets.[9] Although the indirect immunofluorescence staining procedure used in these early experiments is now replaced by antibodies directly conjugated to an ever-increasing list of fluorochromes (also called fluorophores), fluorescein and a 488 nm argon laser used in these initial experiments are still in use. The practice of staining cells from 50 uL of blood is still part of most protocols but the number of target cells analyzed in modern machines has increased by 10x to 100x from the initial 100 lymphocytes/second possible in 1982.[10] Remarkably, at least 3 flow cytometers were commercially available 40 years ago: from Becton-Dickinson's FACS Division (Sunnyvale, CA, USA), Coulter Electronics (Hialeah, FL, USA), and Ortho Diagnostic Systems (Westwood, MA, USA).[11]

Enumeration of various subsets of lymphoid cells in immune disorders dominated the use of flow cytometry in early years, and the use of this technique expanded rapidly during the HIV-AIDS epidemic for counting T-cell subsets. Formal guidelines for the use of a flow cytometry test were first provided by the Centers for Disease Control and Prevention in 1992[12] and then revised in 1994.[13] Both recommendations were based on the availability of the existing state-of-the-art, 2-color flow cytometers and protocols using fluorescein isothiocyanate– and phycoerythrin-labeled antibodies. The availability of 3-color flow cytometers led to a major advance in gating strategy[14,15] in which CD45 versus side scatter was shown to provide better separation of multiple populations of bone marrow cells than the forward scatter versus side scatter plots. This method of "gating" is used in most modern clinical flow cytometry assays. During the last 25 years, there has been a great deal of progress in instrument design, reagent development, and innovations in analysis software for flow cytometry. The use of 8- to 12-color flow cytometers is now routine in most clinical laboratories in the United States. While improving the sensitivity and reliability of flow cytometry assays, this continuous development may have hindered the emergence of a universal consensus among clinical laboratories for a completely standardized assay.[16]

A number of key components/reagents used in clinical flow cytometry have been standardized. The best example is the use of universal nomenclature for monoclonal antibodies adopted since 1984 in which international workshops assign a consensus "clusters of differentiation (CD)" number to all MoAbs reacting with the same antigen molecule. Starting from 15 CD definitions in 1984,[17] today the number of unique, universally accepted CD numbered antibodies exceeds 400 specificities. Lacking a similar consensus in hardware and software architecture and design, there was growing "concern regarding the inconsistent practices and wide variation in styles among laboratories involved in the flow cytometric analysis of leukemias and lymphomas."[18] A consensus conference of clinical hematopathologists, hematologists, and laboratory scientists from United States and Canada was organized in 1995 to improve future practice of clinical flow cytometry, resulting in the US-Canadian consensus recommendations on the immunophenotypic analysis of hematologic neoplasia by flow cytometry.[19–23] In 1997, NCCLS issued guidelines for clinical flow cytometric analysis of leukemia/lymphoma[24] and in 2004 proposed guidelines for quantitative fluorescence calibration and measurement of fluorescence intensity.[25] The second edition of the approved guidelines for leukemia and lymphoma analysis was published in 2007,[26] which was reissued without significant changes in 2017. Separate guidelines for enumeration of immunologically defined cell populations by flow cytometry were also issued by CLSI.[27] Over a decade ago, the US FDA stated its intention to eventually regulate LDTs including flow cytometry assays. Partly in response, the International Council for Standardization of Hematology (ICSH) and the International Clinical Cytometry Society published another series of 5 monographs on the "Validation of Cell-based Fluorescence Assays."[28–32] The bipartisan support in US Congress for a legislation called "Verifying Accurate Leading-edge IVCT Development (VALID) Act," portends increased FDA oversight of all in vitro diagnostic (IVD) products, including LDTs such as flow cytometry assays.[6] In this environment, close adherence to the latest guidance for development and validation of clinical flow cytometry assays described in the latest CLSI document H62 is highly desirable.

DEFINITIONS

CLSI H62 defines 79 terms relevant to clinical flow cytometry. The definition of more than one-third of these terms such as accuracy, calibration, cross-reactivity, internal control, specimen, and so forth do not differ from their common meaning in general scientific, statistical, research, or clinical laboratory usage. Others may have somewhat different meaning from ordinary usage in flow cytometry. Because of limitation of space, it is not possible to provide the full glossary of these terms here. In subsequent sections these CLSI-defined terms will be italicized and underlined and their flow cytometry–specific meaning explained when necessary. However, a review of pp 4 to 13 in the CLSI guidance document H62 is recommended to avoid any ambiguity.

DISCUSSION

An optimally designed and validated clinical flow cytometry assay performed in an appropriately certified clinical laboratory by properly trained personnel will provide accurate information that is easily interpreted by a hematopathologist for the diagnosis of hematolymphoid conditions. Leukemia/lymphoma identification is one of the 29 types of flow cytometry assays listed in CLSI H62, but regardless of assay type, all assay development proceeds in 2 main phases: assay design and assay validation. It is emphasized that only after the assay conditions are completely established during assay design should assay validation begin. Leukemia/lymphoma diagnostic assays can be performed on a broad type of specimens (*matrix*) compared with the singular matrix (usually blood) used for assays such as paroxysmal nocturnal hemoglobinuria evaluation or absolute T-cell counts.

Assay Design

CLSI document H62 suggests 4 basic steps for design phase of a flow cytometry assay: establish the intended use, determine instrument configuration, design the antibody panel, and determine analysis strategy. In addition, before proceeding to validate the assay, "optimization" and "characterization" of the assay is necessary to ensure consistency and efficiency for the clinical use of the assay. Knowledge of basic principles of antigen-antibody reactions, properties of fluorescence and methods of its detection, as well as the operational subsystems of modern flow cytometers, namely fluidics, optics, electronics, and data analysis is essential for rational decision-making when developing flow cytometry assays.

1 .Intended use of the assay: the common applications of clinical flow cytometry assays may be broadly divided into the following:
   a .*Qualitative*/diagnostic assays: these are primarily assays for leukemia/lymphoma diagnosis. These assays must accurately and specifically detect the presence of the abnormal cells and provide a sufficiently detailed immunophenotype of the abnormal population with "*clinical specificity*" to allow correct diagnosis according to the currently accepted classification. Clinical specificity depends on several key factors: reagent properties (highly specific antibodies, reliable *fluorochromes*, appropriate *titration of antibodies*), disease phenotype (well-characterized cellular immunophenotype in literature, availability of biological controls, samples from same or similar diseases), *gating strategy* used for analysis, *spillover* and *compensation*, and correction/avoidance of *interference*.
   b .*Quasi-quantitative* assays: in these assays, the data are continuous and numeric (not *ordinal*) but are not derived from comparison to a standard reference material or true calibration curve. These assays measure proportions of normal cell subsets; capture low level of residual disease after treatment in myeloid and lymphoid malignancies (acute myeloid leukemia, chronic lymphocytic leukemia, myeloma, and others); identify therapeutic targets on abnormal cells before, during, or after treatment with MoAbs; and determine prognostic group based on presence of surface or cytoplasmic markers.

2 .Instrument configuration (flow cytometers and other instruments): the latest Beckman Coulter flow cytometer, Navios Ex, is an 11-color instrument that was approved by the FDA in July 2017, whereas the 12-color BD Lyric was approved in October 2020. Sysmex has recently entered the field after acquisition of Partec GmbH, the German manufacturer of flow cytometers. BioRad flow cytometry instruments are used in many research laboratories. Other optional approved instruments, such as the robotic sample staining system PS10 (Sysmex) or the BD FACSDuet Sample Preparation System and BD lyse/wash assistant provide increased efficiency for the laboratory. Purchase and installation of these instruments requires careful planning and implementation.

Acquisition and analysis software: any clinical flow cytometry analysis software is considered a "medical device" by the FDA and is subject to the same rigorous approval process as the flow cytometers (FDA Quality Systems Regulations 21 CFR § 820). The instrument manufacturer provides dedicated software for data acquisition with variable capabilities for data analysis and display. Third-party analysis software may offer more user-friendly interface and protocols but involve additional purchase price and/or annual licensing fees.

3 .Antibody panel design: this step in assay design offers a bewilderingly high number of possibilities, as the capabilities of the flow cytometers continue to increase. However, the essence of panel design remains the same: include antibodies for antigens that are present and for antigens that are absent on the target cells as well as on other cells in the specimen that have light scatter properties similar to the target cell population. The level of expression for each antigen on normal and abnormal cells is also important. The list of antibodies to be included in the panel can be

assembled based on published immunophenotypes of various hematolymphoid neoplasms and for normal blood and bone marrow cells, but the selection of the correct antibody-fluorochrome combination in the antibody panel is pivotal for the overall success of the assay. Online tools are available from manufacturers of flow cytometers and antibodies, but understanding of the principles of good panel design is essential to allow further optimization of any antibody panel based on actual performance on clinical samples. Fluorochromes have maximum excitation with lasers of different wavelengths and emit maximum number of photons in nonoverlapping wavelengths. This peak emission is measured by the primary photodetector for that fluorochrome (**Table 1**). However, there is also emission of photons of other wavelengths (albeit at lower quantities), producing overlapping emission spectra. The overlapping (or spillover) emission by each fluorochrome is captured by neighboring photodetectors for other fluorochromes (**Fig. 1**). The signal intensity of this *fluorescence spillover* by each fluorochrome in each secondary (spillover) detector is proportional to its signal in the primary detector. This fluorochrome-specific proportion is called *percent spillover*. An instrument capable of detecting N fluorochromes in N detectors produces N-1 spillover signals from each fluorochrome or N x (N-1) total spillover signals, which form the *spillover matrix* for that assay (which is shown in the right side of **Table 1**).

Effects of spillover are corrected by *compensation*: an automated process of applying electronic or mathematical corrections to each spillover detector to eliminate the effect of light signal generated from the spillover fluorochromes simultaneously present on the same cell (**Fig. 2**, left and middle plots). Mathematically inverting the spillover values generates the compensation coefficients for each fluorochrome at each nonprimary detector producing the compensation matrix. However, compensation cannot correct the secondary effect of spillover called *spread* of the signal in the secondary detector. The brighter the fluorescence in the primary detector, the higher its spread in secondary detectors (see **Fig. 2**, right plots). Spread caused by spillover is cumulative and increases the background in the spillover detector; this decreases the sensitivity of detection of cells having dim primary emission in that detector. Based on the emission intensity recorded by the primary detector, fluorochromes can be classified on an ordinal scale (**Table 2**). Because bright fluorochromes cause more spread and reduce sensitivity of detection, the first principle for panel design is to use brighter fluorochromes for weakly expressed antigens and vice versa (**Table 3**). Another useful principle is to distribute the fluorochromes for antigens expressed on the same cells across different lasers. However, in this case the possibility of cross-laser spillover must be considered, particularly if tandem dyes are used (see **Fig. 1**). Tandem dyes present in close proximity may have unexpected quenching effects or show aberrant staining reactivity due to dissociation of the secondary (acceptor) fluorochrome.

Backbone antibody: when the number of antibodies in a panel exceed the maximum number in one tube, the use of backbone antibody/antibodies allows identification of the target cells across different tubes. Assays for detection of minimum residual disease usually require multiple backbone antibodies. Ultimately, panel design is an iterative process, and there may not be a universally acceptable best panel. The panels that work well by providing consistent, accurate, *"fit-for-purpose (FFP)"* results should be used.

Standardized and validated antibody panels were developed by the EuroFlow consortium for 8-color flow cytometers.[33] These panels use an algorithmic approach, starting with an orientation (screening) tube based on clinical impression, followed by the appropriate complete panel. Three "backbone markers" are present in each

Table 1
Proportion of maximum emission with different lasers and spillover percentages for BD FACSCanto-II Flow Cytometer[a]

Fluorochrome	Filter[b]	% of Maximum Emission When Excited by Given Laser[c]			Percent Spillover							
		405 (Violet)	488 (Blue)	633 (Red)	V450	V500	FITC	PE	PerCP-Cy5.5	PE-Cy7	APC	APC-H7
V450	450/50	100	0	0	71.50%	9.10%	x	x	x	x	x	x
V500	510/50	95.1	0.7	0	19.60%	54.80%	59.00%	0.10%	0.40%	1.00%	x	x
FITC	530/30	5.4	88	0	5.30%	27.30%	47.40%	0.40%	0.30%	1.80%	x	x
PE	585/42	6	61.6	0.5	0.50%	9.30%	12.50%	70.40%	0.50%	16.40%	0.20%	0.40%
PerCP-Cy5.5	670 LP	40.6	98.4	10.7	x	x	x	2.50%	90.80%	73.80%	40.50%	86.10%
PE-Cy7	780/60	11.8	61.8	9.5	x	x	x	x	11.90%	60.50%	x	64.50%
APC	660/20	1.1	1.1	71.9	x	0.20%	x	2.50%	6.50%	1.30%	40.20%	6.30%
APC-H7	780/60	5	1.4	35.7	x	x	x	x	11.90%	60.50%	x	64.50%

NOTES: 1. The filters used in front of the primary detector of a fluorochrome match the wavelengths of maximum emission by that fluorochrome. 2. The overall intensity of emission varies with excitation wavelength, but cross-laser excitation is commonly seen. Note that PE-Cy7 and APC-H7 have identical filters but show very different level of total emissions with 488 nm and 633 nm lasers. 3. The overall spectral distribution of emitted light is essentially independent of the excitation wavelength. Thus, the spillover percentages captured by the remaining detectors in this filter configuration remain unchanged for the 3 lasers.

[a] The configuration of fluorochromes and filters are used in the author's laboratory and the online tool "BD Spectrum Viewer" (available at https://www.bdbiosciences.com/en-us/resources/bd-spectrum-viewer) is used to get the data shown in the table. Similar online tools for panel design are available from other manufacturers: https://www.thermofisher.com/us/en/home/life-science/cell-analysis/flow-cytometry/antibodies-for-flow-cytometry/flow-cytometry-panel-builder.html?SID=fr-flowupdated-4 and https://www.biolegend.com/en-us/spectra-analyzer.

[b] The optical properties of the filter placed in front of the photodetector for the designated fluorochrome are indicated in this column: For "band-pass" filters (all except PerCP-Cy5.5), the first number indicates the central wavelength (in nanometers) and the second number indicates the width of the band of wavelengths (in nanometers) across this central wavelength which can pass through. The "LP" (for Long-Pass) filter indicates that all wavelenghts longer than the designated wavelength (in nanometers) can pass through. See also note 1.

[c] The wavelengh (in nanometers) of the light emitted by the particular laser and its percieved color are indicated for the three lasers used in this instrument.

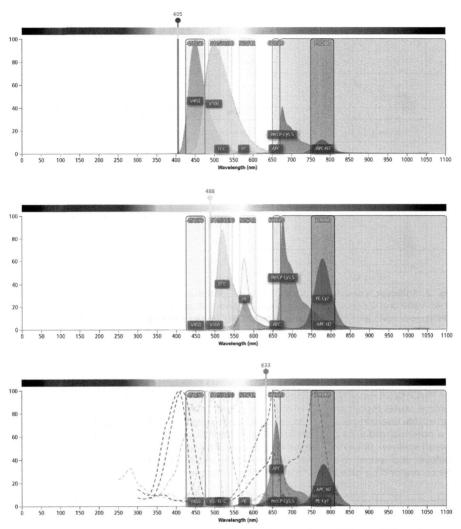

Fig. 1. Lasers, filters, and emission spectra of fluorochromes in FACSCanto-II Flow Cytometer: these images from the online panel design tool, BD Spectrum Viewer, show emission spectra elicited by each of the 3 lasers in this instrument. The overlap between the emissions of neighboring fluorochromes is obvious, and this spillover occurs at a fixed proportion of the fluorochrome's peak emission (which is captured by the primary detector). These images and the corresponding numerical data in Table 1 show that the higher energy violet and blue lasers can elicit some fluorescence from fluorochromes maximally excited by a lower energy laser. This cross-laser excitation adds to the complexity of creating appropriate compensation matrix. (Images courtesy and © Becton, Dickinson and Company. Reproduced with permission.)

8-color tube, and a novel software combines the signals for all nonbackbone antibodies and assigns them to the appropriate cell population determined by the backbone markers, creating potentially unlimited dimensional data. Strict adherence to preanalytical and analytical parameters is required, and a relatively large number of

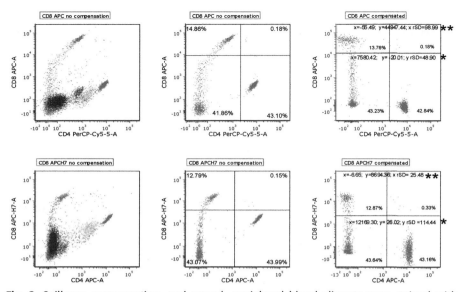

Fig. 2. Spillover, compensation, and spread—peripheral blood aliquots were stained with CD45-V500 and 2 combinations of anti-CD4 and CD8 antibodies—CD4-PerCP-Cy5.5 and CD8-APC (*upper row*) and CD4-APC and CD8-APC-H7 (*lower row*). In all scatter plots CD4 antibody is shown on x-axis and CD8 on y-axis. In both rows the left scatter plots show uncompensated results of all cells, middle plots show same for lymphocytes, and right plots show compensated results for lymphocytes. The values for median fluorescence channel (MFC) in the primary and spillover detector and the robust standard deviation (rSD) in the spillover detector are given for the CD4+ (*asterisk*) and CD8+ (*double asterisk*) populations. The spread of CD8-APC into the PerCP-Cy5.5 detector (*upper right plot*) is significant because the brightness of the fluorochrome causes higher amount of spillover (*upper middle plot*) requiring high compensatory correction. Overcompensation, as indicated by the negative MFC on x-axis for this population, is a potential pitfall in this scenario. The dimmer fluorescence of CD8-APC-H7 leads to less overall spillover (*lower middle plot*) with very little spread (*lower right plot*). Similarly, the spillover and spread of CD4-APC (*lower middle and right plots*, respectively) is higher than the corresponding metrics for CD4-PerCP-Cy5.5 (*upper middle and right plots*).

Table 2	
Relative brightness of fluorochromes expressed as staining index	
Fluorochrome	**Stain Index**
PE	302
APC	278
PE-Cy™7	139
PerCP-Cy™5.5	107
BD Horizon™ V450	85
Pacific Blue™	80
FITC	56
APC-H7	24

Average staining index of peripheral blood cells stained with CD4 antibody conjugated to different fluorochromes and analyzed on the BD BD FACSCanto II.

Modified from "Multicolor Flow Cytometry, Principles of Panel Design", Webinar presented by Mark Edinger. Courtesy and © Becton, Dickinson and Company. Reproduced with permission.

Table 3
Expression level of antigens on human lymphoid subsets

Cell	Antigen	Molecules per Cell
T-cells	TCR	100,000
	CD2	55,000
	CD3	124,000
	CD5	90,000
	CD7	20,000
	CD45	>200,000
CD4+ T-cells	CD4	100,000
	CD28	20,000
CD8+ T-cells	CD8	90,000
	CD28	15,000
B cells	CD19	18,000
	CD20	109,000
	CD21	210,000
	CD22	14,000
	HLA-DR	85,000
	CD11 A	10,000
	CD40	2000
	CD86	16,000
	CD80	2000
Dendritic cells	CD11 A	27,000
	CD40	17,000
	CD80	132,000
	CD86	208,000
Monocytes	CD14	110,000
	CD32	21,000
	CD64	13,000
Neutrophils	CD14	3500
	CD16	225,000
NK cells	CD56	10,000
RBCs	GLY-A	340,000
Basophil	CD22	15,000

Abbreviations: NK, natural killer; RBC, red blood cells.
Adapted from "Multicolor Flow Cytometry, Principles of Panel Design", Webinar presented by Mark Edinger. Courtesy and © Becton, Dickinson and Company. Reproduced with permission.

antibodies are used in EuroFlow panels. These factors may have limited the use of these panels in United States in the past, but the complete and uniform validation available may make them more attractive in coming years.

Additional preanalytical and analytical considerations: the permissible specimen matrix (or matrixes) and optimal conditions for handling and storing each specimen type are specified. The method for obtaining single-cell suspension from solid tissue should be defined to optimize results.[34] The media used for specimen storage and transport, the red cell lysis and removal method, the use of blocking agents, and the fixative used after staining, all must be clearly defined.

All antibodies in the panel need titration. CLSI H62 guidance provides 3 titration methods: signal-to-noise (S/N) ratio, staining index (SI), and staining window (p81). S/N ratio is calculated by dividing the median fluorescence intensity (MFI) of antigen-expressing population by the MFI of the antigen-negative population. This traditional metric of titration is satisfactory for most assays but does not take into consideration the effect of spread or variation specific for the assay conditions (including the cytometer used). The guidance recommends the use of SI, which accounts for effect of spread because it is calculated by dividing the difference between MFI of positive and negative populations by twice the robust standard deviation of the negative population.

4 .Data analysis strategy: manual data analysis based on predefined templates is recommended to ensure uniformity. The gates should include evaluation of acquisition stability by plotting one or more parameters against time, and doublets should be excluded. The quantitative consequences of exclusion of debris and dead cells on proportion of other cells should be recorded. A hierarchical gating strategy is used to identify and isolate populations of interest in a stepwise fashion. Automated, artificial intelligence–based approaches are not endorsed in the CLSI guideline at this time.

Assay optimization: an acquisition template is created for the assay so future sample data can be acquired consistently. Staining time may be optimized before the assay sensitivity is determined for quasi-quantitative assay. Permissible ex vivo time for the samples to ensure adequate viability can be determined.

7 .Assay characterization: this step includes evaluating stability of the antibody cocktails to be prepared for the assay, stability of stained sample before it has to be acquired, specimen stability and optimal storage condition, and identifying appropriate control samples for quality control (QC).

Assay Validation

CLSI H62 guidelines cover assays for research, preclinical laboratories, manufacturers of FDA-cleared in vitro diagnostic devices, and clinical laboratories. The flexibility afforded by an *FFP* approach is integral to formulate a validation plan that best fits the *context of use* and is adequate to satisfy the applicable regulatory requirements. Consideration of potential for risk to patient from erroneous assay result strongly influences the depth and rigor of validation. Minimal and optimal validation requirements for 7 scenarios for flow cytometry assays are provided, of which 3 are primarily relevant for clinical laboratories: CLIA/IMDRF Qualitative Validation (A4), CLIA/IMDRF Quantitative Validation (A5), Laboratory-Initiated Assay Revision (A6).

Validation planning: assay validation should cover all assay matrixes and intended use of the assay. A validation plan is prepared, which lists the following with sufficient identifying details: the purpose of the assay; responsible staff; all parameters to be validated (and explanation for any parameters that cannot be validated); assay method; equipment; software; validation samples; QC material if applicable; the number of samples, replicates, runs, and operators used for each parameter; and the acceptance criteria. Although 10% coefficient of variation (CV) for intraassay precision has been reported for flow cytometry assays, less stringent acceptance criteria may be defined based on the type of assay. In an analogous manner, the requirement that validation samples must be identical to the intended use specimens is relaxed for paucicellular disease states or limited volume specimens such as cerebrospinal fluid, provided a clear explanation for using alternate samples is provided.

A. Validation planning for qualitative assays: leukemia/lymphoma diagnostic assays are qualitative but assays in the same diseases for detection of minimum residual disease, presence and degree of expression of therapeutic targets, residual target cells after treatment, and so forth are quasi-quantitative. Validation of the latter has more stringent steps, which are described later. Qualitative data provide a nominal (disease present or absent) or ordinal (such as mild, moderate, severe) interpretation and ultimately depend on comparison to confirmed clinicopathological diagnosis or/and another accepted reference method for validation. When developing a validation plan for qualitative data the following points should be included:

1. Acceptable specimens and the preanalytical variables.
2. Lower limit of detection (LLoD): the proportion of neoplastic cells reported in flow cytometric report of leukemia or lymphoma is not relevant for clinical decisions but provides a measure of assay robustness by defining the LLoD of certain cell types. Purely diagnostic assays should have LLoD as follows: myelomonocytic cells 0.5%, T cells 1%, B cells 0.1%, and plasma cells 0.1% of total collected cells. To satisfy accepted statistical considerations for rare events, at least 50 target events must be detected for a positive result. Thus, acquiring 50,000 total cells can provide the most stringent, 0.1% sensitivity. Spiking with a known positive sample into a normal specimen and verifying adequate recovery of abnormal cells in acquired events are suggested for detection of LLoD.
3. Accuracy, sensitivity, and specificity of qualitative analysis: if specimens with a confirmed diagnosis tested by the flow assay are available, a 2 x 2 truth table can be constructed to designate each flow cytometry result as true positive, true negative, and so forth. In this process, the calculated values of specificity and sensitivity measure the underlying "clinical or diagnostic accuracy" of the flow cytometry assay, and it is not required to measure the analytical accuracy separately. If suitable abnormal specimens are not available, specimens from normal subjects and those with abnormal conditions in which the cells of interest may be present can be tested by splitting each of several samples and comparing the flow cytometry results with results of an established method or results of morphologic examination. In each specimen the concordance of the nominal results (normal vs abnormal) and presence or absence of each marker tested in the assay should be recorded. A 2 x 2 table showing presence or absence of concordance is constructed, in which the results of the reference method are analogous to "true positive" or "true negative." For both methods at least 20 specimens must be compared and a concordance of greater than 95% should be obtained.
4. Precision: precision for qualitative assay is established to ensure that variations in reagents, instrument, or operator do not affect the results. A suggested rubric for these experiments is to compare the qualitative results for 5 samples, independently tested by 2 operators, each using 2 different instruments. These 20 results (4 results each on 5 specimens) are examined for agreement, and a % concordance is calculated.
5. Sample stability: a minimum of 5 samples are examined at different intervals ex vivo, and result concordance between the shortest and all subsequent intervals is compared. At least one time interval beyond the expected recommendation for maximum stability should be tested.
6. Cocktail stability: results obtained at the "zero" time point are compared for correctness of qualitative interpretation and/or changing mean fluorescence intensity of component antibodies.
7. Assay carryover: this parameter primarily evaluates the potential of abnormal cells from one specimen being detected in the subsequent specimen due to contamination of sample probe used to aspirate the sample. Although this may not be of particular concern in leukemia/lymphoma interpretations and

samples with adequate number of total cells, paucicellular samples such as body fluids require the same stringent precautions used to avoid carryover in high-sensitivity quantitative assays.

8. Linearity and reference intervals: not applicable for qualitative data.

B. Validation planning for quasi-quantitative/semiquantitative data: validation of detection capability, precision, and linearity is critically important in these assays, especially when the assay result may influence treatment decisions in clinical trials or otherwise alter patient care plans. Lacking true reference materials, the emphasis is on a factorial design of validation experiments. Repeated testing by different operators, on different days, and on different flow cytometers is required. The results are validated by interlaboratory comparisons and by using specimens obtained from patients with the same confirmed diagnosis. The necessity for "FFP" flexibility in actual validation protocol is recognized, but explicit documentation is required if any of the recommended steps are abbreviated or omitted in validation.

1. The specificity/selectivity and accuracy of the flow cytometry assay are interrelated and depend on its capability to correctly identify the abnormal cells in a background of normal cells with similar properties in repeated testing under predefined *repeatability conditions*. An example of suggested factorial assay is shown in **Fig. 3**. If after initial evaluation, new literature suggests that the assay may be applied in new disease states, additional validation with minimum of 3 specimens from such a condition should be tested to broaden the specificity of the assay.

2. The *limit of blank* (LoB) provides the foundation for the claimed sensitivity of quasi-quantitative assays. It is defined as the amount of signal detected in the absence of *analyte* (also called measurand). In assays for rare event detection, LoB is the detectable fluorescence signal for the key defining antibody due to nonspecific antibody binding to other cells. For leukemia/lymphoma minimal residual disease (MRD), LoB is established by testing samples from subjects without the disease and samples from patients successfully treated for the disease. The latter allows identification of normal regenerating counterparts and effect of therapy-induced necrosis/apoptosis in the specimen matrix. If seeking approval for the assay as an IVD, additional strategies such as isoclonal blocking by unlabeled antibodies are required. After establishing LoB, the *LLoD* is validated by replicate spiking of normal specimens with serial dilutions, more than 5 or more steps, of an abnormal specimen. The data from these serial spiking experiments are plotted to define the "linearity" of the assay.

3. The *lower limit of quantification (LLoQ)* is established by testing in triplicate 5 or more samples that have been "spiked" near the LLoD. For MRD assays, testing 5 or more samples from previously treated patients with low amount of residual disease may be used as an alternative. In either case, the minimum number of events in the gate created for the abnormal events should be defined based on statistical considerations of Poisson distribution (generally accepted as 20 and 50 events for LLoD and LLoQ, respectively).[35]

4. Precision: 3 to 5 specimens each from the low, mid, and high range of the measurand are tested under the defined reproducibility conditions. Simplified statistical methods provided in the guidance can calculate the CV for these measurements. Setting 10% CV as acceptance criterion for precision is possible for flow cytometry assays on abundant cell populations, which can be easily distinguished from other cell types. Higher level of CV is acceptable for less abundant populations (such as MRD detection) and for populations that do not show a bimodal expression pattern of key identifying antigens.

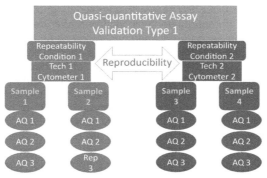

Fig. 3. Suggested factorial design to validate quasi-quantitative assays. This design is suitable for validating clinical assays reporting continuous numerical results, including, but not limited to, assays for minimal residual disease. The factorial design provides data to assess precision under repeatability conditions as well as reproducibility with the least number of repetitions, thus conserving costly reagents and permitting the use of difficult-to-obtain clinical specimens. An assay using the same procedure performed by the same technologist, on the same instrument, and at the same location is considered a "run" under repeatability condition. The precision calculated on results of triplicate aliquots of each sample is the "within-run" precision. By using 4 samples (instead of the 3 samples suggested for establishing precision under repeatability condition) and testing 2 samples under 2 repeatability conditions as shown, the reproducibility of the assay also can be validated. Note that in a laboratory with only one instrument that is used by 2 technologists, an intermediate "within laboratory" precision can be established. When 2 instruments are used as shown, the repeatability of the assay is validated. Of the 4 specimens used, at least 2 should be intended use specimens, preferably at the high and low end of the measurement range. This design is not suitable for regulatory clearance or for approval for in vitro diagnostic devices (assays), and the "type 2" validation matrix shown in the CLSI document H62 should be followed (Tech, technologist operatory, AQ, aliquot) (Based on guidance provided in CLSI document H62).

The selected higher imprecision target should be defined and justified as part of the evaluation.

5. Stability of specimens and reagents (such as antibody cocktails) is established similar to the qualitative assays.
6. Reference intervals: clinical flow cytometry assays intended to be used in clinical decisions should specify the reference intervals. In most cases these are based on published literature, but ideally obtained from the relevant subsets of subjects from local populations seen in the clinical practice.

CLINICAL CARE POINTS: PEARLS AND PITFALLS

- Decision to develop new assay: if the laboratory is already performing flow cytometry assays, survey past sample types and numbers to estimate possible volumes of the new assay. If newly introducing flow cytometry assays, estimate the expected volumes by polling the relevant clinicians. Be mindful of practical conditions such as available technical personnel, instruments, reagent budgets. Survey the clinicians for their expectations for turnaround time and availability of service afterhours and weekends and balance these with workload limits for hematopathologists and technical staff.
- Single-step or 2-step staining protocols: workup of cases with suspected new diagnosis may use a 2-step or 1-step approach depending on the relative cost

of reagents versus labor. In cases with a known diagnosis, the possibility of disease progression, immunophenotypic shift/drift after treatment, and emergence of therapy-induced second malignancy should not be ignored. In both old and new diagnoses, the occurrence of 2 or more abnormal cell populations should be considered and adequately covered in the assay design.

- Spectral flow cytometry: although the conventional methods using peak emission measurements are described in this review, a related technology of *spectral flow cytometry* provides additional flexibility and depth of analysis through the use of up to 44 fluorochromes. Currently for research use only, instruments available from ThermoFisher/Agilent and Sony are being introduced in Asia and Europe for clinical use. When investing in an upgraded conventional flow cytometer, the advances in spectral flow cytometry for clinical use should be kept in mind as a possible alternative *platform*.
- Flow cytometers are precision instruments that require constant and careful maintenance. Initial *installation qualification* and ongoing *operational qualification* are the responsibility of the manufacturer. A preventive maintenance and onsite repair contract with the manufacturer is highly desirable to ensure smooth operations with minimum downtime. The quality and immediate availability of trained service engineers should be assessed as part of the instrument purchase decision.
- Depending on specific circumstances, analysis software may be a significant ongoing expense. However, familiarity by the technical staff to a particular software is a major incentive to continue with the same software. If an alternative software is being considered, a technical expert from the new vendor may be asked to create analysis templates that have parallel paths of analysis steps in the new and old analysis (important for the technical staff) and closely approximate the appearance of the data (important for the hematopathologists).
- When multiple MoAbs reacting with the same antigen are available, the "analyte-specific reagent (ASR)"-grade MoAbs should be used. Use of "research use only (RUO)" MoAb should be reserved for contingencies such as supply chain disruption or overwhelming panel design considerations. A "lot to lot" comparison with previously used antibody for selectivity and titer should be documented with clear explanation for the emergency use circumstances.
- For quasi-quantitative assays for rare cells, precision levels of 10% may not be attainable. In such case, the ability of the assay being FFP to provide clinically relevant results, despite the higher imprecision, should be documented.[36]

CLINICS CARE POINTS

- Decision process to develop new assay should include considerations about prior experience or projected clinical need, practical constraints of availability of trained or trainable technical personnel, budgets for capital and recurring expenses (instruments, reagents, and software), clinical expectations of turnaround time, and ability of technical and professional (hematopathology) staff to fulfill these expectations.

- Single-step or 2-step staining protocols: balance the additional reagent costs of the former against the added work and slower turnaround due to 2-step assay.

- Spectral flow cytometry: although the use of *spectral flow cytometry* is mostly restricted for research in the United States, the deployment of these assays for clinical use in Asia should be kept in mind as a possible alternative *platform*.

- Flow cytometers are precision instruments that require constant and careful maintenance. Initial *installation qualification* and ongoing *operational qualification* are the responsibility of the manufacturer. A preventive maintenance and onsite repair contract with the manufacturer is highly desirable to ensure smooth operations with minimum downtime.

- Cost of analysis software and process for acquiring it (purchase vs annual licensing fees) should be carefully balanced against the advantages familiar to the technical staff as well as to the interpreting pathologists.
- When available, the ASR-grade antibodies should be used. RUO antibodies should be reserved for contingencies such as supply chain disruption or overwhelming panel design considerations.
- For quasi-quantitative assays for rare cells, precision levels of 10% may not be attainable. In such case, the ability of the assay to be FFP to provide clinically relevant results, despite the higher imprecision, should be documented.

ACKNOWLEDGMENTS

The author is thankful for the assistance and input from Mrs. Beverly Williams, MT (ASCP), Analytical Specialist, Clinical Flow Cytometry Lab, Duke Health over the years and for preparing this article.

DISCLOSURE

The authors have nothing to disclose.

REFERENCES

1. Foon KA, Todd RF 3rd. Immunologic classification of leukemia and lymphoma. Blood 1986;68(1):1–31.
2. Harris NL, Jaffe ES, Stein H, et al. A revised European-American classification of lymphoid neoplasms: a proposal from the International Lymphoma Study Group. Blood 1994;84(5):1361–92.
3. Campo E, Jaffe ES, Stein H, et al, editors. WHO classification of Tumours of Haematopoietic and lymphoid tissues. Lyon, France: International Agency for Research on Cancer; 2017.
4. Jaffe ES, Harris NL, Stein H, et al, editors. Pathology and Genetics of Tumours of Haematopoietic and lymphoid tissues. 3 edition. Lyon, France: IARC Press; 2001.
5. Swerdlow SH, Campo E, Harris NL, et al, editors. WHO classification of Tumours of Haematopoietic and Lymhoid tissues. 4 edition. Lyon: International Agency on Research on Cancer; 2008.
6. Genzen JR. Regulation of laboratory-developed tests. Am J Clin Pathol 2019; 152(2):122–31.
7. Clinical and Laboratory Standards Institute (CLSI). Validation of Assays Performed by Flow Cytometry. 1st et. CLSI guideline H62 (ISBN 978-1-68440-128-4 [Print]; ISBN 978-1-68440-129-1 [Electronic]. Clinical and Laboratory Standards Institute, USA, 2021.
8. Kamentsky LA, Melamed MR, Derman H. Spectrophotometer: new instrument for ultrarapid cell analysis. Science 1965;150(3696):630–1.
9. Hoffman RA, Kung PC, Hansen WP, et al. Simple and rapid measurement of human T lymphocytes and their subclasses in peripheral blood. Proc Natl Acad Sci U S A 1980;77(8):4914–7.
10. Ip SH, Rittershaus CW, Healey KW, et al. Rapid enumeration of T lymphocytes by a flow-cytometric immunofluorescence method. Clin Chem 1982;28(9):1905–9.

11. Loken MR, Stall AM. Flow cytometry as an analytical and preparative tool in immunology. J Immunol Methods 1982;50(3):R85–112.
12. Guidelines for the performance of CD4+ T-cell determinations in persons with human immunodeficiency virus infection. MMWR Recomm Rep (Morb Mortal Wkly Rep) 1992;41(RR-8):1–17.
13. Revised guidelines for the performance of CD4+ T-cell determinations in persons with human immunodeficiency virus (HIV) infections. Centers for Disease Control and Prevention. MMWR Recomm Rep (Morb Mortal Wkly Rep) 1994; 43(RR-3):1–21.
14. Borowitz MJ, Guenther KL, Shults KE, et al. Immunophenotyping of acute leukemia by flow cytometric analysis. Use of CD45 and right-angle light scatter to gate on leukemic blasts in three-color analysis. Am J Clin Pathol 1993;100(5):534–40.
15. Stelzer GT, Shults KE, Loken MR. CD45 gating for routine flow cytometric analysis of human bone marrow specimens. Ann N Y Acad Sci 1993;677:265–80.
16. Kalina T. Reproducibility of flow cytometry through standardization: opportunities and challenges. Cytometry 2020;97(2):137–47.
17. Bernard A, Boumsell L. The clusters of differentiation (CD) defined by the first international workshop on human leucocyte differentiation antigens. Hum Immunol 1984;11(1):1–10.
18. U.S.-Canadian. Consensus recommendations on the immunophenotypic analysis of hematologic neoplasia by flow cytometry. Bethesda, Maryland. Cytometry 1997;30(5):213–74.
19. Borowitz MJ, Bray R, Gascoyne R, et al. U.S.-Canadian Consensus recommendations on the immunophenotypic analysis of hematologic neoplasia by flow cytometry: data analysis and interpretation. Cytometry 1997;30(5):236–44.
20. Braylan RC, Atwater SK, Diamond L, et al. U.S.-Canadian Consensus recommendations on the immunophenotypic analysis of hematologic neoplasia by flow cytometry: data reporting. Cytometry 1997;30(5):245–8.
21. Davis BH, Foucar K, Szczarkowski W, et al. U.S.-Canadian Consensus recommendations on the immunophenotypic analysis of hematologic neoplasia by flow cytometry: medical indications. Cytometry 1997;30(5):249–63.
22. Stewart CC, Behm FG, Carey JL, et al. U.S.-Canadian Consensus recommendations on the immunophenotypic analysis of hematologic neoplasia by flow cytometry: selection of antibody combinations. Cytometry 1997;30(5):231–5.
23. Stelzer GT, Marti G, Hurley A, et al. Canadian Consensus recommendations on the immunophenotypic analysis of hematologic neoplasia by flow cytometry: standardization and validation of laboratory procedures. Cytometry 1997;30(5): 214–30.
24. Clinical applications of flow cytometry. Immunophenotyping of leukemic cells. Approved Guideline. Villanova, PA: National Committee for Clinical Laboratory Standards; 1997.
25. CLSI. Fluorescence calibration and quantitation measurements of fluorescence intensity, approved guideline. Villanova, PA: Clinical and Laboratory Standards Institute; 2004.
26. CLSI. Clinical. Flow cytometric analysis of neoplastic hematolymphoid cells; approved guideline. second ed. Wayne, PA: Clinical and Laboratory Standards Institute; 2007.
27. Enumeration CLSI. Of immunologically defined cell populations by flow cytometry. Second ed. Wayne, Pennsylvania: Clinical and Laboratory Standards Institute; 2007. 940 West Valley Road, Suite 1400.

28. Davis BH, Wood B, Oldaker T, et al. Validation of cell-based fluorescence assays: practice guidelines from the ICSH and ICCS - part I - rationale and aims. Cytometry B Clin Cytom 2013;84(5):282-5.
29. Davis BH, Dasgupta A, Kussick S, et al. Validation of cell-based fluorescence assays: practice guidelines from the ICSH and ICCS - part II - preanalytical issues. Cytometry B Clin Cytom 2013;84(5):286-90.
30. Tangri S, Vall H, Kaplan D, et al. Validation of cell-based fluorescence assays: practice guidelines from the ICSH and ICCS - part III - analytical issues. Cytometry B Clin Cytom 2013;84(5):291-308.
31. Barnett D, Louzao R, Gambell P, et al. Validation of cell-based fluorescence assays: practice guidelines from the ICSH and ICCS - part IV - postanalytic considerations. Cytometry B Clin Cytom 2013;84(5):309-14.
32. Wood B, Jevremovic D, Bene MC, et al. Validation of cell-based fluorescence assays: practice guidelines from the ICSH and ICCS - part V - assay performance criteria. Cytometry B Clin Cytom 2013;84(5):315-23.
33. van Dongen JJ, Lhermitte L, Bottcher S, et al. EuroFlow antibody panels for standardized n-dimensional flow cytometric immunophenotyping of normal, reactive and malignant leukocytes. Leukemia 2012;26(9):1908-75.
34. Vallangeon BD, Tyer C, Williams B, et al. Improved detection of diffuse large B-cell lymphoma by flow cytometric immunophenotyping-Effect of tissue disaggregation method. Cytometry B Clin Cytom 2016;90(5):455-61.
35. Rawstron AC, Orfao A, Beksac M, et al. Report of the European Myeloma Network on multiparametric flow cytometry in multiple myeloma and related disorders. Haematologica 2008;93(3):431-8.
36. Kouzegaran S, Siroosbakht S, Farsad BF, et al. Elevated IL-17A and IL-22 regulate expression of inducible CD38 and Zap-70 in chronic lymphocytic leukemia. Cytometry B Clin Cytom 2018;94(1):143-7.

Advances in Monitoring and Prognostication for Lymphoma by Flow Cytometry

Amrit P. Singh, MD, Elizabeth L. Courville, MD*

KEYWORDS

- MRD • Flow cytometry • Immunophenotype • Lymphoma • Immunotherapy
- Chronic lymphocytic leukemia • Prognosis • Clonality

KEY POINTS

- Flow cytometry (FC) is a well-established diagnostic tool in the workup of lymphoma.
- Many prognostic immunophenotypic markers by FC have been explored in chronic lymphocytic leukemia (CLL); fewer exist for other mature lymphomas.
- Robust FC minimal/measurable residual disease assays exist for CLL but not for other mature lymphomas.
- T-cell receptor β constant region 1 evaluation by FC has the potential benefit for diagnosis and monitoring in T cell lymphomas.
- Targeted therapies introduce the potential for loss or downregulation of antigen expression; test interference from therapeutic monoclonal antibodies has been reported.

INTRODUCTION

Lymphomas comprise a heterogeneous group of diseases with variable clinical presentations, pathological features, and prognoses. In lymphoma diagnosis, flow cytometry (FC) can provide a detailed immunophenotypic profile of the lesional material and can provide a surrogate of clonality. Advantages of FC include a rapid turnaround time (within hours) and the ability to provide detailed data on subpopulations of cells. In certain lymphomas that may not have a tissue counterpart, for example, chronic lymphocytic leukemia (CLL), FC may constitute the primary diagnostic method.

Minimal/measurable residual disease (MRD) can be defined as persistent disease present posttherapy using methods more sensitive and specific than morphologic evaluation. Sensitivity levels in MRD can reach between 0.01% and 0.001% abnormal cells depending on the method utilized.[1] In FC, the quality of MRD testing is influenced

Department of Pathology, University of Virginia Health, PO Box 800214, Charlottesville, VA 22908, USA
* Corresponding author.
E-mail address: ec8kk@hscmail.mcc.virginia.edu

Clin Lab Med 43 (2023) 351–361
https://doi.org/10.1016/j.cll.2023.04.010
0272-2712/23/© 2023 Elsevier Inc. All rights reserved.

labmed.theclinics.com

by a number of factors including the amount and quality of the specimen, the staining process (including reagent combinations used), the number of cells evaluated, and the approach to data analysis.[2]

Recent advances in lymphoma treatment, namely targeted therapies such as therapeutic monoclonal antibodies and chimeric antigen receptor (CAR) T-cells, have practical implications for clinical FC.

This article addresses select concepts in monitoring and prognostication by FC in mature lymphomas, with information presented by lymphoma subtype.

Chronic Lymphocytic Leukemia

CLL is common, with diagnostic FC for CLL routine in most clinical FC laboratories. A core FC panel to include CD19, CD20, CD5, CD23, kappa, and lambda was proposed by the European Research Initiative on CLL (ERIC) and European Society for Clinical Cell Analysis harmonization initiative to identify typical CLL.[3] Additional markers that may be helpful in the diagnosis of CLL include CD22, FMC7, CD79b, CD81, CD43, and CD200, with down regulation of CD22, CD81, FMC7, and CD79b, and increased expression of CD43 and CD200 in CLL[3–6] (**Fig. 1**). In CLL, as for all mature B cell lymphomas, monotypic surface light chain expression (either kappa or lambda) can serve as a surrogate for clonality.

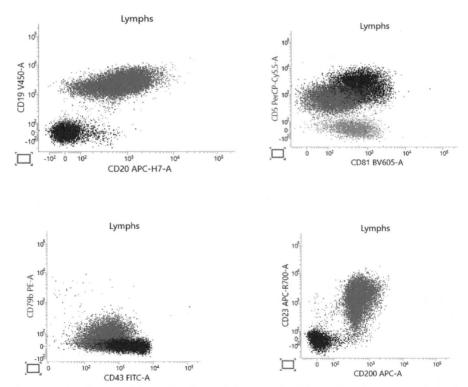

Fig. 1. FC plots from peripheral blood sample involved by CLL. The lymphocyte population is displayed. The neoplastic B cells are shown in red while T cells are shown in blue. The CLL cells are positive for CD5, CD19, CD23, and CD200, with moderate CD43 expression, and dim expression of CD20 and CD81.

A variety of FC prognostic markers have been studied in CLL. Elevated CD38 expression is associated with adverse prognostic factors including advanced disease stage, higher incidence of lymphadenopathy, high-risk cytogenetics, poor response to therapy, and shorter overall survival.[7–9] ZAP-70 expression is associated with poor overall survival and correlates with immunoglobulin heavy chain (IgH) mutational status.[7,8,10] ZAP-70 evaluation by FC can be technically difficult and its use as a surrogate marker for IgH mutational status has become less common.[11] CD49d overexpression predicts inferior overall survival and/or shortened time to treatment.[12–14] There is minimal and conflicting data regarding the prognostic significance of CD200 in CLL.[15,16] Recently, high CD105 surface expression was explored as a potential risk marker and therapeutic target in high-risk CLL.[17]

The CLL International Prognostic Index (CLL-IPI) separates patients into 4 groups with different overall survival at 5 years; it is based on 5 independent prognostic factors: *TP53* deletion and/or mutation, *IGHV* mutational status, serum β_2-microglobulin, clinical stage, and age.[18] Notably, none of the prognostic factors in this model are immunophenotypic markers. In a recent study, authors Giudice and colleagues studied the prognostic significance of expression of 3 surface markers (CD49d, CD38, and CD11c) in conjunction with the CLL-IPI and advocate for an integrated prognostic scoring system.[19]

In the era of novel targeted therapies, current prognostic models for CLL may need to be reassessed because prognostic factors in patients treated with chemoimmunotherapy may not be relevant with novel therapies.[9] In addition, with the development of novel strategies targeting cell surface markers, FC may aid in the identification of potential immunotherapeutic targets on CLL cells for individual patients and may help predict response to targeted therapy based on expression levels.[20,21]

In CLL, undetectable MRD (less than 10^{-4} detectable leukemic cells in peripheral blood or bone marrow) after treatment with chemoimmunotherapy or venetoclax-based regimens seems to be an important predictor of treatment efficacy. The National Comprehensive Cancer network guidelines Version 1.2022 support the integration of MRD assessment as part of response evaluation.[22] Single-tube FC assays for MRD detection in CLL include an 8-color assay (CD19/CD20/CD5/CD43/CD79b/CD81/CD22/CD3) proposed by the ERIC consortium that was able to reliably detect MRD down to 10^{-5}.[23] Alternative FC MRD assays for CLL have been published, including incorporation of CD160, an natural killer cell activating receptor that is also expressed on T-cell subsets, and frequently aberrantly expressed in the neoplastic B cells of CLL,[24] and incorporation of CD43.[25]

Rituximab (anti-CD20 monoclonal antibody) therapy in combination with chemotherapy has been used for decades in the treatment of CLL. Newer anti-CD20 monoclonal antibody agents such as ofatumumab and obinutuzumab have also been introduced.[18] This necessitates FC panels used for monitoring for residual/recurrent disease after therapeutic monoclonal antibody therapy to include alternative strategies (other than CD20 expression) in the identification of CLL cells.

Mantle Cell Lymphoma

Although both are typically composed of CD5-positive monotypic B cells, mantle cell lymphoma (MCL) can usually be distinguished from CLL by additional FC characteristics including brighter expression of CD20, CD22, CD79b, FMC7, and CD81 with typically negative CD23 and CD200, and dimmer CD43 expression. In addition, the expression of monotypic surface light chains in MCL is moderate to bright (in contrast to dim expression in CLL).[26] Other small B cell lymphomas may be CD5 positive, including lymphoplasmacytic lymphoma and splenic marginal zone lymphoma (17% and 22% of cases, respectively, by small case series).[27,28]

Although FC is commonly used in the diagnosis of MCL, its use is not standard for MRD evaluation. In one study of a single-tube, 8-color FC assay (CD20, CD23, CD5, CD19, CD200, CD62 L, CD3, CD45), the sensitivity based on dilutional studies ranged from 2×10^{-4} up to 10^{-2}, not reaching the sensitivity of real-time quantitative polymerase chain reaction (RQ-PCR).[29] In another study using an 8-color 10 antibody panel (CD3/CD14/CD56-[FITC], LAIR-1/CD305-[PE], CD19-[PeCy7], CD5-[PerCPCy5.5], CD11A-[APC], Lambda [Alexa700], Kappa [Pacific Blue], CD45 [V500]), the sensitivity limit was 10^{-4}.[30] PCR-based and next-generation sequencing-based methods of MRD detection in MCL show sensitivities ranging from 10^{-4} to 10^{-5}. The gold standard for monitoring MRD is RQ-PCR amplification of clonal IgH VDJ or IGH-BCL1 rearrangements, with the highest sensitivity, quantitative results, and both highly standardized and widely applicable methods.[31–33]

MCL is frequently treated using anti-CD20 monoclonal antibody regimen and more recently anti-CD19 CAR-T therapy in relapsed or refractory cases.[34,35] As persistent or relapsed disease following therapy may show absent or downregulated expression of these markers, knowledge of such therapy is helpful when designing and interpreting FC panels for monitoring of MCL.

Follicular Lymphoma

CD10 expression by FC aids in the diagnosis of follicular lymphoma (FL), although CD10 expression is not specific for FL, with the differential for a CD10-positive monotypic B cell population by FC including but not limited to diffuse large B cell lymphoma, Burkitt lymphoma, and hairy cell leukemia. Grade 3 FL can present with significantly dimmer CD10 expression than grade 1-2.[36] CD5 expression has been associated with worse outcome in FL.[37,38] In one study, CD5 expression in FL was associated with a higher IPI, higher rate of transformation to diffuse large B cell lymphoma, and shorter progression-free survival. In that study, the CD5 expression by FC was reported to show varying intensity with the majority showing dim partial or moderate expression.[38]

The immune microenvironment of FL has been extensively studied by both FC and immunohistochemical methods.[39] Although there is intriguing literature in this area including studies correlating T-cell subsets with outcomes (eg, refs[40–42]), at the current time, clinical FC evaluation of the T-cell tumor microenvironment in FL is not standard.

Validated and standardized MRD panels for FL do not exist, with MRD evaluation by RQ-PCR considered the gold standard.[43] As for other B-cell lymphomas, therapy for FL frequently includes an anti-CD20 monoclonal antibody. Knowledge of such monoclonal antibody therapy is helpful when designing and interpreting FC panels for monitoring of FL.

Large B Cell Lymphomas

The large B cell lymphomas are a clinically and biologically heterogeneous group of diseases with variable outcomes. Subclassification of large B cell lymphoma typically requires incorporation of morphologic and immunophenotypic features, in conjunction with cytogenetic data and occasionally clinical features. A complete discussion of the subclassification is beyond the scope of this article. In the distinction from B-lymphoblastic leukemia/lymphoma (consists of immature B-lymphoblasts), FC can rapidly provide evidence for a mature B cell process (by lack of expression of CD34 and TdT, bright CD45 expression, and identification of monotypic surface light chains). Bright expression of CD38 by FC has been associated with a *MYC* gene translocation, which may be helpful for rapid preliminary assessment of an aggressive B cell lymphoma.[44]

Many potential prognostic markers have been evaluated in large B cell lymphoma, mainly by immunohistochemical methods.[45–48] The Hans immunohistochemical algorithm (utilizing CD10, BCL6, and MUM1) is widely used as a surrogate for germinal center B cell (GCB) versus non-GCB diffuse large B cell lymphoma.[49] Although CD10 is commonly evaluated by FC in B cell lymphoma, it is our practice to also evaluate by immunohistochemical stain. As examples of other prognostic markers in diffuse large B cell lymphoma (DLBCL), patients with CD5-positive DLBCL often have features associated with aggressive clinical behavior,[50–52] and in a recent study of de novo DLBCL, high CD38 expression by FC was an independent adverse prognostic factor associated with poor clinical outcomes.[53] There is a body of literature regarding the importance of the tumor microenvironment in DLBCL[54,55]; however, at the current time, clinical FC evaluation of the T-cell tumor microenvironment in DLBCL is not standard.

T-cell Lymphoid Proliferations and Lymphomas

T cell lymphoid proliferations and lymphomas represent a diverse group of entities, ranging from indolent to highly aggressive, and include a wide range of clinical presentations and morphologic appearances.[56] FC aids in the appropriate diagnostic classification of T cell lymphoid proliferations/lymphomas by providing an immunophenotyping profile. FC represents a robust method to detect aberrant antigen expression or loss and, in comparison to immunohistochemistry on tissue specimens, is particularly helpful in identifying subtle differences in T-cell antigen expression as well as small subsets of T-cells with immunophenotypic aberrancy.

For decades, T-cell receptor (TCR) gene rearrangement studies have been the primary method to establish T-cell clonality, with a limited number of clinical FC laboratories using assessment of TCR-Vbeta expression to establish clonality.[57,58] TCR-Vbeta analysis by FC uses fluorescently labeled antibody reagents to specific TCR β-chain variable region family members (covering the majority, but not all, of Vbeta domains found in blood T lymphocytes), with a restricted Vbeta-reactivity pattern indicating clonality.[59] In contrast, T-cell receptor β constant region 1 (TRBC1) assessment by FC uses a single fluorescently labeled monoclonal antibody (clone JOVI.1), allowing more widespread adoption among laboratories and easier evaluation of T-cell subset populations. JOVI.1 recognizes one (TRBC1) of 2 mutually exclusive TCR β constant region antigens randomly selected during TCR gene rearrangement, allowing for easy assessment of a restricted reactivity pattern[60] (**Fig. 2**).

The literature on TRBC1-based FC assays has expanded rapidly over the past several years. The method has shown utility in the diagnosis of T-cell large granular lymphocytic leukemia,[60] in the detection of circulating disease in patients with cutaneous T-cell lymphoma,[61,62] and in the diagnosis of T-cell lymphomas including in tissue specimens and body fluids.[63,64] TRBC1-based assays may aid in future FC MRD detection in T-cell receptor alpha-beta (TCRαβ) lymphomas; however, care must be taken to not overinterpret monotypic small T-cell subsets of uncertain significance.[65,66] Similar to Vbeta analysis, TRBC1 assessment is useful in the evaluation of TCRαβ populations, but not TCR gamma-delta populations.

Beyond qualitative immunophenotyping of neoplastic T cells and providing evidence of clonality, FC can also provide semiquantitative data helpful for T-large granular lymphocytic leukemia diagnosis and mycosis fungoides/Sezary syndrome staging.[56] For both these semiquantitative purposes, it is important to recognize that commercial single-platform tests are not widely available for leukemia/lymphoma

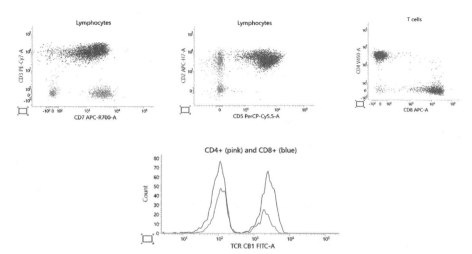

Fig. 2. FC plots from benign peripheral blood sample showing polytypic TRBC1 expression. There are discrete TRBC1-positive and TRBC1-negative subsets for both the CD4+ and CD8+ T cells.

immunophenotyping assays and numerous variables (preanalytic, analytic, and post-analytic) affect both the accuracy and precision of dual platform FC.[67]

Brentuximab vedotin (an antibody-drug conjugate targeting CD30-expressing malignant cells) has been used as a therapeutic agent in patients with relapsed or refractory systemic anaplastic large cell lymphoma (ALCL) as well as other subtypes of relapsed PTCL.[68] This raises the theoretical risk of interference with the detection of CD30+ neoplastic cells by FC after therapy, although documentation of such an interference is not known to the authors. Alemtuzumab (IgG1-kappa monoclonal antibody targeted against CD52) is used in the treatment of T-prolymphocytic leukemia (T-PLL). Artifactual surface kappa light chain restriction has been reported in 2 patients with T-PLL treated with alemtuzumab.[69]

CLINICS CARE POINTS

- FC allows for rapid immunophenotyping, helping to diagnose and distinguish lymphomas.
- In CLL, a variety of flow cytometric prognostic markers have been studied, including CD38, ZAP-70, CD49d, CD200, and CD105, among others. However, none of the prognostic factors in the current CLL-IPI are immunophenotypic markers.
- Robust FC MRD assays exist for CLL, with undetectable MRD an important predictor of treatment efficacy. Single-tube assays have been reported to reliably detect MRD down to 10^{-5}.
- Targeted therapies such as monoclonal antibodies and CAR T-cells affect clinical FC. Treatment-induced changes in CD20 and CD19 expression highlight the need for adaptable FC panels. FC assessment of cell surface marker expression may be helpful in determining potential immunotherapeutic targets.
- In the era of novel targeted therapies, prognostic models for lymphomas may need to be reassessed, as prognostic factors in patients treated with chemoimmunotherapy may not be relevant with novel therapies.

- TRBC1 assessment by FC is becoming standard in the workup of potential T-cell lymphoma/T-cell lymphoproliferative disorders. Their utility in MRD assessment has not been established.

DISCLOSURE

The authors have nothing to disclose.

REFERENCES

1. Cherian S, Soma LA. How I diagnose minimal/measurable residual disease in B lymphoblastic leukemia/lymphoma by flow cytometry. Am J Clin Pathol 2021; 155(1):38–54.
2. Stetler-Stevenson M, Paiva B, Stoolman L, et al. Consensus guidelines for myeloma minimal residual disease sample staining and data acquisition. Cytometry B Clin Cytom 2016;90(1):26–30.
3. Rawstron AC, Kreuzer KA, Soosapilla A, et al. Reproducible diagnosis of chronic lymphocytic leukemia by flow cytometry: an European Research initiative on CLL (ERIC) & European Society for clinical cell analysis (ESCCA) Harmonisation project. Cytometry B Clin Cytom 2018;94(1):121–8.
4. Challagundla P, Medeiros LJ, Kanagal-Shamanna R, et al. Differential expression of CD200 in B-cell neoplasms by flow cytometry can assist in diagnosis, subclassification, and bone marrow staging. Am J Clin Pathol 2014;142(6):837–44.
5. D'Arena G, De Feo V, Pietrantuono G, et al. CD200 and chronic lymphocytic leukemia: biological and clinical relevance. Front Oncol 2020;10:584427.
6. Palumbo GA, Parrinello N, Fargione G, et al. CD200 expression may help in differential diagnosis between mantle cell lymphoma and B-cell chronic lymphocytic leukemia. Leuk Res 2009;33(9):1212–6.
7. Cramer P, Hallek M. Prognostic factors in chronic lymphocytic leukemia-what do we need to know? Nat Rev Clin Oncol 2011;8(1):38–47.
8. Van Bockstaele F, Verhasselt B, Philippe J. Prognostic markers in chronic lymphocytic leukemia: a comprehensive review. Blood Rev 2009;23(1):25–47.
9. Boddu P, Ferrajoli A. Prognostic factors in the era of targeted therapies in CLL. Curr Hematol Malig Rep 2018;13(2):78–90.
10. Liu Y, Wang Y, Yang J, et al. ZAP-70 in chronic lymphocytic leukemia: a meta-analysis. Clin Chim Acta 2018;483:82–8.
11. Best OG, Ibbotson RE, Parker AE, et al. ZAP-70 by flow cytometry: a comparison of different antibodies, anticoagulants, and methods of analysis. Cytometry B Clin Cytom 2006;70(4):235–41.
12. Gooden CE, Jones P, Bates R, et al. CD49d shows superior performance characteristics for flow cytometric prognostic testing in chronic lymphocytic leukemia/small lymphocytic lymphoma. Cytometry B Clin Cytom 2018;94(1):129–35.
13. Bulian P, Shanafelt TD, Fegan C, et al. CD49d is the strongest flow cytometry-based predictor of overall survival in chronic lymphocytic leukemia. J Clin Oncol 2014;32(9):897–904.
14. Shanafelt TD, Geyer SM, Bone ND, et al. CD49d expression is an independent predictor of overall survival in patients with chronic lymphocytic leukaemia: a prognostic parameter with therapeutic potential. Br J Haematol 2008;140(5): 537–46.
15. D'Arena G, Valvano L, Vitale C, et al. CD200 and prognosis in chronic lymphocytic leukemia: conflicting results. Leuk Res 2019;83:106169.

16. Miao Y, Fan L, Wu YJ, et al. Low expression of CD200 predicts shorter time-to-treatment in chronic lymphocytic leukemia. Oncotarget 2016;7(12):13551–62.
17. Greiner SM, Marklin M, Holzmayer S, et al. Identification of CD105 (endoglin) as novel risk marker in CLL. Ann Hematol 2022;101(4):773–80.
18. Hallek M. Chronic lymphocytic leukemia: 2020 update on diagnosis, risk stratification and treatment. Am J Hematol 2019;94(11):1266–87.
19. Giudice V, Serio B, Bertolini A, et al. Implementation of International Prognostic Index with flow cytometry immunophenotyping for better risk stratification of chronic lymphocytic leukemia. Eur J Haematol 2022;109(5):483–93.
20. Paulus A, Malavasi F, Chanan-Khan A. CD38 as a multifaceted immunotherapeutic target in CLL. Leuk Lymphoma 2022;63(10):2265–75.
21. Schilhabel A, Walter PJ, Cramer P, et al. CD20 expression as a possible novel prognostic marker in CLL: application of EuroFlow Standardization technique and normalization procedures in flow cytometric expression analysis. Cancers 2022;14(19):4917.
22. National Comprehensive Cancer Network. Chronic lymphocytic Leukemia/Small Lymphocytic Lymphoma (Version 1.2022). Available at: https://www.nccn.org/guidelines/category_1. Accessed 12 September, 2021.
23. Rawstron AC, Fazi C, Agathangelidis A, et al. A complementary role of multiparameter flow cytometry and high-throughput sequencing for minimal residual disease detection in chronic lymphocytic leukemia: an European Research Initiative on CLL study. Leukemia 2016;30(4):929–36.
24. Farren TW, Sadanand KS, Agrawal SG. Highly sensitive and accurate assessment of minimal residual disease in chronic lymphocytic leukemia using the novel cd160-ROR1 assay. Front Oncol 2020;10:597730.
25. Dowling AK, Liptrot SD, O'Brien D, et al. Optimization and validation of an 8-color single-tube assay for the sensitive detection of minimal residual disease in B-cell chronic lymphocytic leukemia detected via flow cytometry. Lab Med 2016;47(2):103–11.
26. Qiu L, Xu J, Tang G, et al. Mantle cell lymphoma with chronic lymphocytic leukemia-like features: a diagnostic mimic and pitfall. Hum Pathol 2022;119:59–68.
27. Lin P, Molina TJ, Cook JR, et al. Lymphoplasmacytic lymphoma and other non-marginal zone lymphomas with plasmacytic differentiation. Am J Clin Pathol 2011;136(2):195–210.
28. Hsu A, Kurt H, Zayac AS, et al. CD5 expression in marginal zone lymphoma predicts differential response to rituximab or bendamustine/rituximab. Leuk Lymphoma 2022;63(1):31–42.
29. Chovancova J, Bernard T, Stehlikova O, et al. Detection of minimal residual disease in mantle cell lymphoma-establishment of novel eight-color flow cytometry approach. Cytometry B Clin Cytom 2015;88(2):92–100.
30. Cheminant M, Derrieux C, Touzart A, et al. Minimal residual disease monitoring by 8-color flow cytometry in mantle cell lymphoma: an EU-MCL and LYSA study. Haematologica 2016;101(3):336–45.
31. Jung D, Jain P, Yao Y, et al. Advances in the assessment of minimal residual disease in mantle cell lymphoma. J Hematol Oncol 2020;13(1):127.
32. Ladetto M, Tavarozzi R, Pott C. Minimal residual disease in mantle cell lymphoma: methods and clinical significance. Hematol Oncol Clin North Am 2020;34(5):887–901.
33. Pott C. Minimal residual disease detection in mantle cell lymphoma: technical aspects and clinical relevance. Semin Hematol 2011;48(3):172–84.

34. Armitage JO, Longo DL. Mantle-cell lymphoma. N Engl J Med 2022;386(26): 2495–506.
35. Wang M, Munoz J, Goy A, et al. KTE-X19 CAR T-cell therapy in relapsed or refractory mantle-cell lymphoma. N Engl J Med 2020;382(14):1331–42.
36. Ray S, Craig FE, Swerdlow SH. Abnormal patterns of antigenic expression in follicular lymphoma: a flow cytometric study. Am J Clin Pathol 2005;124(4): 576–83.
37. Miyoshi H, Sato K, Yoshida M, et al. CD5-positive follicular lymphoma characterized by CD25, MUM1, low frequency of t(14;18) and poor prognosis. Pathol Int 2014;64(3):95–103.
38. Li Y, Hu S, Zuo Z, et al. CD5-positive follicular lymphoma: clinicopathologic correlations and outcome in 88 cases. Mod Pathol 2015;28(6):787–98.
39. Wahlin BE, Aggarwal M, Montes-Moreno S, et al. A unifying microenvironment model in follicular lymphoma: outcome is predicted by programmed death-1– positive, regulatory, cytotoxic, and helper T cells and macrophages. Clin Cancer Res 2010;16(2):637–50.
40. Wahlin BE, Sander B, Christensson B, et al. CD8+ T-cell content in diagnostic lymph nodes measured by flow cytometry is a predictor of survival in follicular lymphoma. Clin Cancer Res 2007;13(2 Pt 1):388–97.
41. Wu H, Tang X, Kim HJ, et al. Expression of KLRG1 and CD127 defines distinct CD8(+) subsets that differentially impact patient outcome in follicular lymphoma. J Immunother Cancer 2021;9(7):e002662.
42. Magnano L, Martinez A, Carreras J, et al. T-cell subsets in lymph nodes identify a subgroup of follicular lymphoma patients with favorable outcome. Leuk Lymphoma 2017;58(4):842–50.
43. Pott C, Bruggemann M, Ritgen M, et al. MRD detection in B-cell non-Hodgkin lymphomas using ig gene rearrangements and chromosomal translocations as targets for real-time quantitative PCR. Methods Mol Biol 2019;1956:199–228.
44. Alsuwaidan A, Pirruccello E, Jaso J, et al. Bright CD38 expression by flow cytometric analysis is a biomarker for double/triple Hit lymphomas with a moderate sensitivity and high Specificity. Cytometry B Clin Cytom 2019;96(5):368–74.
45. Li S, Young KH, Medeiros LJ. Diffuse large B-cell lymphoma. Pathology 2018; 50(1):74–87.
46. Chastain EC, Duncavage EJ. Clinical prognostic biomarkers in chronic lymphocytic leukemia and diffuse large B-cell lymphoma. Arch Pathol Lab Med 2015; 139(5):602–7.
47. Xie Y, Bulbul MA, Ji L, et al. p53 expression is a strong marker of inferior survival in de novo diffuse large B-cell lymphoma and may have enhanced negative effect with MYC coexpression: a single institutional clinicopathologic study. Am J Clin Pathol 2014;141(4):593–604.
48. Hu S, Xu-Monette ZY, Tzankov A, et al. MYC/BCL2 protein coexpression contributes to the inferior survival of activated B-cell subtype of diffuse large B-cell lymphoma and demonstrates high-risk gene expression signatures: a report from the International DLBCL Rituximab-CHOP Consortium Program. Blood 2013;121(20): 4021–31, quiz 4250.
49. Hans CP, Weisenburger DD, Greiner TC, et al. Confirmation of the molecular classification of diffuse large B-cell lymphoma by immunohistochemistry using a tissue microarray. Blood 2004;103(1):275–82.
50. Alinari L, Gru A, Quinion C, et al. De novo CD5+ diffuse large B-cell lymphoma: adverse outcomes with and without stem cell transplantation in a large, multicenter, rituximab treated cohort. Am J Hematol 2016;91(4):395–9.

51. Thakral B, Medeiros LJ, Desai P, et al. Prognostic impact of CD5 expression in diffuse large B-cell lymphoma in patients treated with rituximab-EPOCH. Eur J Haematol 2017;98(4):415–21.

52. Yamaguchi M, Seto M, Okamoto M, et al. De novo CD5+ diffuse large B-cell lymphoma: a clinicopathologic study of 109 patients. Blood 2002;99(3):815–21.

53. Wada F, Shimomura Y, Yabushita T, et al. CD38 expression is an important prognostic marker in diffuse large B-cell lymphoma. Hematol Oncol 2021;39(4):483–9.

54. Coutinho R, Clear AJ, Mazzola E, et al. Revisiting the immune microenvironment of diffuse large B-cell lymphoma using a tissue microarray and immunohistochemistry: robust semi-automated analysis reveals CD3 and FoxP3 as potential predictors of response to R-CHOP. Haematologica 2015;100(3):363–9.

55. Gomez-Gelvez JC, Salama ME, Perkins SL, et al. Prognostic impact of tumor microenvironment in diffuse large B-cell lymphoma uniformly treated with R-CHOP chemotherapy. Am J Clin Pathol 2016;145(4):514–23.

56. WHO Classification of Tumours Editorial Board. Haematolymphoid tumours Internet; beta version ahead of print. Lyon (France): International Agency for Research on Cancer; 2022 cited 2022 Dec 1. (WHO classification of tumours series, 5th ed.; vol. 11). Available at: https://tumourclassification.iarc.who.int/chapters/63. In.

57. Morice WG, Kimlinger T, Katzmann JA, et al. Flow cytometric assessment of TCR-Vbeta expression in the evaluation of peripheral blood involvement by T-cell lymphoproliferative disorders: a comparison with conventional T-cell immunophenotyping and molecular genetic techniques. Am J Clin Pathol 2004;121(3):373–83.

58. Novikov ND, Griffin GK, Dudley G, et al. Utility of a Simple and robust flow cytometry assay for rapid clonality testing in mature peripheral T-cell lymphomas. Am J Clin Pathol 2019;151(5):494–503.

59. Langerak AW, van Den Beemd R, Wolvers-Tettero IL, et al. Molecular and flow cytometric analysis of the Vbeta repertoire for clonality assessment in mature TCRalphabeta T-cell proliferations. Blood 2001;98(1):165–73.

60. Horna P, Olteanu H, Jevremovic D, et al. Single-antibody evaluation of T-cell receptor beta constant chain monotypia by flow cytometry facilitates the diagnosis of T-cell large granular lymphocytic leukemia. Am J Clin Pathol 2021;156(1):139–48.

61. Martin-Moro F, Martin-Rubio I, Garcia-Vela JA. TRBC1 expression assessed by flow cytometry as a novel marker of clonality in cutaneous alphabeta T-cell lymphomas with peripheral blood involvement. Br J Dermatol 2022;187(4):623–5.

62. Horna P, Shi M, Jevremovic D, et al. Utility of TRBC1 expression in the diagnosis of peripheral blood involvement by cutaneous T-cell lymphoma. J Invest Dermatol 2021;141(4):821–829 e822.

63. Berg H, Otteson GE, Corley H, et al. Flow cytometric evaluation of TRBC1 expression in tissue specimens and body fluids is a novel and specific method for assessment of T-cell clonality and diagnosis of T-cell neoplasms. Cytometry B Clin Cytom 2021;100(3):361–9.

64. Waldron D, O'Brien D, Smyth L, et al. Reliable detection of T-cell clonality by flow cytometry in mature T-cell neoplasms using TRBC1: implementation as a reflex test and comparison with PCR-based clonality testing. Lab Med 2022;53(4):417–25.

65. Munoz-Garcia N, Lima M, Villamor N, et al. Anti-TRBC1 antibody-based flow cytometric detection of T-cell clonality: Standardization of sample preparation and diagnostic implementation. Cancers 2021;13(17):4379.

66. Shi M, Jevremovic D, Otteson GE, et al. Single antibody detection of T-cell receptor alphabeta clonality by flow cytometry rapidly identifies mature T-cell neoplasms and monotypic small CD8-positive subsets of uncertain significance. Cytometry B Clin Cytom 2020;98(1):99–107.
67. Horna P, Wang SA, Wolniak KL, et al. Flow cytometric evaluation of peripheral blood for suspected Sezary syndrome or mycosis fungoides: International guidelines for assay characteristics. Cytometry B Clin Cytom 2021;100(2):142–55.
68. Horwitz SM, Ansell S, Ai WZ, et al. T-cell lymphomas, version 2.2022, NCCN clinical practice guidelines in oncology. J Natl Compr Canc Netw 2022;20(3): 285–308.
69. Chen PP, Tormey CA, Eisenbarth SC, et al. False-positive light chain clonal restriction by flow cytometry in patients treated with alemtuzumab: potential pitfalls for the misdiagnosis of B-cell neoplasms. Am J Clin Pathol 2019;151(2):154–63.

Flow Cytometry in Diagnosis, Prognostication, and Monitoring of Multiple Myeloma and Related Disorders

Mikhail Roshal, MD, PhD*, Qi Gao, DCLS, MLS ASCP(CM)

KEYWORDS

- Multi-myeloma • Flow cytometry • Measurable residual disease (MRD)
- Plasma cells

KEY POINTS

- Measurable disease analysis is critical for monitoring disease response and is strongly predictive of treatment outcomes in multi-myeloma.
- Early data shows promise for MRD-driven treatment strategies.
- Flow cytometric MRD analysis in myeloma must be carefully designed for optimal sam collection, adequate cell numbers, proper informative marker selection, and analysis strategies.

OVERVIEW OF PLASMA CELL NEOPLASMS AND OTHER DISORDERS WITH CLONAL PLASMA CELL EXPANSIONS

Primary plasma cell neoplasms are a group of disorders characterized by the proliferation of clonal plasma cells. These entities can be broadly divided into predominantly localized (plasmacytoma of the bone, extraosseous plasmacytoma) and those presenting with a diffuse marrow involvement (non-IgM monoclonal gammopathy of unknown significance (MGUS), IgM MGUS, plasma cell type, and multiple myeloma (MM)). Primary AL light chain amyloidosis, as well as plasma cell neoplasms associated with paraneoplastic syndromes POEMS (Polyneuropathy, Organomegaly, Endocrinopathy, Monoclonal protein, Skin changes),[1,2] TEMPI (Telangiectasias, Elevated Erythropoietin, and Erythrocytosis, Monoclonal Gammopathy, Perinephric Fluid Collections, and Intrapulmonary Shunting),[3,4] AESOP (adenopathy and extensive skin patch overlying a plasmacytoma)[5] which result from the secretion of abnormal immunoglobulins by plasma cells, may also be grouped with the primary plasma cell neoplasms.[1,2]

The authors have no relevant conflicts of interest to disclose.
Department of Pathology and Laboratory Medicine, Memorial Sloan Kettering Cancer Center
* Corresponding author. Department of Pathology and Laboratory Medicine, Memorial Sloan Kettering Cancer Center, 1275 York Avenue, New York, NY 10065.
E-mail address: roshalm@mskcc.org

Clin Lab Med 43 (2023) 363–375
https://doi.org/10.1016/j.cll.2023.05.003
0272-2712/23/© 2023 Elsevier Inc. All rights reserved.

MM is thought to arise from years to decades of clonal evolution and MGUS preceding myeloma in nearly all patients.[3,4] MM is the most common symptomatic plasma cell neoplasm and accounts for approximately 13% of all lymphoid cancers in the Western world.[5,6] While MM is most often diagnosed in the bone marrow, virtually every organ in the body can be involved either at presentation or in disease progression. MM is further stratified as either smoldering (asymptomatic) or symptomatic.[1,2] Precise classification schemas based on extensive clinical and biological evidence are available.[1,2]

A range of other neoplasms may present with plasma cell expansions. These neoplasms must be distinguished from the primary plasma cell neoplasms for proper clinical intervention. Many low-grade B cell neoplasms, such as marginal zone lymphoma and lymphoplasmacytic lymphoma, but also others may present with simultaneous expansions of both clonal B and plasma cell components. More aggressive B lineage neoplasms such as plasmablastic lymphoma and primary effusion B-cell lymphoma among others, as well as post-transplant lymphoproliferative disorders can show clonal plasma cells. Angioimmunoblastic T cell lymphoma, while formally a T cell neoplasm, is often associated with clonal B and/or plasma cell expansions. These expansions can progress to B cell neoplasms with a marked plasmacytic component.[7–9] Finally, rare entities such as HHV8-associated lymphoproliferative disorders may present with light chain restricted (lambda), but not clonal plasma cell expansions.[10]

ROLE OF FLOW CYTOMETRY IN THE DIAGNOSTIC EVALUATION OF PLASMA CELL EXPANSIONS

Flow cytometry plays a critical role in the initial evaluation of suspected neoplasms with a plasma cell component. At Memorial Sloan Kettering Cancer Center (MSKCC), the flow cytometry evaluation protocol includes evaluation for both B and plasma cell components in the bone marrow, bony lesions, and/or blood and B, T, and plasma cell components in the lymphoid tissue. Such evaluations are generally prompted by either discovery of monoclonal immunoglobulin in the serum (with or without other neoplastic signs) or the morphologic discovery of plasma cell/plasmacytic proliferation. **Fig. 1** presents the common scenarios for workup and outcome considerations. The presence of a neoplastic B cell component in association with plasma cells sharing the same light chain restriction should prompt the consideration of B cell lymphoma with plasmacytic differentiation. In low-grade B cell neoplasms, plasma cell components tend to lack many overt myeloma-associated abnormalities such as expression of CD56 and/or CD117 and losses of expression of CD45 and CD19, although the latter two occasionally occur in B cell lymphomas. The typical phenotypic differences are illustrated in **Fig. 2**. If the phenotype of the plasma cells lacks these abnormal features and is associated with a B cell expansion sharing the light chain restriction, the diagnosis of B cell lymphoproliferative neoplasm with plasmacytic differentiation is highly likely. If, on the other hand, plasma cells show a frank myeloma-like phenotype, the probable diagnosis would be coincident B and plasma cell neoplasms despite sharing the same light chain type. In either case, morphologic, clinical, and molecular genetic/cytogenetic evaluation is needed to confirm the original impression. The presence of AITL-like (CD4+, PD1+, surface CD3+/−, CD5+, CD7+/−) T cells in association with clonal B and/or plasma cell components should prompt further consideration of AITL. More aggressive B cell lymphomas with plasmacytic/plasmablastic differentiation pose further diagnostic challenges as they occasionally may have phenotypes like those found in MM. The presence of a B cell component is helpful in such cases,

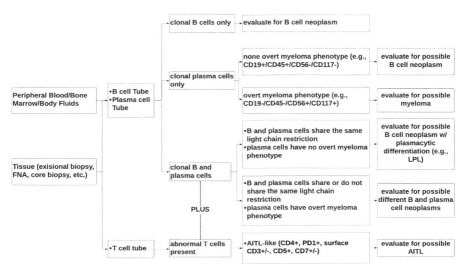

Fig. 1. MSKCC workflow for suspected plasma cell neoplasms.

but the ultimate diagnosis requires an extensive clinicopathologic correlation that is beyond the scope of the review.

The presence of the isolated plasma cell component with a myeloma-like phenotype generally argues for a primary plasma cell neoplasm in the proper clinicopathologic context. Conversely, light chain restricted plasma cell expansion showing normal expression of CD19, CD45, and without CD56 or CD117 is not strong evidence of plasma cell neoplasm and should still prompt consideration of B cell lymphoma or even a light chain restricted non-neoplastic expansion.

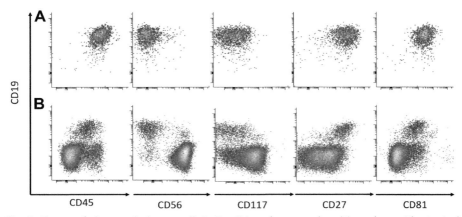

Fig. 2. Exams of abnormal plasma cells in B cell lymphoma and multi-myeloma. The typical phenotypes of abnormal plasma cells in B cell lymphoma with plasmacytic differentiation and multi-myeloma differ. Plasma cells associated with B cell lymphoma (*A*) tend to show a relatively normal phenotype including normal expression of CD19, CD27, CD45, and CD81, without CD56 or CD117, while multi-myeloma plasma cells (*B*) tend to have multi abnormalities. Kappa light chain expressing plasma cells are shown in blue, while lambda light chain expressing plasma cells are shown in red.

Flow cytometry alone usually does not distinguish between primary plasma cell neoplasms as there is a considerable degree of overlap in immunophenotypes of these entities and quantitation of bone marrow plasma cells by flow cytometry in bone marrow is usually a significant underestimate compared to biopsy. The presence of a significant number of polytypic plasma cells in the background tends to be associated with lower-risk MGUS and a less aggressive clinical course in multi-myeloma.[11] However, the finding is also relatively common in AL light chain amyloidosis and POEMS syndrome.

Finally, flow cytometry of the peripheral blood is poised to play a critical role in the confirmation of the diagnosis of a rare but extremely aggressive plasma cell leukemia which may arise either *de-novo* or as a transformation of myeloma. Recent data from the Catalan[12] and Mayo Clinic[13] groups showed that patients with greater than 5% clonal plasma cells in the peripheral blood have markedly poor outcomes like those with circulating plasma cells greater than 20%. This prompted the international myeloma working group (IMWG) to redefine a plasma cell cutoff from 20% to 5% of the white blood cells for the diagnosis of plasma cell leukemia in the peripheral blood.[14] Even a lower (2%) cutoff for plasma cell leukemia has been proposed based on inferior outcomes and aggressive disease course.[15] This, in turn, leads to an increase in the prevalence of plasma cell leukemia in patients with myeloma. While the criteria are based on cytomorphologic assessment, the difficulties in morphologic plasma cell enumeration in peripheral blood and the need for the confirmation of the clonal nature of the plasma cells will almost certainly play an increasing role in plasma cell leukemia evaluations. Notably, unlike bone marrow evaluations, plasma cell enumeration in the peripheral blood is accurate compared to cytomorphologic assessment.[16]

ROLE OF FLOW CYTOMETRY IN THE PROGNOSTICATION OF PLASMA CELL NEOPLASMS AT DIAGNOSIS

Flow cytometry plays a role in upfront risk stratification in primary plasma cell neoplasms. Solitary plasmacytoma of the bone is defined in part by the absence of myeloma-defining clinical signs. In particular, the monoclonal plasma cells must be less than 10%. However, recent studies have demonstrated that the presence of even a low detectable bone marrow infiltration by flow cytometry leads to a high risk of progression to overt myeloma.[17] In particular, the study showed that 71% of patients with detectable low-level bone marrow infiltration by flow cytometry developed myeloma with a median time of progression of 26 months, whereas only 8% of patients without detectable marrow involvement did so. Of interest, no such association was seen in patients with solitary extraosseous plasmacytomas. This may be related to the relatively low rate of progression of extraosseous plasmacytoma.[18,19]

Newer risk stratification schemas for smoldering myeloma and MGUS do not include bone marrow flow cytometry.[20,21] Nonetheless, the presence of greater than 95% of clonal plasma cells within the plasma cell compartment by flow cytometry has been linked to the increased risk for progression to symptomatic disease.[11]

Recently the more sensitive flow cytometric techniques allowed for the measurement of circulating plasma cells in the peripheral blood. In a study of patients with smoldering myeloma, the presence of higher-than-average levels of abnormal circulating plasma cells (>0.015%) could potentially substitute for bone marrow biopsy plasma cell quantitation in risk prediction models.[22]

The presence of increased circulating plasma cells at diagnosis is also a risk factor for symptomatic myeloma outcomes. Both 4-year progression-free (PFS) and overall survival (OS) were negatively impacted in patients showing greater than 0.07% circulating abnormal plasma cells (hazard ratio of 2.61 for both outcome measures).

ROLE OF MEASURABLE RESIDUAL DISEASE IN THE ASSESSMENT OF TREATMENT RESPONSE IN MULTIPLE MYELOMA

While highly sensitive MRD detection methods have rightly attracted recent attention, flow cytometry also plays a role in the routine assessment of post-therapy marrow with even a relatively high number of plasma cells. For instance, our group has reviewed historical data on patients receiving extended lenalidomide maintenance therapy. A substantiation proportion of these patients showed elevated levels of plasma cells in the bone marrow in the range of 5% to 20%.[23] Morphologic assessment of the clonal, partially clonal versus polyclonal nature of these plasma cells is challenging and often unreliable for technical reasons. For instance, morphologic and immunohistochemical assessment alone produced many false positives for persistent disease. Flow cytometry allowed for correct response determination in these patients with the majority falling into the stringent comte response category (MRD-) despite greater than 5% plasma cells in the bone marrow. It is therefore imperative not to use morphology for screening sams for flow cytometry under most circumstances.

Deep MRD determination has become exceptionally important in managing patients with myeloma. The need arose because of the greatly improved expanded arsenal of therapeutic options for myeloma. These treatments now routinely produce disease reduction levels significantly below those that can be detected by conventional techniques, including morphology, fluorescence in situ hybridization, or even earlier iterations of flow cytometric MRD assessment.[24–26] Many of these patients however still have a low level of abnormal plasma cells that can be detected by the more sensitive methods. Thanks to these new therapeutic options, patients are living longer, have many more response assessments, and can switch therapies should the initial approach prove less effective over time.[27,28] The new IMWG criteria for therapy response are a recognition of this reality.[29] A sensitivity of 10^{-5} or lower for MRD testing is now a part of the requirement for the adequate assessment of drug response and disease status while on treatment.

Prospective clinical trials and metanalysis of pooled data from multi trials have firmly established a strong prognostic role of MRD evaluation in predicting progression-free and overall survival in patients with myeloma.[30–35] The most recent combined analysis of 4 trials in different therapeutic settings showed an impressive hazard ratio of 0.2 for progression-free survival with 3–4-year follow-up using MRD sensitivity of 10^{-5}.[30] This association holds regardless of specific therapy, although different therapies produced different rates of MRD negativity.[30,35] Importantly, sensitive MRD determination is far superior to morphologic and serologic remission assessment in predicting the outcome. A pooled analysis of Spanish trials has demonstrated that the achievement of comte remission by morphologic and serologic criteria was not superior to lesser responses unless accompanied by MRD negativity.[34] Outside of the sim binary determination of MRD positivity versus negativity, the quantitative depth of response provides additional prognostic information in those patients with low but detectable levels of MRD.[36]

While achieving MRD negativity is associated with superior outcomes, many patients nonetheless relapse after a period of MRD negativity. Loss of MRD negativity is associated with inferior outcomes.[32,37–41] IMWG defined sustained MRD negativity criterion defined by requires MRD negativity measured at least 12 months apart.

However, recent studies show that sustained MRD for at least 6 months also provides additional diagnostic information.[32,39]

While the prognostic role of MRD in myeloma is now exceptionally well established, important clinical questions remain. The fundamental question is whether such prognostic information is clinically actionable to improve the outcomes of MRD-positive patients and potentially de-intensify therapy for those who achieve a durable MRD negativity. Preliminary data from retrospective studies suggests that both may be possible.[42] In a retrospective analysis, the discontinuation of therapy upon the achievement of MRD during the maintenance phase of treatment was not associated with inferior PFS compared to the patients in whom treatment was continued. Importantly, patients who did not achieve MRD negativity and who were further treated with intensification or change in therapy showed superior PFS compared to those in whom no change in therapy was made. The data is retrospective and therefore should be confirmed in a well-designed clinical trial. Prospective studies are being designed to address tailored MRD-guided therapy approaches.[43,44]

Given the clear and overwhelming evidence for the association of MRD status (both sustained and single point) with outcomes, and the possible utility of using MRD to change therapy, there is a significant movement to utilize MRD as a meaningful clinical endpoint for drug registration trials.[45] If accepted by regulatory authorities, such an approach could expedite the "readout" of myeloma therapy trials.

Finally, an assessment of plasma cells in stem cell graft products in patients undergoing autologous transplants for myeloma has attracted considerable attention.[46] Sensitive flow cytometry can show the presence of contaminating neoplastic plasma cells in the grafts. The presence of neoplastic plasma cells is associated with inferior transplant outcomes. However, it is less clear that the finding provides independent prognostic information compared to established disease status assessment techniques including circulating plasma cell assessment outside of the graft.

QUANTITATIVE ASPECTS OF MEASURABLE RESIDUAL DISEASE ASSESSMENT

Specific aspects of flow cytometry assay validation are covered elsewhere in the issue (see Anand Shreeram Lagoo's article, "How to Design and Validate a Clinical Flow Cytometry Assay," in this issue). Recent CLSI guideline H62 provides an excellent and detailed guide as well.[47] Each MRD assay must have a well-validated limit of detection (LOD) and a lower limit of quantitation (LLOQ). For an excellent and detailed overview of the topic, the reader is referred to a recent review.[48] The minimum precision required for adequate quantitation is determined by the lower limit of quantitation. For MRD assays in general, a variation of 20% to 30% is considered acceptable. The LLOQ may be equivalent to or higher than the LOD.

LOD may be best understood as a minimum signal (number of events) that can be consistently distinguished from a normal background in the same matrix under the testing conditions. The concept is closely linked to the limit of blank (LOB). LOB can be estimated by running 5 to 10 normal sams with and without spike-in with very low numbers of abnormal cells at the proposed detection limit. The abnormal events can be gated and any events in the normal (blank) sams falling within the "abnormal" gate would be calculated as a part of the matrix background. LOB can then be calculated as a $mean_{blank} + 1.645(Standard Deviation (SD)_{blank})$

LOD can then be calculated as $LOB + 1.645(SD_{low\ concentration\ sam})$.[49]

The maximal obtainable precision of an assay for LLOQ is determined by Poisson counting statistics where the SD of the assay can be estimated as

$SD=\sqrt{n}$, where n is the number of events in the population of interest. The preferred measure of variability the coefficient of variation (CV) can be obtained by SD/n or $CV=\sqrt{n}/n$. Therefore at least 25 events would be required to obtain a CV of 20% and roughly 11 events would be needed for a CV of 30%. In practice, precision tends to be significantly reduced due to biological sam variation and sam processing. LLOQ therefore must be empirically validated on sams with varying phenotypes in the same matrix as used for clinical testing under the same conditions.

With these calculations in mind, it can now be understood why the at least $2*10^6$ cells are required for the sensitivity of $1/10^5$. In practice, 5 to 10 million cells are obtained for plasma cell MRD analysis with obtainable sensitivities of $1/10^5 - 2/10^6$. For instance, the EuroFlow plasma cell MRD assay claims a sensitivity of $2*10^{-6}$ with 10 million cells acquired[50] and the published Memorial Sloan Kettering assay shows a sensitivity of $3*10^{-6}$ with 6 million cells analyzed.[51,52] The input cell number for the assays should be at least 2-3-fold higher (12–30 million) because of cell losses during sam processing. Such cell numbers can only routinely be obtained via cell concentration and are not consistently achievable via staining unconcentrated sams of up to 400 µL.[50] Some laboratories stain multi unconcentrated marrow sams from the same patient and pool them for analysis to obtain the required cell numbers. This approach may be a better fit in some laboratory workflows but may increase reagent costs and instrument usage[53,54]

SAMPLE COLLECTION

Bone marrow usually provides the highest concentration of abnormal plasma cells in the context of multi-myeloma. While peripheral blood usually contains abnormal plasma cells at diagnosis, the proportion is markedly lower compared to the bone marrow.[55] At follow-up, the circulating abnormal plasma cells may still be detected in a proportion of patients; however, the detection shows markedly lower sensitivity for patients with MRD positivity as compared to bone marrow analysis or even serologic studies.[56] It follows that the hemodilution of the bone marrow sams can markedly affect the sensitivity of bone marrow analysis. A study from NIH/NCI has shown that plasma cells are reduced at least 30-fold in hemodiluted versus minimally -hemodiluted bone marrows.[57] To obtain the desired number of cells without marked hemodilution, 2 to 4 mL of first-pull anticoagulated (EDTA) bone marrow should be provided to the testing laboratory. A recent study showed that a technical first pull (marrow pull after needle repositioning) could achieve similar results.[58] It was our experience that a real (rather than repositioned) first pull can be obtained and is desirable when the sam is collected rapidly and shared for morphologic and flow cytometric assessment (data not shown).

Modern flow cytometry panels also allow for at least a qualitative assessment of the extent of hemodilution in the analysis and reporting phase. An illustration is shown in **Fig. 3**. Assessment for the presence of immature B cells, nucleated red blood cells, mast cells, and maturing (CD117+) myeloid progenitors can allow the analyst to evaluate if the sam consists predominantly of blood or marrow elements. This is critical for sams with no detectable disease as hemodilution leads to increased false negative results.

FLOW CYTOMETRIC PANEL DESIGN

Both normal and neoplastic plasma cells show significant immunophenotypic heterogeneity necessitating significant multixing to be able to separate normal from abnormal plasma cells in nearly all patients. Very few short (2–4 antigen) phenotypes are entirely specific for neoplastic plasma cells. For exam, while the CD45 and CD19

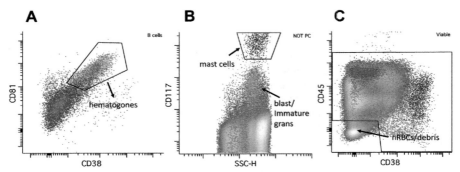

Fig. 3. Built-in quality control for hemodilution in bone marrow evaluation for residual multi-myeloma. Immature B cells (hematogones) (*A*, light blue), mast cells (*B*, purple), immature myeloid precursors (*B*, yellow), and nucleated red cells (*C*, *arrow*) can be measured to assess the extent of hemodilution.

negative CD56 positive phenotype is indeed relatively common in plasma cell neoplasm, it is shared by a subset of normal plasma cells.[59,60] This is illustrated in **Fig. 4**. Therefore additional abnormalities would be important to detect even in this canonical phenotype. EuroFlow investigators have shown that a panel targeting antigen combination of CD19, *CD27*, CD45, CD56, *CD81*, and CD117, along with cytoplasmic light chain assessment, allowed for the separation of virtually all myeloma plasma cells from their normal counterparts in diagnostic sams.[50,61] Moreover, the investigators showed that all these antigens had added value to the panel. Therefore, these

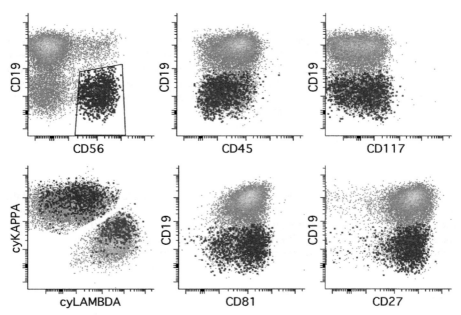

Fig. 4. Normal plasma cells can show CD56 positive phenotype with loss of CD19 and CD45. Plasma cells showing kappa light chain expression and shown in blue, while those showing lambda light chain expression are shown in red. Note CD56 positive normal plasma cells (emphasized) showing normal polytypic light chain expression.

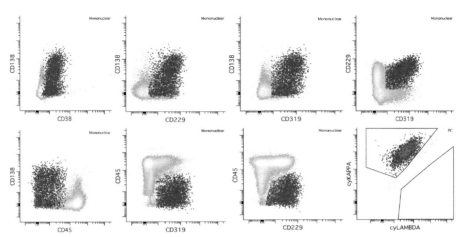

Fig. 5. Exam of the use of redundant lineage antigens for plasma cell gating in the absence of CD38. Abnormal plasma cells (*blue*) lacking anti-CD38 reactivity post-treatment can be identified using combinations of anti-CD138, CD319, CD229, and light chains.

antigens along with the gating reagents targeting CD38 and CD138 are now considered obligatory for optimal panel design.[29,59]

TARGETED THERAPY

Approaches to multiple myeloma MRD in the era of targeted therapy have recently been reviewed by our group.[62] Briefly, the introduction of ant-CD38 therapies has necessitated alternative plasma cell gating strategies to overcome both steric hindrances by the therapeutic antibody and the reduction of CD38 cell surface expression. Euroflow group introduced a multi-epitope anti- CD38 formulation that appears to partially overcome the steric hindrance problem but does not address the marked reduction of CD38 expression seen in some patients with myeloma under therapy. Alternative gating reagents have been explored, with CD319 and CD229 emerging as the most promising targets.[63,64] Utilization of either or both these antigens improves the sensitivity of the myeloma MRD panels in anti–CD38-treated patients. MSKCC has introduced both antigens in the current iteration of the 12-color single-tube panel (**Fig. 5**).

Flow cytometry is also used to assess the presence of immunotherapy targets such as BCMA, GPRC5D, and CD229 on the cell surface.[65–67] Such targets may have relatively low antigen density on the cell surface, making proper antibody clone selection, use of very bright fluorochromes, and minimizing background critically important for proper assessment.

FUNDING

National Cancer Institute (NCI) Core Grant (P30 CA008748).

CLINICS CARE POINT

- Flow cytometry is critical for diagnosis, prognostication, and follow-up of multi-myeloma

REFERENCES

1. Alaggio R, Amador C, Anagnostopoulos I, et al. The 5th edition of the world Health Organization classification of Haematolymphoid tumours: lymphoid neoplasms. Leukemia 2022;36(7):1720–48.
2. Campo E, Jaffe ES, Cook JR, et al. The international consensus classification of mature lymphoid neoplasms: a report from the clinical advisory Committee. Blood 2022;140(11):1229–53.
3. Landgren O, Kyle RA, Pfeiffer RM, et al. Monoclonal gammopathy of undetermined significance (MGUS) consistently precedes multi myeloma: a prospective study. Blood 2009;113(22):5412–7.
4. Weiss BM, Abadie J, Verma P, et al. A monoclonal gammopathy precedes multi myeloma in most patients. Blood 2009;113(22):5418–22.
5. Kyle RA, Rajkumar SV. Multi myeloma. N Engl J Med 2004;351(18):1860–73.
6. Kazandjian D. Multi myeloma epidemiology and survival: a unique malignancy. Semin Oncol 2016;43(6):676–81.
7. Attygalle AD, Kyriakou C, Dupuis J, et al. Histologic evoluticn of angioimmunoblastic T-cell lymphoma in consecutive biopsies: clinical correlation and insights into natural history and disease progression. Am J Surg Pathol 2007;31(7):1077–88.
8. Balague O, Martinez A, Colomo L, et al. Epstein-Barr virus negative clonal plasma cell proliferations and lymphomas in peripheral T-cell lymphomas: a phenomenon with distinctive clinicopathologic features. Am J Surg Pathol 2007;31(9):1310–22.
9. Huppmann AR, Roullet MR, Raffeld M, et al. Angioimmunoblastic T-cell lymphoma partially obscured by an Epstein-Barr virus-negative clonal plasma cell proliferation. J Clin Oncol 2013;31(2):e28–30.
10. Wang HW, Pittaluga S, Jaffe ES. Multicentric Castleman disease: where are we now? Semin Diagn Pathol 2016;33(5):294–306.
11. Perez-Persona E, Vidriales MB, Mateo G, et al. New criteria to identify risk of progression in monoclonal gammopathy of uncertain significance and smoldering multi myeloma based on multiparameter flow cytometry analysis of bone marrow plasma cells. Blood 2007;110(7):2586–92.
12. Granell M, Calvo X, Garcia-Guinon A, et al. Prognostic impact of circulating plasma cells in patients with multi myeloma: implications for plasma cell leukemia definition. Haematologica 2017;102(6):1099–104.
13. Ravi P, Kumar SK, Roeker L, et al. Revised diagnostic criteria for plasma cell leukemia: results of a Mayo Clinic study with comparison of outcomes to multi myeloma. Blood Cancer J 2018;8(12):116.
14. Fernandez de Larrea C, Kyle R, Rosinol L, et al. Primary plasma cell leukemia: consensus definition by the International Myeloma Working Group according to peripheral blood plasma cell percentage. Blood Cancer J 2021;11(12):192.
15. Jelinek T, Bezdekova R, Zihala D, et al. More than 2% of circulating tumor plasma cells Defines plasma cell leukemia-like multi myeloma. J Clin Oncol 2022;JCO2201226.
16. Bezdekova R, Jelinek T, Kralova R, et al. Necessity of flow cytometry assessment of circulating plasma cells and its connection with clinical characteristics of primary and secondary plasma cell leukaemia. Br J Haematol 2021;195(1):95–107.
17. Paiva B, Chandia M, Vidriales MB, et al. Multiparameter flow cytometry for staging of solitary bone plasmacytoma: new criteria for risk of progression to myeloma. Blood 2014;124(8):1300–3.
18. Finsinger P, Grammatico S, Chisini M, et al. Clinical features and prognostic factors in solitary plasmacytoma. Br J Haematol 2016;172(4):554–60.

19. Nakaya A, Tanaka H, Yagi H, et al. Retrospective analysis of plasmacytoma in Kansai myeloma Forum Registry. Int J Hematol 2020;112(5):666–73.

20. Kyle RA, Durie BG, Rajkumar SV, et al. Monoclonal gammopathy of undetermined significance (MGUS) and smoldering (asymptomatic) multi myeloma: IMWG consensus perspectives risk factors for progression and guidelines for monitoring and management. Leukemia 2010;24(6):1121–7.

21. Mateos MV, Kumar S, Dimopoulos MA, et al. International Myeloma Working Group risk stratification model for smoldering multi myeloma (SMM). Blood Cancer J 2020;10(10):102.

22. Termini R, Zihala D, Terpos E, et al. Circulating tumor and immune cells for minimally Invasive risk stratification of smoldering multi myeloma. Clin Cancer Res 2022;28(21):4771–81.

23. Zamarin D, Devlin SM, Arcila ME, et al. Polyclonal immune activation and marrow plasmacytosis in multi myeloma patients receiving long-term lenalidomide therapy: incidence and prognostic significance. Leukemia 2013;27(12):2422–4.

24. Diamond BT, Rustad E, Maclachlan K, et al. Defining the undetectable: the current landscape of minimal residual disease assessment in multi myeloma and goals for future clarity. Blood Rev 2021;46:100732.

25. Landgren O, Iskander K. Modern multi myeloma therapy: deep, sustained treatment response and good clinical outcomes. J Intern Med 2017;281(4):365–82.

26. Landgren O, Owen RG. Better therapy requires better response evaluation: paving the way for minimal residual disease testing for every myeloma patient. Cytometry B Clin Cytometry 2016;90(1):14–20.

27. Binder M, Nandakumar B, Rajkumar SV, et al. Mortality trends in multi myeloma after the introduction of novel therapies in the United States. Leukemia 2022; 36(3):801–8.

28. Costello CL. Newly diagnosed multi myeloma: making sense of the menu. Hematology Am Soc Hematol Educ Program 2022;2022(1):539–50.

29. Kumar S, Paiva B, Anderson KC, et al. International Myeloma Working Group consensus criteria for response and minimal residual disease assessment in multi myeloma. Lancet Oncol 2016;17(8):e328–46.

30. Cavo M, San-Miguel J, Usmani SZ, et al. Prognostic value of minimal residual disease negativity in myeloma: combined analysis of POLLUX, CASTOR, ALCYONE, and MAIA. Blood 2022;139(6):835–44.

31. Munshi NC, Avet-Loiseau H, Rawstron AC, et al. Association of minimal residual disease with superior survival outcomes in patients with multi myeloma: a meta-analysis. JAMA Oncol 2017;3(1):28–35.

32. San-Miguel J, Avet-Loiseau H, Paiva B, et al. Sustained minimal residual disease negativity in newly diagnosed multi myeloma and the impact of daratumumab in MAIA and ALCYONE. Blood 2022;139(4):492–501.

33. Landgren O, Devlin S, Boulad M, et al. Role of MRD status in relation to clinical outcomes in newly diagnosed multi myeloma patients: a meta-analysis. Bone Marrow Transplant 2016;51(12):1565–8.

34. Lahuerta JJ, Paiva B, Vidriales MB, et al. Depth of response in multi myeloma: a pooled analysis of three PETHEMA/GEM clinical trials. J Clin Oncol 2017;35(25): 2900–10.

35. de Tute RM, Rawstron AC, Gregory WM, et al. Minimal residual disease following autologous stem cell transplant in myeloma: impact on outcome is independent of induction regimen. Haematologica 2016;101(2):e69–71.

36. Rawstron AC, Gregory WM, de Tute RM, et al. Minimal residual disease in myeloma by flow cytometry: independent prediction of survival benefit per log reduction. Blood 2015;125(12):1932–5.

37. Paiva B, Manrique I, Dimopoulos MA, et al. MRD dynamics during maintenance for improved prognostication of 1280 myeloma patients in TOURMALINE-MM3 and -MM4 trials. Blood 2022;141(6):579–91.

38. Avet-Loiseau H, San-Miguel J, Casneuf T, et al. Evaluation of sustained minimal residual disease negativity with daratumumab-combination Regimens in relapsed and/or Refractory multi myeloma: analysis of POLLUX and CASTOR. J Clin Oncol 2021;39(10):1139–49.

39. de Tute RM, Pawlyn C, Cairns DA, et al. Minimal residual disease after autologous stem-cell transplant for patients with myeloma: prognostic significance and the impact of lenalidomide maintenance and molecular risk. J Clin Oncol 2022; 40(25):2889–900.

40. Diamond B, Korde N, Lesokhin AM, et al. Dynamics of minimal residual disease in patients with multi myeloma on continuous lenalidomide maintenance: a single-arm, single-centre, phase 2 trial. Lancet Haematol 2021;8(6):e422–32.

41. Mohan M, Kendrick S, Szabo A, et al. Clinical implications of loss of bone marrow minimal residual disease negativity in multi myeloma. Blood Adv 2022;6(3): 808–17.

42. Martinez-Lopez J, Alonso R, Wong SW, et al. Making clinical decisions based on measurable residual disease improves the outcome in multi myeloma. J Hematol Oncol 2021;14(1):126.

43. Korde N, Mastey D, Tavitian E, et al. Tailored treatment to MRD response: a phase I/II study for newly diagnosed multi myeloma patients using high dose twice-weekly carfilzomib (45 and 56 mg/m(2)) in combination with lenalidomide and dexamethasone. Am J Hematol 2021;96(6):E193–6.

44. Royle KL, Coulson AB, Ramasamy K, et al. Risk and response adapted therapy following autologous stem cell transplant in patients with newly diagnosed multi myeloma (RADAR (UK-MRA Myeloma XV Trial): study protocol for a phase II/III randomised controlled trial. BMJ Open 2022;12(11):e063037.

45. Anderson KC, Auclair D, Adam SJ, et al. Minimal residual disease in myeloma: application for clinical Care and new drug registration. Clin Cancer Res 2021; 27(19):5195–212.

46. Cengiz Seval G, Beksac M. Is quantification of measurable clonal plasma cells in stem cell grafts (gMRD) clinically meaningful? Front Oncol 2022;12:800711.

47. CLSI. Clinical Laboratory Standards Institute; 2021.

48. Sommer U, Eck S, Marszalek L, et al. High-sensitivity flow cytometric assays: considerations for design control and analytical validation for identification of Rare events. Cytometry B Clin Cytom 2021;100(1):42–51.

49. Armbruster DA, Pry T. Limit of blank, limit of detection and limit of quantitation. Clin Biochem Rev 2008;29(Suppl 1):S49–52.

50. Flores-Montero J, Sanoja-Flores L, Paiva B, et al. Next Generation Flow for highly sensitive and standardized detection of minimal residual disease in multi myeloma. Leukemia 2017;31(10):2094–103.

51. Roshal M, Flores-Montero JA, Gao Q, et al. MRD detection in multi myeloma: comparison between MSKCC 10-color single-tube and EuroFlow 8-color 2-tube methods. Blood Adv 2017;1(12):728–32.

52. Royston DJ, Gao Q, Nguyen N, et al. Single-tube 10-Fluorochrome analysis for efficient flow cytometric evaluation of minimal residual disease in plasma cell myeloma. Am J Clin Pathol 2016;146(1):41–9.

53. Soh KT, Tario JD Jr, Hahn TE, et al. Methodological considerations for the high sensitivity detection of multi myeloma measurable residual disease. Cytometry B Clin Cytom 2020;98(2):161–73.
54. Soh KT, Wallace PK. Monitoring of measurable residual disease in multi myeloma by multiparametric flow cytometry. Curr Protoc Cytom 2019;90(1).
55. Garces JJ, Cedena MT, Puig N, et al. Circulating tumor cells for the staging of patients with newly diagnosed transplant-eligible multi myeloma. J Clin Oncol 2022; 40(27):3151–61.
56. Sanoja-Flores L, Flores-Montero J, Puig N, et al. Blood monitoring of circulating tumor plasma cells by next generation flow in multi myeloma after therapy. Blood 2019;134(24):2218–22.
57. Manasanch EE, Salem DA, Yuan CM, et al. Flow cytometric sensitivity and characteristics of plasma cells in patients with multi myeloma or its precursor disease: influence of biopsy site and anticoagulation method. Leuk Lymphoma 2015; 56(5):1416–24.
58. Foureau DM, Paul BA, Guo F, et al. Standardizing clinical workflow for assessing minimal residual disease by flow cytometry in multi myeloma. Clin Lymphoma Myeloma Leuk 2023;23(1):e41–50.
59. Stetler-Stevenson M, Paiva B, Stoolman L, et al. Consensus guidelines for myeloma minimal residual disease sam staining and data acquisition. Cytometry B Clin Cytom 2016;90(1):26–30.
60. Tembhare PR, Yuan CM, Venzon D, et al. Flow cytometric differentiation of abnormal and normal plasma cells in the bone marrow in patients with multi myeloma and its precursor diseases. Leuk Res 2014;38(3):371–6.
61. Flores-Montero J, de Tute R, Paiva B, et al. Immunophenotype of normal vs. myeloma plasma cells: toward antibody panel specifications for MRD detection in multi myeloma. Cytometry B Clin Cytom 2016;90(1):61–72.
62. Gao Q, Chen X, Cherian S, et al. Mature B- and plasma-cell flow cytometric analysis: a review of the impact of targeted therapy. Cytometry B Clin Cytom 2023; 104(3):224–42.
63. Pojero F, Flores-Montero J, Sanoja L, et al. Utility of CD54, CD229, and CD319 for the identification of plasma cells in patients with clonal plasma cell diseases. Cytometry B Clin Cytom 2016;90(1):91–100.
64. Soh KT, Tario JD Jr, Hahn T, et al. CD319 (SLAMF7) an alternative marker for detecting plasma cells in the presence of daratumumab or elotuzumab. Cytometry B Clin Cytom 2021;100(4):497–508.
65. Mailankody S, Devlin SM, Landa J, et al. GPRC5D-Targeted CAR T cells for myeloma. N Engl J Med 2022;387(13):1196–206.
66. Radhakrishnan SV, Luetkens T, Scherer SD, et al. CD229 CAR T cells eliminate multi myeloma and tumor propagating cells without fratricide. Nat Commun 2020;11(1):798.
67. Salem DA, Maric I, Yuan CM, et al. Quantification of B-cell maturation antigen, a target for novel chimeric antigen receptor T-cell therapy in Myeloma. Leuk Res 2018;71:106–11.

Advances in Acute Myeloid Leukemia Classification, Prognostication and Monitoring by Flow Cytometry

Fabienne Lucas, MD, PhD, Christopher B. Hergott, MD, PhD*

KEYWORDS

- Acute myeloid leukemia • AML • Genomic profiling • Immunophenotype
- Flow cytometry • Minimal residual disease • Measurable residual disease • MRD

KEY POINTS

- Acute myeloid leukemia (AML) immunophenotyping can complement genomic classification and allows monitoring of therapeutic efficacy.
- Refinements in AML immunophenotype/genotype correlations have yielded clinically and prognostically relevant biomarkers.
- Measurable residual disease (MRD) monitoring has become an indispensable tool for prognostication and clinical management.
- Efforts to standardize MRD assays will improve reproducibility and permit clearer comparisons between laboratories and treatment approaches.

INTRODUCTION

The categorization of acute myeloid leukemia (AML) into subsets with specific biological characteristics and clinical outcomes is guided by morphologic, cytogenetic, and molecular studies.[1] New classification systems continually evolve to account for advances in our understanding of pathogenetic mechanisms and to better integrate information from new diagnostic modalities.[2–5] Flow cytometric analysis remains an essential tool with immediate diagnostic and prognostic importance. The full scope of flow cytometry's role in AML blast identification, lineage assignment, and aberrancy pattern identification are beyond the scope of this article and are well reviewed elsewhere.[6] Here, we focus on recent advances in genotype-immunophenotype correlation, the dissection of immunophenotypically ambiguous AML cases, and flow

Department of Pathology, Brigham and Women's Hospital, 75 Francis Street, Boston, MA 02115, USA
* Corresponding author.
E-mail address: Christopher_Hergott@DFCI.HARVARD.EDU

Clin Lab Med 43 (2023) 377–398
https://doi.org/10.1016/j.cll.2023.04.005
0272-2712/23/© 2023 Elsevier Inc. All rights reserved.

cytometric measurable residual disease (MRD) — often referred to as minimal residual disease — monitoring.

Several recurring immunophenotype/genotype correlations for AML are already well established, as we will summarize below.[1-3,6] In these situations, flow cytometric findings can inform immediate treatment decisions (ie, before genetic information is available) and guide subsequent diagnostic evaluation. These associations and their effects on biological and clinical behaviors have been refined further in recent years, often incorporating additional molecular alterations illuminated by next-generation sequencing (NGS). Moreover, several clinically tractable strategies to classify leukemias with overlapping or ambiguous immunophenotypes more accurately have recently been proposed, and we will discuss their merits herein. For patients receiving AML-directed therapy, the technical capacity for flow cytometry to detect MRD continually improves. However, limited comparability and harmonization between treatment centers has hampered its clinical utility, especially for patients transferring care.[7] Recent European LeukemiaNet (ELN) recommendations promise to enhance the availability and reproducibility of MRD assessments,[8-10] and we will discuss these guidelines below. Collectively, these advances position flow cytometry to remain a powerful diagnostic and management tool for patients with AML and will enable the innovation of novel biomarkers and treatment strategies.

ADVANCES IN ACUTE MYELOID LEUKEMIA PHENOTYPE/GENOTYPE CORRELATION

Although blasts in AML commonly share core immunophenotypic features, certain immunophenotypic patterns correlate closely with recurrent genetic alterations.[1-3,6] Flow cytometry profiles can therefore predict genomic classifications in many instances, and specific surface markers (or combinations) may help stratify genetically defined AML with respect to underlying biology and clinical behavior. **Table 1** summarizes well-established immunophenotypic features associated with key genetic alterations in AML. These associations have been further refined for several subgroups, and clinically tractable strategies to differentiate leukemias with overlapping immunophenotypes more accurately have been proposed.

Acute Myeloid Leukemia with t(8;21) (q22;q22)/RUNX1::RUNX1T1

The immunophenotypic correlates of AML with t(8;21) (q22;q22)/*RUNX1::RUNX1T1* are well established (see **Table 1**).[1] To distinguish t(8;21) AML from other subtypes, Shang and colleagues[11] integrated phenotypic aberrancies of blasts and background populations into a clinically tractable scoring system. Key features included high-intensity CD34 expression and aberrant CD19, cytoplasmic CD79a (cCD79a), and CD56 expression on blasts, coexpression of CD56 on neutrophils (especially immature neutrophils) and altered granulocyte maturity. A score of at least 3 points achieved a sensitivity, specificity, positive predictive value (PPV), and negative predictive value (NPV) of 0.86, 0.90. 0.91, and 0.84, respectively, for detecting t(8;21). Wang and colleagues[12] further explored the therapeutic and prognostic implications of aberrant CD19 expression in the context of co-occurring *KIT* mutations, which are present in a subset of t(8;21) AML and confer adverse prognostic implications.[13] In their study, pathogenic *KIT* mutations (particularly at D816) conferred a higher relapse risk irrespective of CD19 status, and this risk was higher still in CD19-negative patients (60% cumulative incidence [CI] in 3 years).[12] Inversely, CD19-positive patients without *KIT* mutations showed the lowest risk of relapse (10% 3-year CI), suggesting that CD19 immunophenotype is an important modifier of genetic risk prediction.

Table 1
Acute myeloid leukemia immunophenotypic profiles and aberrancy patterns per 2016 World Health Organization diagnostic categories[1]

Acute Myeloid Leukemia with Recurrent Genetic Abnormalities

AML with t(8;21) (q22;q22.1); *RUNX1::RUNX1T1*	• High-intensity expression of CD34, HLA-DR, MPO, CD13 • Relatively weak expression of CD33 • Maturation asynchrony (eg, coexpression of CD34 and CD15) • Aberrant expression of B-cell antigens CD19, cCD79a • Occasionally terminal deoxynucleotidyl transferase (TdT)-positive (weak) • *KIT* activating mutations are associated with aberrant expression of CD56 with relatively lower CD19 expression
AML with inv(16) (p13.1q22) or t(16;16) (p13.1;q22); *CBFB::MYH11*	• Complex immunophenotype with multiple blast populations: ○ CD34, CD117, CD13, CD33, CD15, CD65, MPO (granulocytic) ○ CD34, CD117, CD11b, CD11c, CD4,CD64, CD36, lysozyme (monocytic) • Maturation asynchrony • Expression of CD2
APL with *PML::RARA*	• High SSC • Homogeneous bright CD33, CD64, MPO • Often CD117+ (might be weak) • Heterogeneous CD13 (often decreased) • Low to absent CD15 (typically positive in normal promyelocytes) • Absence of CD34, HLA-DR, leukocyte integrins CD11a, CD11b, CD18, CD65 • Microgranular variant: ○ Lower SSC ○ More likely to express variable CD34 and CD2 (associated with *FLT3*-ITD) ○ Uniform CD13, CD64
AML with t(9;11) (p21.3;q23.3); *KMT2A::MLLT3*	• Children: ○ Strong expression of CD33, HLA-DR, CD65, CD4 ○ Low expression of CD34, CD13, CD14 • Adults: ○ Markers of monocytic differentiation: CD14, CD4, CD11b, CD11c, CD64, CD36, lysozyme ○ Variable CD34, CD117, CD56
AML with t(6;9) (p23;q34.1); *DEK::NUP214*	• Nonspecific myeloid immunophenotype: ○ Positive for MPO, CD117, CD34, HLA-DR, CD9, CD13, CD33, CD15, CD38, CD123 ○ Occasionally positive for CD64, TdT • Basophil clusters: ○ Positive for CD123, CD33, CD38 ○ Negative for HLA-DR

(continued on next page)

Table 1
(continued)

AML with inv(3) (q21.3q26.2) or t(3;3) (q21.3;q26.2); *GATA2::MECOM*	• Positive for CD34, CD33, CD13, CD117, HLA-DR • Often positive for CD38 • Aberrant CD7 expression • Occasionally aberrant megakaryocytic marker expression: CD41, CD61 • High CD34 expression more common with inv(3) than with t(3;3)
AML (megakaryoblastic) with (1;22) (p13.3;q13.1); *RBM15::MKL1*	• Expression of $\geq$1 platelet glycoprotein: CD41, CD61 (cCD41, cCD61 more specific and sensitive than sCD41, sCD61), CD42b • Positive for CD36 (not specific) • Can express CD13, CD33 • Often negative for CD45, CD34, HLA-DR • Negative for MPO, TdT, lymphoid markers
AML with *BCR::ABL1*	• Expression of CD34, CD13, CD33 • Aberrant expression of CD19, CD7, TdT
AML with gene mutations	

AML with mutated *NPM1*	• Commonly positive for CD117, CD123
	• "APL-like":
	  ○ High CD33 expression, MPO+
	  ○ Often low to absent HLA-DR, CD34
	  ○ Variable (often low) CD13 expression
	• Subtype with immature myeloid immunophenotype
	• Subtype with monocytic immunophenotype: CD36+, CD64+, CD14+

AML with biallelic mutation of *CEBPA*	• High/homogeneous expression of CD34, CD117, HLA-DR • Asynchronous maturation (concomitant high expression of CD15, CD65, CD64, cMPO) • Can express CD7, CD56
AML with mutated *RUNX1*	• Expression of CD13, CD34, HLA-DR • Variable expression of CD33, monocytic markers, MPO
AML with myelodysplasia-related changes	• Variable immunophenotypes, aberrant CD13, CD33, CD56 and/or CD7 common • Multilineage dysplasia: decreased HLA-DR, CD117, FLT3 (CD135), CD38 • Increased CD14 related to poor prognosis • High-risk patients, monosomal karyotypes: increased CD11b • Aberrations of chromosomes 5 and 7: CD34, TdT, CD7 • Prior MDS: blasts with only subset CD34+, stem-cell immunophenotype (low expression of CD38 and/or HLA-DR) • Increased populations with stem-cell immunophenotype: high-risk cytogenetics, poor outcome
Therapy-related myeloid neoplasms	No specific immunophenotypic findings

(continued on next page)

Table 1 (continued)	
AML, not otherwise specified	
AML without maturation	• Positive for MPO and ≥ one myeloid-associated antigens (CD13, CD33, CD117) • Frequently positive for CD34, HLA-DR, occasionally for CD11b • No expression of granulocytic (CD15, CD65) or monocytic maturation markers (CD14, CD64) • Subset with aberrant expression of CD7, CD2, CD4, CD19, CD56
AML with minimal differentiation	• Express early hematopoietic-associated antigens CD34, CD38, HLA-DR (CD38 and/or HLA-DR may be decreased) and ≥2 myeloid-associated markers, usually CD13, CD117, often CD33 • Lack myeloid and monocytic maturation and differentiation markers: CD11b, CD15, CD14, CD64, CD36, CD65 • May be positive for MPO (rare cells), CD7 and nuclear TdT (favorable prognostic marker)
AML with maturation	• Express HLA-DR, CD34, CD117, ≥1 myeloid-associated antigen (CD13, CD33, CD65, CD11b, CD15), and evidence of granulocytic differentiation. • Monocytic markers (CD14, CD36, CD64) usually absent • Occasionally aberrant expression of CD7 • Rarely aberrant expression of CD56, CD2, CD19, CD4 (CD4 might be restricted to most immature blasts)
Acute myelomonocytic leukemia	• Several populations of blasts variably expressing HLA-DR, myeloid antigens CD13, CD33, CD65, and CD15 and markers of monocytic differentiation (CD14, CD64, CD11b, CD11c, CD4, CD36, CD68, CD163, lysozyme) • Characteristic of monocytic differentiation: coexpression of CD15, CD36, strong CD64 • Immature blasts positive for CD34 and/or CD117 • Occasionally aberrant expression of CD7
Acute monoblastic and monocytic leukemia	• Variably expression of myeloid antigens CD13, CD33 (often very bright), CD15, CD65 • Occasionally CD34+ • Frequently HLA-DR+ • ≥ 2 markers of monocytic differentiation: CD14, CD4, CD11b, CD11c, CD64 (bright), CD68, CD36 (bright), lysozyme • MPO more frequently positive in acute monocytic than in acute monoblastic leukemia • Occasionally aberrant expression of CD7, CD56
Pure erythroid leukemia	• Positive for CD71, E-cadherin (more specific and expressed in early forms), CD36 (also positive in monocytes and megakaryocytes) • Positive for glycophorin, hemoglobin A (unless poorly differentiated erythroblasts), CD117 • Usually negative for HLA-DR, CD34 • May show partial expression of megakaryocyte markers CD41, CD61

(continued on next page)

Table 1 (continued)	
Acute megakaryoblastic leukemia	• Expression of ≥ 1 platelet glycoprotein: CD41, CD61 (cCD41, cCD61 more specific and sensitive than sCD41, sCD61), CD42b • Positive for CD36 (not specific) • Can express CD13, CD33 • Often negative for CD45, CD34, HLA-DR • Negative for MPO, markers of granulocytic differentiation • Occasionally aberrant expression of CD7
Acute basophilic leukemia	• Positive for CD13, CD33, CD123, CD203c, CD11b, CD9 • May express CD34, HLA-DR • Negative for other monocytic markers, CD117 • Occasionally aberrant expression of CD22 and/or TdT
Acute panmyelosis with myelofibrosis	If material available for cytometric assessment: • Phenotypic heterogeneity with varying degrees of expression of myeloid-associated antigens CD13, CD33, CD117 • Positive for CD34 • Negative for MPO

Adapted from Swerdlow SH, Campo E, Pileri SA, et al. The 2016 revision of the World Health Organization classification of lymphoid neoplasms. Blood. 2016;127(20):2375–2390.

Acute Promyelocytic Leukemia and Mimics

Flow cytometric analysis, together with cytomorphology, is essential for the prompt diagnosis and treatment of AML with t(15;17) (q24.1;q21.2)/*PML::RARA* (acute promyelocytic leukemia [APL]). Although both the hypergranular and microgranular variants are characterized by abnormal promyelocytes, morphologic and immunophenotypic distinction from mimics can be challenging (eg, *NPM1*-mutated, other AML with monocytic differentiation, *KMT2A*-rearranged AML). Characteristics facilitating this distinction are summarized in **Table 2**. Among established markers CD34, HLA-DR, and CD11b, the combined absence of all 3 yielded a higher specificity and PPV and a similar sensitivity for APL compared with absence of any 2 of these antigens.[14] Similarly, quantification of CD117, CD13, CD56, CD64, and myeloperoxidase (MPO) expression together achieved significantly higher area-under-the-curve, sensitivity, and specificity for APL (0.98, 92%, 93%, respectively) compared with individual markers alone.[15] In addition, several studies identified CD9, a member of the tetraspanin protein family expressed by leukocytes,[16] as a useful diagnostic and prognostically favorable marker for APL.[17–19]

Several strategies have been explored to distinguish APL from AML subtypes with APL-like immunophenotypes. One study used radar plots to discriminate classic APL, microgranular APL, and *NPM1*-mutated AML.[20] Classic APL was characterized by significantly higher expression of CD2, CD13, and CD64, lack of monocyte-associated markers (apart from CD64), the presence of a prominent CD11c + population, and absent expression of HLA-DR and CD15. In contrast, higher positivity for CD11b, CD11c, CD15, CD36, and HLA-DR, low blast SSC, admixed monocytes, and a prominent CD11c + population were characteristic of *NPM1*-mutated AML. A multicenter study demonstrated that an APL-like immunophenotype is present in approximately 30% of *NPM1*-mutated AML, whereas blasts in remaining patients showed monocytic or

Table 2
Immunophenotypic profiles to distinguish acute promyelocytic leukemia from nonacute promyelocytic leukemia leukemias with similar morphology or antigen expression

AML Subtype	Frequent Characteristics

APL	• Combination of features:
	  ◦ Triple-negative (absence of CD34, HLA-DR, CD11b)[14]
	  ◦ MPO ($\geq$97% events), CD117 ($\geq$49% events), CD13 ($\geq$88% events), CD64 ($\geq$42% events), CD56 ($\leq$25% events)[15]
	  ◦ Higher blast expression of CD64, CD2, and CD13, lack of monocytic population, no prominent CD11c + population, absent expression of HLA-DR and CD15[20]
	• Role of CD9:
	  ◦ CD9+ CD11b− HLADR−[17]
	  ◦ CD9+ CD64+[18]
	  ◦ CD9 as favorable prognostic marker[19]

NPM1-mutated AML	• Higher positivity for CD11b, CD11c, CD15, CD36, HLA-DR on blasts, low blast side scatter, presence of monocytes, prominent CD11c population[20] • Rarely positive for CD13, CD64, CD2[22]
APL-like *NPM1*-mutated AML[21]	• Expression of CD117, CD33, CD38, CD123, MPO • Lack of CD34, HLA-DR, CD11b, CD64, CD2, CD7, CD14, CD19
Monocytic *NPM1*-mutated AML[21]	• Negative for CD34 • Positive for HLA-DR, CD4, CD64 • "Double-negative" CD34/HLA-DR phenotype very rare

KMT2A rearranged AML	• Rarely positive for CD13, CD64, CD2; minimal MPO[22]
	• 5 different immunophenotypic groups[28]:
	  ◦ Immature monocytic: bright CD64, increased expression of CD117, CD15, CD34; substantial loss of CD14, CD13, CD36
	  ◦ Mature monocytic: positive for CD64, CD14, CD36, CD4, dimCD15; negative for CD117 or CD34
	  ◦ APL-like: positive for CD117, CD13, CD33; negative for CD34, HLA-DR; lower side scatter; lack of abundant cytoplasmic granules/MPO
	  ◦ Myelomonocytic: myeloblasts and monocytic blasts each represent $\geq$20% of blast population or simultaneously express monocytic and granulocytic markers; often aberrant CD56
	  ◦ Myeloblastic: positive for CD117, CD13, CD33; variably positive for CD34, HLA-DR, MPO

AML with t(8;16) (p11;p13)[56]	• Monocytic/myelomonocytic differentiation • Erythrophagocytosis • Bright expression of CD45 • High side scatter overlapping with maturing myeloid elements • Positive for CD13, CD33, CD64, HLA-DR (in 4/5 cases) • Variable expression of CD11b, CD14 • Negative for CD34 and CD117

"myeloid" (ie, absence of monocytic) differentiation.[21] Most monocytic *NPM1*-mutated AML cases were positive for CD33, CD11b, CD4, and CD64, variably positive for HLA-DR and CD117, and negative for CD34. A CD34/HLA-DR double-negative phenotype was more common among "myeloid" *NPM1*-mutated AML. Importantly, these immunophenotypically defined *NPM1* subgroups carried different *TET2*, *IDH1/2*, and *DNMT3A* comutation profiles and showed significant differences in clinical outcome, with APL-like immunophenotype associating with significantly longer relapse-free and overall survival. More recently, Fang and colleagues compared patients with APL to those with *NPM1*-mutated AML with APL-like immunophenotypes. They suggested that expression of CD2 and/or CD34, along with uniform CD13 and CD64 copositivity, makes the diagnosis of *NPM1*-mutated AML unlikely, and is more consistent with microgranular APL.[22] *NPM1* mutation might also be presaged by significantly higher expression of CD123 (interleukin-3 receptor alpha chain) on blasts compared with other AML subtypes.[23,24] The immunophenotypic correlates of co-occurring *FLT3*-ITD mutations are less clear. In one study, a combination of CD123/CD25/CD34/CD99 was strictly associated with *FLT3*-ITD mutations in the context of *NPM1*-mutated AML.[25] In contrast, a prospective large-scale study did not identify any *FLT3*-associated immunophenotype,[26] and the addition of CD123 and C-type lectin domain family 12 member A (CLEC12A)/low C-type lectin-like molecule-1 (CLL-1) to CD34 and CD117 had limited utility in predicting *FLT3* and *NPM1* mutation status.[27] Together, these findings suggest that immunophenotypic correlates of *FLT3* mutation have limited clinical utility at present.

An analysis of patients with *KMT2A*-rearranged AML identified 5 discrete immunophenotypic groups that correlated with laboratory characteristics such as total leukocyte and monocyte counts and blast frequency.[28] In addition, there was an enrichment of t(11;19) (q23;p13.1)/*ELL::KMT2A* and t(9;11) (p22;q23)/*MLLT3::KMT2A* rearrangements in patients with the mature monocytic immunophenotype, whereas t(9;11) (p22;q23)/*MLLT3::KMT2A* was identified most frequently in patients with immature monocytic, APL-like, and myelomonocytic phenotypes. Myeloblasts with t(6;11) (q27;q23)/*AFDN::KMT2A* more often exhibited a typical CD34+ CD117+ CD13+ CD33+ HLA-DR + phenotype without overt aberrancies. Mutations involving the RAS pathway or *PTPN11, ASXL1*, or *FLT3* mutations occurred in subsets of patients with all immunophenotypes except APL-like, where no such mutations were detected. Importantly, at the time of relapse, changes in immunophenotypic subtype were observed in almost half of all patients.

Acute Myeloid Leukemia with Mutations of CCAAT/Enhancer Binding Protein Alpha

AML with biallelic mutation of CCAAT/enhancer binding protein alpha (*CEBPA*) is prognostically favorable but molecular detection can be challenging.[29] This entity's immunophenotype is well-defined (see **Table 1**). In addition, low side scatter, decreased CD65 and higher CD64 expression in mature neutrophils, high CD64 and low CD36 expression on monocytes, and left-shifted erythroid elements with low expression of CD36 and CD71 have been described.[30] In one cohort, a classifier incorporating blast (CD34, CD117, CD7, CD15, CD65), neutrophil (SSC, CD64), monocytic (CD14, CD64), and erythroid (CD117) expression profiles correctly identified all cases of AML with biallelic *CEBPA* mutation (100% specificity and sensitivity).[30] Another scoring system assigned one point each for expression of HLA-DR, CD7, CD13, CD15, CD33, CD34, along with one point for the absence of CD14.[31] This system yielded a significant correlation between a score of 6 or greater and the presence of biallelic *CEBPA* mutation, with aberrant CD7 being the most important marker. Together, these approaches are useful in prompting targeted molecular evaluation, such as PCR-based fragment-length analysis or Sanger sequencing.[29] Although concurrent mutations are well described and have varying effects on outcome,[13,29,32] their effect on immunophenotype is less well explored. For example, in the study by Manelli and colleagues,[30] mutations of *TET2* and *GATA2* genes did not alter the immunophenotypic profile. As single in-frame basic leucine zipper (bZIP) *CEBPA*-mutations have been found to define the favorable prognostic group (independent of monoallelic or biallelic status), the definition of AML with *CEBPA* mutation has been expanded to include biallelic and single bZIP region mutations in the most recent World Health Organization (WHO) classification system,[2] and refined to AML with in-frame bZIP *CEBPA* mutations in the International Consensus Classification (ICC) guidelines.[3] Studies on potentially associated immunophenotypes are not yet available.

Acute Myeloid Leukemia Associated with Plasmacytoid Dendritic Cell Proliferations

Plasmacytoid dendritic cells (pDCs) are emerging as a cell subset with complex immunologic and pathogenic roles.[33] They are characterized by coexpression of CD123 and HLA-DR and the absence of classic lineage markers. As they mature, pDCs exhibit progressive loss of CD34 and CD117 with gradual upregulation of CD4, CD36, and CD303. AML with accompanying pDC proliferations has emerged as a subgroup with inferior outcomes.[34–38] Both blasts and pDCs frequently show *RUNX1* mutations, pointing toward a shared progenitor origin.[34,36] The proposed new WHO classification system therefore includes clonal pDC diseases in "dendritic cell and histiocytic neoplasms" as "plasmacytoid dendritic cell neoplasm/mature plasmacytoid dendritic cell proliferation associated with myeloid neoplasm" (MPDCP).[2] The immunophenotype of pDCs from patients with pDC-AML is variable, likely reflecting different maturation stages. The cells are positive for CD45, CD123, HLA-DR, and CD4 at levels comparable to normal pDCs, with variable expression of CD303, CD304, CD2, cTCL1, CD38, CD22, CD13, CD33, CD7, CD25, CD117, CD11b, CD14, and CD15.[34–36,38] In one series, CD2 expression was observed more frequently in *RUNX*1 wild type compared with mutated patients.[38] Some studies observed CD56 and cTdT on pDCs in subsets of patients.[34,37,38] AML blast phenotypes varied between studies but included monocytic differentiation features, variable CD123, and expression of lineage-discordant antigens such as CD2, cCD3, CD5, CD7, CD10, CD19, and cCD79.[34,36] In contrast, pDC (cTCL1, CD303, CD304, CD56) or classic DC lineage markers (CD1c, CD11c) were absent.

Phenotype/Karyotype Correlations

Associations between phenotype and survival have been described in patients with AML with normal karyotypes. The absence of dysplastic features as determined by a flow cytometry score correlated with significantly higher complete remission rates and longer survival compared with patients showing dysplasia.[39] In contrast, normal karyotype patients with AML exhibiting coexpression of CD25 and CD123 on blasts exhibited lower remission rates following induction and shorter overall survival compared with patients lacking these markers. This behavior may be explained by a positive association with *FLT3* mutations and a negative association with *NPM1* mutation among cases coexpressing CD25 and CD123.[40]

Chromosome 7 aberrations in AML are strongly indicative of antecedent myelodysplasia and predictive of inferior outcome. Both monosomy 7 and del(7q) have been found to be accompanied by immunophenotypic alterations that include expression of CD13, CD14, and CD64.[41] In this study, increased CD14 expression on maturing granulocytic cells was significantly more frequent in myeloid neoplasms with monosomy 7 than in those with del(7q). This included cases with normal blast frequencies and cases with fewer than 3 other immunophenotypic abnormalities observed on myeloid populations, suggesting that increased CD14 expression on maturing granulocytic cells may be particularly helpful in identifying monosomy 7.

In summary, these efforts have advanced phenotype/genotype correlations in AML, revealing several immunophenotypic biomarkers relevant for diagnosis and prognosis. Ongoing efforts will explore the immunophenotypic profiles of recently refined AML classes, promising growing utility for flow cytometry in the years to come.

ADVANCES IN MEASURABLE RESIDUAL DISEASE MONITORING FOR ACUTE MYELOID LEUKEMIA
General Practices and Challenges

The assessment of remission status and relapse risk relies on the monitoring and accurate quantification of residual leukemia populations. The prognostic value and clinical utility of MRD is supported by numerous studies,[9,42,43] including a recent meta-analysis of 81 publications with 11,151 patients with AML where achievement of MRD negativity was associated with superior disease-free and overall survival across age groups, AML subtypes, time of MRD assessment, specimen source, and MRD detection methods.[44] Estimated 5-year disease-free survival and OS rates were 64% and 68%, respectively, for patients with negative MRD. For those with positive MRD, 5-year disease free survival was 25% and overall survival was 34%. Positive MRD refers to the presence of a leukemia population above assay-specific or laboratory-specific thresholds. However, negative results do not necessarily indicate absence of disease, as leukemic populations might still be present at levels below the lower limit of detection of the assay.

Flow cytometry-based MRD detection relies on defining and quantifying blast immunophenotypes and abnormalities; general assay principles are described elsewhere.[6,7,45] In brief, it centers on the identification of leukemia-associated immunophenotypes (LAIPs)—ideally established in a diagnostic sample—and/or different from normal (DfN) immunophenotypes, in which deviancy from normal phenotypic patterns is assessed.[6,7,45] The latter has the advantage of being able to detect aberrant clones despite immunophenotypic shifts over time but requires extensive knowledge of normal differentiation profiles. Flow cytometric MRD assessments are therefore challenging to interpret. In addition, MRD assays are technically complex and therefore most often available within specialized laboratories. Direct comparisons between laboratories are often difficult because protocols, analysis methodologies, and reporting strategies often vary.

MRD can also be assessed by molecular methods. Quantitative real-time polymerase chain reaction (qPCR) is most commonly used but digital PCR and NGS platforms are increasingly adopted alternatives. Error-corrected sequencing is emerging as a particularly useful tool for MRD detection because tagging individual DNA molecules with unique molecular identifiers can limit base calling errors, particularly at lower variant allele fractions. Flow cytometric and molecular approaches possess distinct advantages and disadvantages (**Table 3**). MRD assessment and monitoring by both techniques is included as a standard into the 2017[46] and recently updated 2022[8] ELN recommendations for diagnosis and management of adult AML.

Updated Flow Cytometry Measurable Residual Disease Recommendations

Recently, new and revised recommendations for both standardized flow cytometric and molecular MRD analysis, MRD thresholds, definition of MRD response, and suggestions for clinical implications were established.[9] Tettero and colleagues[10] further outlined the technical aspects of cytometry-based MRD, including general principles, sample preparation, and analytical requirements. An integrative summary of these updated flow cytometry recommendations for harmonized LAIP/DfN MRD detection, analysis, and reporting is provided in **Table 4**. Per these recommendations, all patients

Table 3
Methods for the detection of measurable residual disease in acute myeloid leukemia

Modality	Principle	Advantages	Disadvantages
Flow cytometry	Assessment of blast immunophenotype, aberrancies and normal background populations (LAIP and DfN)	• Widely available technique • Fast turnaround time • Applicable to ~90% of patients with AML • Can provide absolute quantification • Allows discrimination of live/dead cells	• Lower sensitivity (10^{-3} to 10^{-4}) • Historically limited assay standardization • Historically limited report standardization • Potential overlap with immunophenotype of background or regenerating marrow populations • Blasts might exhibit phenotypic shifts during treatment or at relapse/recurrence • Emergence of subclones
Real-time quantitative PCR (qPCR)	Monitoring of specific mutations and chimeric gene fusions	• Easily standardized • Can be multiplexed • Higher sensitivity (10^{-3}–10^{-5})	• Applicable to ~50% of patients with AML • Time intensive and labor intensive
Digital PCR	Specific mutations	• More sensitive than qPCR (10^{-5}) • Less labor-intensive	• Requires validation
NGS	Gene panels	• High sensitivity (10^{-2}–10^{-4})	• Costly • Time intensive and labor intensive • Threshold has not been defined for individual mutations; NGS-MRD positivity is provisionally defined as $\geq 0.1\%$ variant allele frequency, excluding mutations related to CH and germline mutations

Table 4
European LeukemiaNet technical recommendations for flow cytometry based measurable residual disease assessment

Sampling, Sample Preparation, and Preanalytical Phase

Sample	MRD should be assessed from the first pull of a bone marrow aspirate
Choice of anticoagulant	• EDTA, heparin, and sodium citrate are acceptable (validation of stability required) • EDTA may induce a change of expression patterns of antigens • For MDS, heparin is generally recommended

Sample transportation and criteria for acceptability	• Preferred interval between bone marrow (BM) aspiration and processing: 3 d
	• Stored undiluted, in ambient conditions
	  ○ For samples stored at ambient temperature >3d, the MRD report should make a specific note of potentially compromised cell viability
	• Testing for viability, stability, and overall quality is recommended, especially in samples >72 h, by viability dye or initial plotting of forward scatter (FSC) vs side scatter (SSC)
	  ○ MRD analysis can be performed in suboptimal samples but should be accompanied by a comment on sample quality in the report

Sample processing	• Stain-lyse-wash (SLW): clearer separation between positive and negative events
	• Lyse-wash-stain-wash (LWSW): more reproducible labeling conditions, volume is constant for a given quantity of cells, fewer artifacts due to concentration of leukocytes
	• Lysis solutions:
	  ○ Ammonium chloride (NH_4Cl): minimal effects on WBC counts, but unavoidable cell loss.
	  ○ Lysis buffers: may contain additional chemicals that alter light scatter properties of leukocytes (cell death, cell shrinkage, loss of granulation)
	• No specific lysis protocol recommended but laboratories should ensure that selected solution maintains optimal scatter properties and mean fluorescent intensity
	• Additional sample fixation is not recommended

Hemodilution	• Should routinely be assessed and reported as part of the MRD assay but no consensus on specific methodology due to varying needs of individual laboratories • When present, repeat BM evaluation should be requested within 2 wk to avoid unreliable MRD results • Helpful formulas/approaches to detect hemodilution: ○ Comparison to peripheral blood: bone marrow purity = [1-(erythrocytes BM/erythrocytes PB) × (leukocytes PB/leukocytes BM)] × 100% predicted bone marrow purity = [1 – (lymphocytes by flow/lymphocytes PB) × (leukocytes PB/leukocytes by flow)] × 100%

(continued on next page)

Table 4 (*continued*)	
	○ Comparison to CD10, CD34+ cells and plasma cells: PB contamination index = −3.052 + 0.065 × (% CD10+ neutrophils) − 0.609 × (%CD34+) −2.008 × (%plasma cells) ○ Comparison to CD16+ cells: normalized blast count = (80%/% dim CD16) × blast count ○ Comparison to CD117+ mast cells: suggested blood contamination if mast cell population (CD117+) ≤ 0.002% ○ Proportion of mature neutrophils: suggested blood contamination if mature neutrophils >90% • Change of denominator to primitive/progenitor fraction (ie, based on CD34, CD117, or CD133)
Analytical	
Cytometer settings and set-up	• Standardized flow cytometer settings are crucial • Daily cytometer calibration checks and use of calibration beads are strongly advised • Automated compensation is more robust, and manual compensation is strongly discouraged
Sample acquisition	• Principles of rare events acquisition apply • The gating syntax should include FSC vs time and doublet exclusion plots ○ Monitors for fluidic instability, shear turbulence or disturbances ○ A high pressure or flow rate can lead to technical issues • The assay sensitivity depends on the number of relevant events acquired: ○ The standard for determining MRD negativity is the acquisition of >500 000 CD45+ cells and ≥100 viable cells in the blast compartment assessed for the best aberrancy(ies) available ○ Increasing the number of analyzed cells may improve sensitivity, allow monitoring of minority clones ○ Negativity should be confirmed with all tubes
Controls	• Bone marrow samples collected during surgical procedures, from healthy donor, or patients with solid or hematological malignancies without marrow involvement are suitable • At least 10 are required with a preference of age-matched controls; a larger number and variety of samples will minimize the risk of false-positive control samples ○ "Stressed" normal differentiation ○ CH of indeterminate potential ○ Obvious outliers >2 SD, should be excluded • Should be repeated every time the assay methodology is modified

(*continued on next page*)

Table 4 (continued)	
Analysis and interpretation	

General principles	• For clinical decision-making, MRD assessment should be performed with a qualified assay following the guidelines for rare events
	• Implementation of a minimum required set of tubes/fluorochromes combination is a prerequisite
	• When available, comparison to a diagnostic sample should be made
	• An integrated diagnostic LAIP and DfN strategy is recommended that incorporates the following monoclonal antibodies:
	  ○ 3 to 5 core MRD markers: CD45, CD34, CD117, CD13, CD33, HLA-DR, cMPO
	  ○ CD56, CD7
	  ○ Myeloid maturation markers CD11b, CD15, CD64, CD65
	  ○ Monocytic markers CD14, CD36, CD64, CD4, CD38, CD11c
	  ○ CD38, CD64, CD11b, and CD4 can be helpful if leukemic stem cell markers (eg, CD56, CD7, CD45RA) are aberrantly expressed or in cases with monocytic differentiation
	  ○ Megakaryocytic markers CD41, CD61, CD36
	  ○ Erythroid markers CD235e, CD71, CD36
	• There is no agreement to minimal percentage of LAIP that should be present at diagnosis to select a given marker for MRD monitoring during therapy

Gating strategy	• Check for fluidic alterations using FSC-Height or FSC-Area versus TIME • Eliminate debris and check for viability • Discriminate singlets vs doublets (eg, FSC-A versus FSC-H) to exclude cell aggregates • Define WBC in a CD45/SSC plot • Identify blasts • Define immunophenotype and aberrancies • Confirm complete inclusion of the leukemic population in each gate by using a density plot display • Backgate LAIP cells on CD45, CD34, and SSC/FSC plots

Regenerating bone marrow	Immunophenotypic abnormalities may reflect transient features of regenerating or "stressed" hematopoiesis
	• Several sources can be used to investigate regeneration:
	  ○ After completion of consolidation therapy with no subsequent emerging leukemia
	  ○ After stem cell transplantation
	  ○ LAIP-negative patients with no subsequent relapse
	  ○ Patients treated with myelosuppressive chemotherapy for other malignancies not involving bone marrow
	• Markers/marker combinations that may be transiently expressed in regenerating BM:
	  ○ CD25
	  ○ CD22
	  ○ CD15

(continued on next page)

Table 4 (continued)	
	○ CD34-CD117+HLA-DR+ • The report should comment on this possibility and note that a repeat sample in 2–4 wk, if clinically indicated, may be informative
Software	No recommendations made
Threshold defining positivity	• May depend on the time point of sample collection, treatment schedule and AML subtype • In general, after 2 cycles of intensive chemotherapy, the threshold of 0.1% on a denominator of 500,000–1,000,000 CD45+ cells expressing relevant events is the used as a prognostic factor in AML for outcome and for clinical decisions
Assay performance	The following characteristics need to be considered: • LOB = maximum number of LAIP cells measured in samples lacking leukemia (such as normal or regenerating BM or samples not stained with the antibody of interest) ○ LOB = mean blank + 1.645(SD blank) • Limit of detection (LOD): minimal number of LAIP cells that can accurately be distinguished above background ○ LOD = LOB + 1.645(SD low positive) ○ Ideally established by measuring 10 samples with a very low positive LAIP in triplicate ○ The LOD of DfN gates is estimated in the same manner • Lower limit of quantitation (LLOQ) is the lowest LAIP% that can be reliably quantified relative to a defined acceptance criterion and is equal to or higher than LOD ○ A coefficient of variation (CV) of <30% is proposed to confirm acceptable LLOQ
Reporting	• The final MRD assay result is reported as "MRD-positive" or "MRD-negative" • "Technical MRD" <0.1% threshold with appearance of residual or emerging leukemic populations may also be described to alert the clinician in case monitoring closely with short follow-up is advisable • Concerns and limitations regarding number of events, sample quality, cell viability, or hemodilution should be noted

with AML should be monitored using a flow cytometry-based MRD assay after 2 cycles of chemotherapy, at the end of consolidation, and before stem cell transplantation (if pursued), whereas evaluation during follow-up is currently considered exploratory (**Fig. 1**). However, molecular MRD assessment (by qPCR or dPCR) is recommended for patients with AML with subtype-defining genetic alterations such as *RUNX1-RUNX1T1*, *CBFB-MYH11*, *PML-RARA*, or mutated *NPM1*.

At present, NGS-based techniques are considered supportive but not sufficient for MRD monitoring. The concordance between flow cytometry and NGS-MRD panels is high overall, and NGS-MRD might be especially helpful when a clear LAIP is lacking or cannot be differentiated from background hematopoiesis.[9] In a single-institution study, NGS and flow cytometry MRD were concordant in 80% of paired tests, whereas in 18%, NGS was positive and flow cytometry negative.[47] Molecular findings in

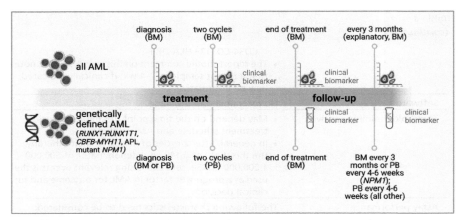

Fig. 1. Currently recommended algorithm of MRD assessment and use of MRD as a clinical biomarker to inform treatment decisions/modifications.

discrepant cases frequently included mutations associated with clonal hematopoiesis (CH, eg, *DNMT3A, TET2, ASXL1*), highlighting that the presence of residual CH does not necessarily signify residual leukemia. A comparison between an MRD flow cytometry assay and an error-corrected 34-gene NGS-MRD panel in another study demonstrated that at the end of induction, NGS-MRD identified more than 80% of cases identified by flow cytometry, whereas flow cytometry identified 50% identified by NGS.[48] The PPV, NPV, and accuracy for relapse were 71%, 58%, and 67% for NGS, and 75%, 48%, and 60% for flow cytometry, respectively. Patients MRD positive by both techniques had significantly inferior outcomes compared with patients negative by both modalities but no significant survival differences were observed between patients positive by just one method and those negative by both.

Advances in MRD detection and interpretation have also begun to reshape the treatment response criteria and clinical recommendations for AML.[6] MRD-based complete response (CR) criteria are now expanded to include "CR with partial hematologic recovery" (CRh) and "CR with incomplete hematologic recovery" (CRi) without MRD (ie, MRD is below a defined threshold by flow cytometry or qPCR). CRh is defined as "absolute neutrophil count $\geq 0.5 \times 10^9$/L and platelet count $\geq 50 \times 10^9$/L," whereas the hematologic parameters for CRi are "residual neutropenia $<1.0 \times 10^9$/L or thrombocytopenia $<100 \times 10^9$/L," all in the absence of G-CSF or transfusion support for 7 days before the assessment. Both require that all other CR criteria are met (ie, bone marrow blasts <5%, absence of circulating blasts, absence of extramedullary disease). It is encouraged to monitor improvements in blood counts to reflect the best hematologic response achieved before commencement of subsequent treatment. Moreover, response without MRD should be confirmed by another assessment at least 4 weeks hence.

MRD thresholds and time points for MRD assessments require further exploration and validation. Although currently defined as less than 0.1% of CD45-expressing cells with the target immunophenotype, MRD levels less than 0.1% may still indicate active disease.[9] However, a recent analysis suggested that flow cytometric MRD negativity after the first cycle of therapy is highly concordant with MRD status after cycle 2, implying that earlier management decisions based on first-cycle MRD results may reduce unnecessary allogeneic donor searches and costs in some circumstances.[49]

CHALLENGES AND OPEN QUESTIONS

The studies described above have significantly advanced our understanding of the immunophenotypic biomarkers of genetic alterations and elucidated their importance for AML diagnosis and prognosis. In the years ahead, flow cytometry will remain an essential tool to further refine newly introduced types of AML. Moreover, flow cytometry will support ongoing research and clinical studies dedicated to identifying novel therapeutic targets that could also serve as better biomarkers or targets for MRD assessments. Promising strategies include antigens predominantly or disproportionately expressed on leukemic stem cells and blasts such as CLL-1, CD244, and CD99, and aberrantly expressed antigens such as CD123, CD47, CD96 (TACTILE-1), CD157, or IL1RAP.[42,50,51]

To improve diagnostic accuracy, facilitate MRD monitoring, and discover new associations or biomarkers, flow cytometry will increasingly be complemented by high-dimensional analysis algorithms and comparisons to reference databases. For example, the EuroFlow Consortium's Infinicyt Compass enables recognition of complex immunophenotypic patterns by incorporating simultaneous measurements of the mean fluorescence values from 8 different markers and 2 scatter parameters into a PCA algorithm.[52] Aanei and colleagues[53] constructed Compass databases using well-defined AML WHO diagnostic categories and prospectively evaluated their utility in AML analysis. New AML cases were classified based on scores assigned for standard deviations, and then compared with their final diagnosis integrating morphologic, cytogenetic, and molecular findings. This approach was particularly suited to exclude recurrent genetic abnormalities such as AML with t(8;21), t(15;17), inv(16)/t(16;16), and KMT2A. It also allowed the identification of NPM1-mutant AML cases with an APL-like immunophenotype and confirmed aberrant expression of makers in AML subtypes as described above.

A recent prospective study used a standardized EuroFlow AML/MDS panel and multidimensional analysis strategies to compare databases of normal samples with new AML cases and created reference images of LAIPs for successive MRD monitoring.[26] Three hundred and ten different LAIPs were identified and classified into compartments based on the maturation stage in which they are found and correlated with AML-WHO subtypes. These compartments were enriched for specific mutations, for example, the common myeloid progenitor compartment included all cases of AML with CBFβ-MYH11, RUNX1-RUNX1T1, biallelic mutations of CEBPA, mutated RUNX1, BCR-ABL, and DEK-NUP214, confirming that the most specific immunophenotypes are found in the most immature compartments. For MRD monitoring, a cutoff of 0.01% residual leukemia by flow cytometry was found to correlate closely with risk of relapse and differentiate most accurately between different progression-free survival groups, with high concordance between flow cytometry and qPCR-MRD results.

However, the independent prognostic relevance of flow cytometry MRD in relation to baseline genetic profiles, expression of antigens, and specific treatment approaches remains unclear. In a subgroup of 189 patients with AML enrolled in the Eastern Cooperative Oncology Group (ECOG) - American College of Radiology Imaging Network (ACRIN) E1900 trial, MRD-negative patients were more likely to have favorable cytogenetic alterations compared with MRD-positive patients, and MRD status had a significant impact on OS among patients with favorable but not unfavorable cytogenetic risk groups.[54] DNMT3A R882 was the only mutation class significantly associated with the presence of flow cytometry MRD, whereas NPM1, FLT3-ITD, and DNMT3A R882 were significantly associated with CD25 positivity.

Importantly, a higher rate of MRD-positivity was found in CD25+ compared with CD25-patients, and CD25 expression and MRD status were independently associated with OS, irrespective of age, WBC count, and cytogenetic risk. Additional studies are needed to validate these findings. Of note, certain pathogenic alterations, such as RUNX1-RUNX1T1, might persist at very-low levels even after curative treatment.[53,55] Similarly, the presence of residual CH does not necessarily signify residual leukemia. These caveats hamper the specificity of molecular MRD and emphasize that continued inclusion of LAIP-based MRD detection may provide a more accurate representation of clinical outcomes.

Together, comprehensive and reproducible yet context-appropriate interpretation strategies are essential. Updated clinical and technical recommendations will continue to improve the reproducibility of flow cytometry-based MRD assays and harmonize diagnostic and treatment approaches. However, it remains to be seen which standards and practices become most essential to achieving accurate and reliable MRD results for the broader community. Individual laboratories will need to balance these recommendations with their own local and national regulations. Moreover, published guidelines need not dictate individual laboratories' behavior so comprehensively as to restrain ongoing innovation and improvement. Inversely, laboratories involved in MRD testing must clearly communicate assay performance criteria, instrumentation and reagents used, antibodies/antibody combinations, and gating and analysis strategies because these are frequent sources of intralaboratory and interlaboratory variabilities.[10]

CLINICS CARE POINTS

- Immunophenotypic profiles can identify underlying genomic alterations and be useful to highlight prognostically relevant differences within subgroups of genetically defined AML.
- Novel diagnostic subtypes often show characteristic immunophenotypes but further validation is required to establish flow cytometry as diagnostic or biologic classifiers.
- Immunophenotypic MRD assessment is a complex process, requiring specific experience and rigorous method validation.
- Laboratories involved in MRD detection must provide information on methodology, tissue source, and minimum assay sensitivity for their assays and may benefit from standardized protocols.
- The combination of new molecular technologies with advanced flow cytometry and improved computational tools will ultimately allow more definite risk stratifications and inform treatment strategies.

DISCLOSURE

The authors have nothing to disclose.

FUNDING

C.B. Hergott is funded by a Society of '67 Scholar Award from the Association of Pathology Chairs, a Young Investigator Grant from the Academy of Clinical Laboratory Physicians and Scientists, and by NIH 5T32CA251062. F. Lucas is funded by a Young Investigator Grant from the Academy of Clinical Laboratory Physicians and Scientists.

REFERENCES

1. Swerdlow SH, Campo E, Pileri SA, et al. The 2016 revision of the World Health Organization classification of lymphoid neoplasms. Blood 2016;127(20): 2375–90.
2. Khoury JD, Solary E, Abla O, et al. The 5th edition of the World Health Organization classification of haematolymphoid tumours: myeloid and histiocytic/dendritic neoplasms. Leukemia 2022;36(7):1703–19.
3. Arber DA, Orazi A, Hasserjian RP, et al. International consensus classification of myeloid neoplasms and acute leukemias: integrating morphologic, clinical, and genomic data. Blood 2022;140(11):1200–28.
4. Alaggio R, Amador C, Anagnostopoulos I, et al. The 5th edition of the World Health Organization classification of haematolymphoid tumours: lymphoid neoplasms. Leukemia 2022;36(7):1720–48.
5. Campo E, Jaffe ES, Cook JR, et al. The International consensus classification of mature lymphoid neoplasms: a report from the clinical advisory committee. Blood 2022;140(11):1229–53. https://doi.org/10.1182/blood.2022015851. Erratum appears in Blood 2023;141(4):437.
6. Chen X, Cherian S. Acute myeloid leukemia immunophenotyping by flow cytometric analysis. Clin Lab Med 2017;37(4):753–69.
7. Chen X, Wood BL. Monitoring minimal residual disease in acute leukemia: technical challenges and interpretive complexities. Blood Rev 2017;31(2):63–75.
8. Döhner H, Wei AH, Appelbaum FR, et al. Diagnosis and management of AML in adults: 2022 recommendations from an international expert panel on behalf of the ELN. Blood 2022;140(12):1345–77.
9. Heuser M, Freeman SD, Ossenkoppele GJ, et al. 2021 update on MRD in acute myeloid leukemia: a consensus document from the European LeukemiaNet MRD Working Party. Blood 2021;138(26):2753–67.
10. Tettero JM, Freeman S, Buecklein V, et al. Technical Aspects of flow cytometry-based measurable residual disease quantification in acute myeloid leukemia: experience of the european leukemiaNet MRD working party. HemaSphere 2022;6(1):e676.
11. Shang L, Chen X, Liu Y, et al. The immunophenotypic characteristics and flow cytometric scoring system of acute myeloid leukemia with t(8;21) (q22;q22); RUNX1-RUNX1T1. Int J Lab Hematol 2019;41(1):23–31.
12. Wang B, Yang B, Ling Y, et al. Role of CD19 and specific KIT-D816 on risk stratification refinement in t(8;21) acute myeloid leukemia induced with different cytarabine intensities. Cancer Med 2021;10(3):1091–102.
13. Sadigh S, Kim AS. Molecular pathology of myeloid neoplasms. Surg Pathol Clin 2021;14(3):517–28.
14. Rahman K, Gupta R, Singh MK, et al. The triple-negative (CD34-/HLA-DR-/CD11b-) profile rapidly and specifically identifies an acute promyelocytic leukemia. Int J Lab Hematol 2018;40(2):144–51.
15. Tran VT, Phan TT, Mac H-P, et al. The diagnostic power of CD117, CD13, CD56, CD64, and MPO in rapid screening acute promyelocytic leukemia. BMC Res Notes 2020;13(1):394.
16. Reyes R, Cardeñes B, Machado-Pineda Y, et al. Tetraspanin CD9: a key regulator of cell adhesion in the immune system. Front Immunol 2018;9:863.
17. Ren F, Zhang N, Xu Z, et al. The CD9+ CD11b- HLA-DR- immunophenotype can be used to diagnose acute promyelocytic leukemia. Int J Lab Hematol 2019; 41(2):168–75.

18. Mosleh M, Mehrpouri M, Ghaffari S, et al. Report of a new six-panel flow cytometry marker for early differential diagnosis of APL from HLA-DR negative Non-APL leukemia. Scand J Clin Lab Invest 2020;80(2):87–92.
19. Siraj F, Tanwar P, Singh A, et al. Analysing "tear-drop" prints of acute promyelocytic leukemia (APML): immunophenotypic prognostication of APML by FCM. Am J Blood Res 2021;11(4):446–57.
20. Gupta M, Jafari K, Rajab A, et al. Radar plots facilitate differential diagnosis of acute promyelocytic leukemia and NPM1+ acute myeloid leukemia by flow cytometry. Cytometry B Clin Cytom 2021;100(4):409–20.
21. Mason EF, Hasserjian RP, Aggarwal N, et al. Blast phenotype and comutations in acute myeloid leukemia with mutated NPM1 influence disease biology and outcome. Blood Adv 2019;3(21):3322–32.
22. Fang H, Wang SA, Hu S, et al. Acute promyelocytic leukemia: immunophenotype and differential diagnosis by flow cytometry. Cytometry B Clin. Cytom 2022; 102(4):283–91.
23. Bras AE, de Haas V, van Stigt A, et al. CD123 expression evels in 846 acute leukemia patients based on standardized immunophenotyping. Cytometry B Clin. Cytom 2019;96(2):134–42.
24. Perriello VM, Gionfriddo I, Rossi R, et al. CD123 is consistently expressed on NPM1-mutated AML Cells. Cancers 2021;13(3):496.
25. Angelini DF, Ottone T, Guerrera G, et al. A leukemia-associated CD34/CD123/CD25/CD99+ immunophenotype Identifies FLT3-mutated clones in acute myeloid leukemia. Clin Cancer Res 2015;21(17):3977–85.
26. Piñero P, Morillas M, Gutierrez N, et al. Identification of leukemia-associated immunophenotypes by databaseguided flow cytometry provides a highly sensitive and reproducible strategy for the study of measurable residual disease in acute myeloblastic leukemia. Cancers 2022;14(16):4010.
27. Herborg LL, Nederby L, Brøndum RF, et al. Antigen exoression varies significantly between molecular subgroups of acute myeloid leukemia patients: clinical applicability is hampered by establishment of relevant cutoffs. Acta Haematol 2021;144(3):275–84.
28. Konoplev S, Wang X, Tang G, et al. Comprehensive immunophenotypic study of acute myeloid leukemia with KMT2A (MLL) rearrangement in adults: a single-institution experience. Cytometry B Clin Cytom 2022;102(2):123–33.
29. Mendoza H, Podoltsev NA, Siddon AJ. Laboratory evaluation and prognostication among adults and children with CEBPA-mutant acute myeloid leukemia. Int J Lab Hematol 2021;43(S1):86–95.
30. Mannelli F, Ponziani V, Bencini S, et al. CEBPA–double-mutated acute myeloid leukemia displays a unique phenotypic profile: a reliaole screening method and insight into biological features. Haematologica 2017;102(3):529–40.
31. Marcolin R, Guolo F, Minetto P, et al. A simple cytofluorimetric score may optimize testing for biallelic CEBPA mutations in patients with acute myeloid leukemia. Leuk Res 2019;86:106223.
32. Hergott CB, Kim AS. Molecular diagnostic testing for hematopoietic neoplasms. Clin Lab Med 2022;42(3):325–47.
33. Roussel X, Garnache Ottou F, Renosi F. Plasmacytoid dendritic cells, a novel target in myeloid neoplasms. Cancers 2022;14(14):3545.
34. Xiao W, Chan A, Waarts MR, et al. Plasmacytoid dendritic cell expansion defines a distinct subset of RUNX1-mutated acute myeloid leukemia. Blood 2021; 137(10):1377–91.

35. Hamadeh F, Awadallah A, Meyerson HJ, et al. Flow cytometry identifies a spectrum of maturation in myeloid neoplasms having plasmacytoid dendritic cell differentiation. Cytometry B Clin Cytom 2020;98(1):43–51.
36. Zalmaï L, Viailly P-J, Biichle S, et al. Plasmacytoid dendritic cells proliferation associated with acute myeloid leukemia: phenotype profile and mutation landscape. Haematologica 2020;106(12):3056–66.
37. Huang Y, Wang Y, Chang Y, et al. Myeloid neoplasms with elevated plasmacytoid dendritic cell differentiation reflect the maturation process of dendritic cells. Cytom Part J Int Soc Anal Cytol 2020;97(1):61–9.
38. Wang W, Xu J, Khoury JD, et al. Immunophenotypic and molecular features of acute myeloid leukemia with plasmacytoid dendritic cell differentiation are distinct from blastic plasmacytoid dendritic cell neoplasm. Cancers 2022;14(14):3375.
39. Mannelli F, Bencini S, Piccini M, et al. Multilineage dysplasia as assessed by immunophenotype in acute myeloid leukemia: a prognostic tool in a genetically undefined category. Cancers 2020;12(11):E3196.
40. Aref S, Azmy E, Ibrahim L, et al. Prognostic value of CD25/CD123 pattern of expression in acute myeloid leukemia patients with normal cytogenetic. Leuk Res Rep 2020;13:100203.
41. Chen X, Wood BL, Cherian S. Immunophenotypic features of myeloid neoplasms associated with chromosome 7 abnormalities. Cytometry B Clin Cytom 2019; 96(4):300–9.
42. Bewersdorf JP, Shallis RM, Boddu PC, et al. The minimal that kills: why defining and targeting measurable residual disease is the "Sine Qua Non" for further progress in management of acute myeloid leukemia. Blood Rev 2020;43:100650.
43. Shallis RM, Pollyea DA, Zeidan AM. The complete story of less than complete responses: the evolution and application of acute myeloid leukemia clinical responses. Blood Rev 2021;48:100806.
44. Short NJ, Zhou S, Fu C, et al. Association of measurable residual disease with survival outcomes in patients with acute myeloid leukemia: a systematic review and meta-analysis. JAMA Oncol 2020;6(12):1890–9.
45. Wood BL. Acute myeloid leukemia minimal residual disease detection: the difference from normal approach. Curr Protoc Cytom 2020;93(1):e73.
46. Döhner H, Estey E, Grimwade D, et al. Diagnosis and management of AML in adults: 2017 ELN recommendations from an international expert panel. Blood 2017;129(4):424–47.
47. McGowan P, Hyter S D, Cui W, et al. Comparison of flow cytometry and next-generation sequencing in minimal residual disease monitoring of acute myeloid leukemia: one institute's practical clinical experience. Int J Lab Hematol 2022; 44(1):118–26.
48. Patkar N, Kakirde C, Shaikh AF, et al. Clinical impact of panel-based error-corrected next generation sequencing versus flow cytometry to detect measurable residual disease (MRD) in acute myeloid leukemia (AML). Leukemia 2021; 35(5):1392–404.
49. Tettero JM, Al-Badri WKW, Ngai LL, et al. Concordance in measurable residual disease result after first and second induction cycle in acute myeloid leukemia: an outcome- and cost-analysis. Front Oncol 2022;12:999822.
50. Weeda V, Mestrum SGC, Leers MPG. Flow cytometric identification of hematopoietic and leukemic blast cells for tailored clinical follow-up of acute myeloid leukemia. Int J Mol Sci 2022;23(18):10529.
51. Ali A, Vaikari VP, Alachkar H. CD99 in malignant hematopoiesis. Exp Hematol 2022;106:40–6.

52. Lhermitte L, Mejstrikova E, van der Sluijs-Gelling AJ, et al. Automated database-guided expert-supervised orientation for immunophenotypic diagnosis and classification of acute leukemia. Leukemia 2018;32(4):874–81.

53. Aanei C-M, Veyrat-Masson R, Selicean C, et al. Database-guided analysis for immunophenotypic diagnosis and follow-up of acute myeloid leukemia with recurrent genetic abnormalities. Front Oncol 2021;11:746951.

54. Ganzel C, Sun Z, Baslan T, et al. Measurable residual disease by flow cytometry in acute myeloid leukemia is prognostic, independent of genomic profiling. Leuk Res 2022;123:106971.

55. Liu F-J, Cheng W-Y, Lin X-J, et al. Measurable residual disease detected by multiparameter flow cytometry and sequencing improves prediction of relapse and survival in acute myeloid leukemia. Front Oncol 2021;11:677833.

56. Aqil B, Gao J, Stalling M, et al. Distinctive flow cytometric and mutational profile of acute myeloid leukemia with t(8;16)(p11;p13) translocation. Am J Clin Pathol 2022;157(5):701–8.

Advances in Flow Cytometry for Mixed Phenotype and Ambiguous Leukemias

Jason H. Kurzer, MD, PhD[a],*, Olga K. Weinberg, MD[b]

KEYWORDS

• Mixed phenotype acute leukemia • Flow cytometry • Genetics • Classification

KEY POINTS

• Classification of mixed phenotype acute leukemia has evolved to include fewer lineage specific markers with an emphasis on expression intensity.
• New entities with defined genetic alterations have been introduced in recently updated classifications.
• Multiparameter flow cytometry should include panels that fully evaluate the lineage specific markers and use fluorochromes that allow for appropriate comparison of intensities.

INTRODUCTION

Acute leukemias are typically classified by their unique lineage, either acute lymphoblastic leukemia (ALL) or acute myeloid leukemia (AML). In contrast, acute leukemias of ambiguous lineage (ALAL), which include mixed phenotype acute leukemia (MPAL) and acute undifferentiated leukemia (AUL), are leukemias that cannot be ascribed to a single lineage.[1–9] MPAL includes those leukemias with more than one single lineage blast population (bilineal, **Fig. 1**) as well as those with a single blast population with expression of various lineage-associated markers (biphenotypic, **Fig. 2**). AUL, on the other hand, is made up of leukemias that fail to demonstrate clear lineage commitment. MPAL makes up ~3% of acute leukemia, whereas acute undifferentiated leukemia is rarer still.[5,10–13]

The Fifth Edition of the World Health Organization (WHO) classification of hematolymphoid tumors divides ALAL into 2 broad categories: ALAL with defining genetic abnormalities and ALAL, immunophenotypically defined.[1] The defining genetic abnormalities include MPAL with *BCR::ABL1*, MPAL with *KMT2A* rearrangements, MPAL with *ZNF384* rearrangement, and ALAL with *BCL11B* rearrangement.

[a] Department of Pathology, Stanford University School of Medicine, 300 Pasteur Drive, H1524B, Stanford, CA 94305-5324, USA; [b] Department of Pathology, University of Texas Southwestern, Medical Center, 5323 Harry Hines Boulevard, Dallas, TX 75390-9072, USA
* Corresponding author.
E-mail address: kurzer@stanford.edu

Clin Lab Med 43 (2023) 399–410
https://doi.org/10.1016/j.cll.2023.04.006   labmed.theclinics.com
0272-2712/23/© 2023 Elsevier Inc. All rights reserved.

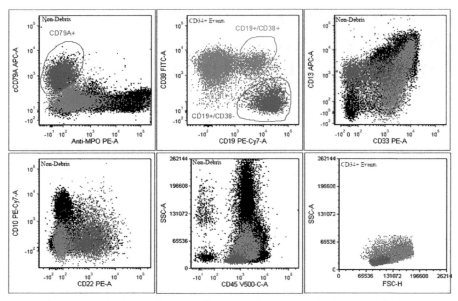

Fig. 1. Bilineal acute leukemia (B/myeloid MPAL with *BCR::ABL1*). The CD34+ blasts separate into at least 2 populations, a B-lymphoblast population (*red/violet*) with low forward scatter that expresses CD79a, CD19, CD22, dim CD45, CD13, and CD33 (*partial, dim*) and lacks CD38 and MPO and a myeloid population (*light blue*) with variably high forward scatter that lacks CD19 but expresses dim/partial CD38, MPO, and variable CD13/CD33. A third population (*orange*) is intermediate in nature, with expression of CD19, CD38, CD33, and moderate CD45, and displays high forward scatter. CD34-negative cells are represented in black.

Immunophenotypically defined ALAL includes MPAL (B/myeloid), MPAL (T/myeloid), MPAL (B/T), MPAL (B/T/myeloid), MPAL (T/megakaryocytic), ALAL, NOS, and AUL.

HISTORY

Although bilineal and biphenotypic leukemias are included in the umbrella category of MPAL in the World Health Organization classification and International Consensus Classification of hematopoietic neoplasms, historically the focus has been on how

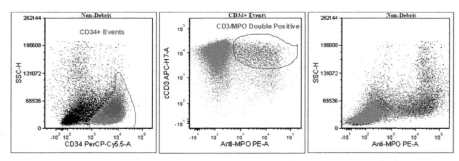

Fig. 2. Biphenotypic acute leukemia (T/myeloid MPAL). CD34+ blasts (*light blue*) are composed of primarily T lymphoblasts with cytoplasmic CD3; however, there is a subset (*red/violet*) with double expression of cytoplasmic CD3 and MPO. MPO expression is greater than 50% that of background neutrophils.

best to categorize biphenotypic leukemias.[1,14] Initial classification systems used a scoring system whereby certain lineage markers were assigned points, with the diagnosis of biphenotypic acute leukemia dependent on a certain score summation.[15–17] The first prominent scoring system was put forth by Catovsky and colleagues **(Table 1)**.[16] This system was then modified by the European Group for the Immunological Characterization of Leukemias (EGIL) **(Table 2)**, which was subsequently endorsed by the third edition of the WHO Classification of Tumors and Lymphoid Tissues.[17,18]

When biphenotypic leukemias and bilineal leukemias were combined within the MPAL category, the WHO eliminated a scoring system and sought to simplify the diagnosis by reducing the specific markers necessary to ascribe a lineage to biphenotypic leukemias in the fourth edition of the classification system.[19] Specifically, myeloid lineage is assigned when blasts express the enzyme, myeloperoxidase (MPO), or at least 2 of the of the following monocytic markers: nonspecific esterase, CD11c, CD14, CD64, or lysozyme. For T-lineage, blasts must express CD3 on the surface or within the cytoplasm. Assignment of B-lineage requires blasts express CD19, with strong CD19 expression requiring strong expression of at least one other B-lineage marker and weak CD19 expression requiring 2 of these markers. Revisions to the fourth edition as well as the fifth edition have essentially maintained these criteria, while contextualizing further the degree of expression **(Table 3)**.[1,20,21]

Ultimately, lineage assessment has important implications for therapy selection. Currently, MPAL is frequently treated with ALL-based therapy coupled with stem cell transplant at first remission.[22,23] Indeed, although terminology such as "lineage-specific" is frequently used to imply these markers are specific to a normal hematopoietic lineage, the data underpinning much of the original marker criteria are based on how frequently these markers associate with a "disease" (eg, AML or ALL) as conceived in the French American British classification system.[7,24] As such, an apparent goal in classification of MPAL is to assure that those diseases that may benefit best from AML-based therapy or ALL-based therapy remain classified as AML or ALL, respectively. Consequently, careful assessment of flow markers by flow cytometry is essential. Moreover, as immunotherapies such as chimeric antigen receptor T-cell therapy and bispecific T-cell engagers begin to be used in the treatment of MPAL, flow cytometry will likely become invaluable for assessing suitability and response to therapy.[25] In parallel, as the molecular/cytogenetic bases for MPAL become more apparent and therapies become increasingly targeted toward these molecular abnormalities (eg, kinase inhibitors for *BCR::ABL1* MPAL), the conception of MPAL based on "lineage"/"disease" is likely to evolve as well.

DISCUSSION
Assigning Myeloid Lineage to Biphenotypic Mixed Phenotype Acute Leukemia

Myeloperoxidase has long been considered the most specific marker for myeloid lineage leukemias.[26] Before the routine use of flow cytometry in the diagnosis of acute leukemias, cytochemical staining for Sudan Black/MPO with a cutoff of 3% was the primary means of diagnosing AML.[24] For biphenotypic acute leukemias, MPO was weighted high in all scoring systems and, with certain exceptions and caveats (discussed later), is sufficient alone to ascribe myeloid lineage in the WHO classification system.[1,16,17,27]

CD117 (c-Kit receptor) can be found expressed on early myeloid precursors as well as early monocytic precursors.[27–29] CD13 (aminopeptidase N) and CD33 (sialic acid–binding immunoglobulinlike protein) are detected in early myeloid precursors as well,

Table 1 Catovsky scoring system			
Points	B-Lineage	T-Lineage	Myeloid Lineage
2	cCD22, cμ chain	cCD3	MPO
1	CD10, CD19, CD24	CD2, CD5, TCR rearr. (β or δ chain)	CD33, CD13 m/c, CD14 m/c, AML morphology, or cytochemistry (other than MPO)
0.5	TdT; IgH rearr.	TdT, CD7	CD11b, CD11c, CD15

A case is considered biphenotypic when scores for both myeloid and lymphoid lineages are greater than or equal to 2 points.

undergoing increased and/or decreased expression as myeloid cells mature into granulocytic, monocytic, and dendritic cells.[30,31] The EGIL system incorporated use of CD117, CD13, and CD33 for assigning myeloid lineage; however, the WHO removed them in favor of a simpler, more specific use of markers. More recently, the WHO has recognized a form of T-lymphoblastic leukemia with earlier immunophenotypic properties, termed early T-cell precursor (ETP) lymphoblastic leukemia, as a diagnostic entity.[21,32] As this entity is partly defined by the additional expression of one or more myeloid markers (including CD117, CD13, CD33, CD11b, and CD65) as well as the stem cell markers (CD34 and HLA-DR), it would not be possible to distinguish this entity from MPAL if CD117, CD13, or CD33 were included as lineage defining markers for biphenotypic MPAL. As described later, however, molecular/cytogenetic data continue to blur the lines between these entities.

Flow cytometry in the assignment of myeloid lineage

Despite the 3% cutoff for cytochemical staining for MPO, there exists no blast percentage cutoff for MPO by flow cytometry. To provide standardization, groups have attempted to provide cutoffs, including greater than 10%, greater than 13% compared with isotype controls, and greater than 20% to 28% expression compared with background lymphocytes.[33–35] Despite these studies, the definition of MPAL in the fourth and fifth editions of the WHO has no set threshold for the percentage of blasts that must be positive for MPO by flow cytometry. Indeed, although bilineal MPAL is defined as a composite of 2 or more blast populations that aggregate to 20% blasts, there is no minimum percentage for either blast component.[1,19,21] Nevertheless, small immature MPO + blasts must demonstrate some immunophenotypic aberrancy to discriminate them from normal myeloid precursors.[1,36]

In contrast to percent blast cutoffs, the current emphasis of the WHO classification system is toward interpreting the marker expression in light of the intensity of lineage markers, with stronger expression comparable with background populations signifying greater commitment to a lineage.[1] To this end, in order to standardize flow cytometric interpretation of MPO based on internal positive and negative control populations, the fifth edition of the WHO has clarified that the intensity of MPO expression on blasts must exceed 50% of the background mature neutrophils.[1] This criteria has been shown to reduce MPAL classifications (by third edition WHO criteria) by greater than 50%.[37]

Excluding leukemic cases with weak MPO expression from the diagnosis of MPAL results in their classification as lymphoblastic leukemias with isolated weak expression of MPO (isoMPO). Indeed, the fourth and fifth editions of the WHO have stressed that cases of acute leukemia with a B-lymphoblastic immunophenotype with isoMPO are best classified as B-cell acute lymphoblastic leukemia (B-ALL), as MPO messenger

Table 2
The European Group for the Immunological Characterization of Leukemias scoring system

Points	B-Lineage	T-Lineage	Myeloid Lineage
2	CD79a, cIgM, cCD22	CD3, TCR-α/β, TCR-γδ	MPO, lysozyme
1	CD19, CD10, CD20	CD2, CD5, CD8, CD10	CD13, CD33, CDw65, CD117
0.5	TdT, CD24	TdT, CD7, CD1a	CD14, CD15, CD64,

A case is considered biphenotypic when scores for both myeloid and lymphoid lineages are >2 points.

RNA can frequently be detected in B-ALL.[1,21,38] Some reports suggest B-ALL expressing MPO carries a worse prognosis; however, this finding is controversial.[39–42] On account of this, a recent study was performed on isolated dim MPO expression (<50% of background neutrophils) in adult leukemias of otherwise B-ALL immunophenotype, which revealed that these patients had similar overall and leukemia-free survivals as B-ALL patients and worse survival compared with other patients with MPAL and AML, supporting the threshold cutoff recommendations of the WHO.[43]

Assigning T-Lineage to Biphenotypic Mixed Phenotype Acute Leukemia

The most specific marker for T-lineage leukemias is currently CD3.[44–46] Other T-cell markers, including CD2, CD4, CD5, CD7, CD8, TCR α/β have been used in prior scoring systems, with CD3 receiving the most weight.[16,17,27] However, CD2 and CD7 are commonly found expressed on blasts for leukemias that otherwise are consistent with AML, while CD4 is expressed on early granulocytic precursors and on monocytic and dendritic precursors.[46–50] As such, the WHO classification system utilizes only CD3 to assign T-lineage to blasts expressing mixed lineage antigens.[1,19,21]

Flow cytometry in the assignment of T-lineage

Similar to the scenario of B-ALL with isolated dim MPO expression, it has been recognized that certain leukemias with a predominantly AML-immunophenotype occasionally express dim cytoplasmic CD3.[47,51,52] The WHO has therefore historically restricted T-lineage assignment for MPAL to those cases where the brightest blastic cCD3 expression is comparable to normal T-cells.[19,21] The 5th edition of the WHO has clarified that blasts must show cytoplasmic CD3 expression that is >50% of background T-cells, similar to the MPO requirement for myeloid lineage.[1] Accordingly, it is recommended that assessment of CD3 by flow cytometry be performed with strong fluorochromes, such as phycoerythrin (PE), APC, or BV. Use of a bright fluorochrome

Table 3
The World Health Organization fifth edition scoring system

Myeloid	MPO (intensity ≥ 50% background mature neutrophils) OR Evidence of monocytic differentiation: ≥ 2 of NSE, CD11c, CD14, CD64, or lysozyme
B-lineage	CD19 (intensity ≥ 50% of background normal lymphocytes) and ≥1 strongly expressed marker: CD79a, cCD22, or CD10 OR CD19 (intensity ≤ 50% of background normal B lymphocytes) and ≥2 strongly expressed markers: CD79a, cCD22, or CD10
T-lineage	cCD3 (intensity ≥ 50% of background mature T lymphocytes) or surface CD3

allows a wider range of emission intensities, allowing for adequate comparison of leukemic expression of CD3 to that of background T-cells.

Assigning B-Lineage to Biphenotypic Mixed Phenotype Acute Leukemia

The most specific marker for B-lineage leukemias is CD19; however, it is not sufficient for lineage assignment in the EGIL or WHO classification systems.[1,17,53] Although CD19 is detected in most of the B-ALLs, the detection of CD19 in a subset of AML, including t(8;21) (q22;q22)-rearranged AML, precludes its use as the sole lineage assignment marker.[54,55] Additional B-lineage markers used by the EGIL scoring system include CD79a, cytoplasmic immunoglobulin M, cytoplasmic CD22, CD10, CD20, terminal deoxynucleotidyl transferase (TdT), and CD24.[17] CD79a is expressed early in B cells and is retained through plasmacytic differentiation; however, its expression is not unique to acute leukemias of B-lineage.[56–61] CD10 is similarly expressed early in B-cell development; however, it is detected in fewer cases of B-ALL than CD19 and is detected in a subset of T-cell acute lymphoblastic leukemia (T-ALL), making it less sensitive and specific than CD19.[54] Cytoplasmic expression of CD22 was historically detected in 99% of B-ALL and not identified in AML or T-ALL, but its expression in basophils and dendritic cells makes it less specific for assigning B-lineage.[46,62] TdT is present in both immature B- and T-cell precursors; however, it can be detected in a subset of otherwise straightforward AMLs, making it less useful for ascribing lymphoid versus myeloid lineage.[63–65]

Flow cytometry in the assignment of B-lineage

Similar to myeloid and T-lineage assignment, the WHO has emphasized the strength of antigen expression for B-lineage assignment. Expression of CD19 is required, but additional markers are required depending on the relative intensity of CD19 expression. Again, the WHO endorses a relative comparison to normal cells, defining "strong" CD19 expression as exceeding, at least in part, 50% of normal B-cell progenitors.[1] In this setting, only one additional B-lineage marker is required among CD10, CD22, or CD79a (CD79a cannot be used if T-lineage is under consideration). If the blasts express CD19 at less than 50% normal B cells, then 2 of these additional markers are required. In addition to flow cytometry, immunohistochemistry may be used, in which case PAX5 may potentially be used, pending further research.

FLOW CYTOMETRIC EVALUATION OF NEWLY DESCRIBED ACUTE LEUKEMIAS OF AMBIGUOUS LINEAGE ENTITIES

The fifth edition of the WHO classification system recognizes 2 new entities with defined genetic alterations, MPAL with *ZNF384* rearrangements and ALAL with *BCL11B* rearrangements. Although *ZNF384* rearrangements have been identified in B-ALL, Alexander and colleagues characterized them in the setting of pediatric B/myeloid MPAL at a rate of 48% of B/myeloid MPAL.[13] Gene expression profiling suggests *ZNF384*-rearranged MPAL more closely resembles B-ALL than AML, with a maturation profile that is more mature than most B/myeloid MPAL but less mature than most B-ALL.[13]

A study of a handful of *ZNF384*-rearranged MPALs suggests they tend to express CD19 and CD22 on most of the blasts, whereas expression of CD10 tends to be more variable, with many cases showing minimal CD10 expression.[66] CD20 expression tends to be negative or expressed on a minority of blasts. The myeloid component tends to be a minor component of the leukemia, typically defined by MPO expression, and with CD13, CD33, and CD15 frequently coexpressed. CD117 is typically not expressed, whereas conversely, CD34 frequently is positive.[66] Additional markers frequently seen in most of the blasts include CD45 and HLA-DR.

The newly described *BCL11B*-rearranged MPAL tends to present as T/myeloid MPAL and expresses CD34, CD117 (weak), cCD3, CD2, CD7, CD11b (weak to negative), CD13, CD15, CD133, MPO (variable), and TdT and lacks CD1a, CD5, CD8, CD33, and CD65.[67] Of note, *BCL11B*-rearranged ETP is also described, with a similar immunophenotype except, definitionally, for the expression of MPO.[67] Further research will be necessary to determine whether the new 50% MPO intensity threshold will affect the classification of these entities as well as whether distinguishing ETP and T/Myeloid MPAL with *BCL11B* rearrangements is even clinically meaningful.

Flow Cytometry in the Diagnosis of Acute Leukemias of Ambiguous Lineage

Reagents and panel design

In performing multiparameter flow cytometry to assign lineage to leukemic blasts, it is important to develop tubes and panels that fully evaluate the aforementioned markers and use fluorochromes that allow for appropriate comparison of intensities. As the antibodies per tube increase, it is likely that tandem-fluorochromes will be used. The use of tandem fluorochromes raises potential problems associated with general degradation as well as diminished fluorescence due to permeabilization and fixation of cells, and therefore avoidance of light and care in storage/handling must be taken when using these reagents.[68]

Lineage assignment is heavily dependent on examination of intracellular markers (MPO, cCD3, cCD22, CD79a). Although large fluorochromes (PE and PE-tandem dyes) pose a theoretical problem for use in interrogating intracellular targets, it has been reported that most large dyes do work well for this purpose.[69] Nevertheless, proper validation and assessment of the effects of permeabilization and fixation should be performed for any panel using tandem fluorochromes for the lineage-specific intracellular markers.

Panel design for the assessment of lineage requires thorough testing to ensure coverage of all necessary markers without introducing interpretative error due to inherent artifacts (eg, spectral overlap, fluorochrome degradation, and so forth). Of note, the EuroFlow consortium has established a validated 8-color antibody tube for the diagnosis of acute leukemias, termed the acute leukemia orientation tube (ALOT).[70] The ALOT is a screening tube composed of cCD3 (*PacB*), sCD3 (*APCH7*), CD45 (*PacO*), CyMPO (*FITC*), CyCD79a (*PE*), CD34 (*PerCPCy5.5*), CD19 (*PECy7*), and CD7 (*APC*), which allows an initial assessment of blast lineage and allows for further assessment with a more directed panel of antibodies (eg, B-ALL, T-ALL, and AML/myelodysplastic syndrome panels). Subsequently, many commercial preparations have been released based on this tube composition.

ALAL is rare, with, no as of yet, well-defined treatment. Nevertheless, minimal residual disease (MRD) testing is likely to become a more used modality in assessing treatment response. Laboratories will need to determine if they will adapt established ALL- and AML-oriented MRD panels or validate new, more blended panels for the purpose of tracking MPAL MRD. The challenges will include designing standardized tubes in the face of rare, heterogeneous leukemias, as well as choosing compensatory markers to maintain the utility of the assay in the face of immunotherapy that targets one or more of the panel markers.

Interpretation

Of note, one must avoid making a diagnosis of MPAL based solely on flow cytometric immunophenotyping. The WHO restricts MPAL diagnoses to those that cannot be ascribed other defined entities, such as AML with *RUNX1::RUNX1T1*; AML, myelodysplasia-related; or blast crisis chronic myeloid leukemia.

Advances in analysis

Renowned ALAL experts, Béné and Porwit, have published on their use of the Flow-SOM package for the interpretation of mixed phenotype acute leukemias.[9,71] This R-based visualization tool allows users to perform self-organizing map clustering and minimal spanning trees on cytometry data. Using unsupervised clustering of 10 merged normal bone marrow controls analyzed for TdT, MPO, CD2, HLA-DR, CD19, cCD79a, CD34, CD33, cCD3, CD45, and side scatter (SSC), Béné and colleagues generated a reference plot composed of 16 cell subsets for this MPAL-oriented panel. This reference plot was then used to readily reveal atypical mixed phenotype populations within patients with MPAL and proved more capable of identifying unique subsets than conventional flow cytometry.[9]

SUMMARY

The diagnosis of acute leukemia of ambiguous lineage continues to evolve, with increasing focus on a handful of lineage-specific markers. Flow cytometry is essential for the diagnosis of these rare leukemias, with the WHO stressing the importance of the overall intensity of lineage-specific markers in relation to each other in order to standardize diagnoses and, by extension, treatments. Moreover, novel entities, including MPAL with *ZNF384* rearrangements and ALAL with *BCL11B* rearrangements, have been added to the list of ambiguous leukemias, both of which seem to show characteristic flow cytometric immunophenotypes. Detecting the aberrant marker expression and fluorescence intensities of these leukemias is aided by an increasing number of tube antibodies, which in turn requires careful validation to maximize sensitivity and reduce error. Finally, further advances in flow cytometry are on the horizon not only from the analytical realm but from the interpretative side as well, as artificial intelligence tools, such as FlowSOM, become more widely applied.

CLINICS CARE POINTS

- As the diagnosis of MPAL requires integration of flow cytometric, cytochemical, cytogenetic, and potentially molecular data avoid making a diagnosis of mixed phenotype acute leukemia without ruling out other defined entities that take precedence in classification.

- Acute leukemias that express CD34, CD117 (weak), cCD3, CD2, CD7, CD11b (weak to negative), CD13, CD15, CD133, MPO (variable), and TdT and lack CD1a, CD5, CD8, CD33, and CD65 raise suspicion for *BCL11B* rearrangements and, depending on the intensity of MPO expression, may qualify as T/myeloid MPAL (if strong) or ETP ALL (if dim to negative).

- Flow panels must have lineage markers coupled to fluorochromes with sufficient dynamic range for adequate comparison to background normal precursors.

DISCLOSURE

The authors have no conflicts of interest to disclose.

REFERENCES

1. Khoury JD, Solary E, Abla O, et al. The 5th edition of the World Health organization classification of haematolymphoid Tumours: myeloid and histiocytic/dendritic neoplasms. Leukemia 2022;36(7):1703–19.

2. Weinberg OK, Arber DA. Mixed-phenotype acute leukemia: historical overview and a new definition. Leukemia 2010;24(11):1844–51.
3. Béné MC, Porwit A. Acute leukemias of ambiguous lineage. Semin Diagn Pathol 2012;29(1):12–8.
4. Porwit A, Béné MC. Acute leukemias of ambiguous origin. Am J Clin Pathol 2015; 144(3):361–76.
5. Wolach O, Stone RM. Mixed-phenotype acute leukemia: current challenges in diagnosis and therapy. Curr Opin Hematol 2017;24(2):139.
6. Charles NJ, Boyer DF. Mixed-phenotype acute leukemia: diagnostic criteria and pitfalls. Arch Pathol Lab Med 2017;141(11):1462–8.
7. Kurzer JH, Weinberg OK. Acute leukemias of ambiguous lineage: clarification on lineage specificity. Surg Pathol Clin 2019;12(3):687–97.
8. Porwit A, Béné MC. Multiparameter flow cytometry applications in the diagnosis of mixed phenotype acute leukemia. Cytometry B Clin Cytom 2019;96(3):183–94.
9. Béné MC, Porwit A. Mixed phenotype/lineage leukemia: has anything changed for 2021 on diagnosis, classification, and treatment? Curr Oncol Rep 2022; 24(8):1015–22.
10. Yan L, Ping N, Zhu M, et al. Clinical, immunophenotypic, cytogenetic, and molecular genetic features in 117 adult patients with mixed-phenotype acute leukemia defined by WHO-2008 classification. Haematologica 2012;97(11):1708–12.
11. Shi R, Munker R. Survival of patients with mixed phenotype acute leukemias: a large population-based study. Leuk Res 2015;39(6):606–16.
12. Matutes E, Pickl WF, Van't Veer M, et al. Mixed-phenotype acute leukemia: clinical and laboratory features and outcome in 100 patients defined according to the WHO 2008 classification. Blood 2011;117(11):3163–71.
13. Alexander TB, Gu Z, Iacobucci I, et al. The genetic basis and cell of origin of mixed phenotype acute leukaemia. Nature 2018;562(7727):373–9.
14. Arber DA, Orazi A, Hasserjian RP, et al. International Consensus classification of myeloid neoplasms and acute leukemias: integrating morphologic, clinical, and genomic data. Blood 2022;140(11):1200–28.
15. Mirro J, Kitchingman G. The morphology, cytochemistry, molecular characteristics and clinical significance of acute mixed-lineage leukaemia. In: Scott C, editor. Leukaemia cytochemistry and diagnosis: principles and practice. West Sussex, England: Ellis Horwood; 1989. p. 155–79.
16. Catovsky D, Matutes E, Buccheri V, et al. A classification of acute leukaemia for the 1990s. Ann Hematol 1991;62(1):16–21.
17. Bene MC, Castoldi G, Knapp W, et al. Proposals for the immunological classification of acute leukemias. European group for the immunological characterization of leukemias (EGIL). Leukemia 1995;9(10):1783–6.
18. Jaffe ES, Harris NL, Stein H, et al. In: *WHO classification of tumours of haematopoietic and lymphoid tissues*. 3rd edition. Lyon Cedex, France: International Agency for Research on Cancer Press; 2001.
19. Swerdlow SH, Campo E, Harris NL, et al, editors. WHO classification of tumours of haematopoietic and lymphoid tissues. 4th edition. Lyon Cedex, France: International Agency for Research on Cancer; 2008.
20. Arber DA, Orazi A, Hasserjian R, et al. The 2016 revision to the World Health Organization classification of myeloid neoplasms and acute leukemia. Blood 2016; 127(20):2391–405.
21. Swerdlow SH, Campo E, Harris NL, et al, editors. WHO classification of tumours of haematopoietic and lymphoid tissues. Revised 4th edition. Lyon Cedex, France: International Agency for Research on Cancer; 2017.

22. Wolach O, Stone RM. How I treat mixed-phenotype acute leukemia. Blood 2015; 125(16):2477–85.

23. Wolach O, Stone RM. Optimal therapeutic strategies for mixed phenotype acute leukemia. Curr Opin Hematol 2020;27(2):95–102.

24. Bennett JM, Catovsky D, Daniel MT, et al. Proposals for the classification of the acute leukaemias. French-American-British (FAB) co-operative group. Br J Haematol 1976;33(4):451–8.

25. El Chaer F, Ali OM, Sausville EA, et al. Treatment of CD19-positive mixed phenotype acute leukemia with blinatumomab. Am J Hematol 2019;94(1):E7–8.

26. Buccheri V, Shetty V, Yoshida N, et al. The role of an anti-myeloperoxidase antibody in the diagnosis and classification of acute leukaemia: a comparison with light and electron microscopy cytochemistry. Br J Haematol 1992;80(1):62–8.

27. Bene MC, Bernier M, Casasnovas RO, et al. The reliability and specificity of c-kit for the diagnosis of acute myeloid leukemias and undifferentiated leukemias. The European Group for the Immunological Classification of Leukemias (EGIL). Blood 1998;92(2):596–9.

28. Yarden Y, Kuang WJ, Yang-Feng T, et al. Human proto-oncogene c-kit: a new cell surface receptor tyrosine kinase for an unidentified ligand. EMBO J 1987;6(11): 3341–51.

29. Ashman LK, Cambareri AC, To LB, et al. Expression of the YB5.B8 antigen (c-kit proto-oncogene product) in normal human Bone Marrow. Blood 1991;78(1):30–7.

30. Mina-Osorio P. The moonlighting enzyme CD13: old and new functions to target. Trends Mol Med 2008;14(8):361–71.

31. Laszlo GS, Estey EH, Walter RB. The past and future of CD33 as therapeutic target in acute myeloid leukemia. Blood Rev 2014;28(4):143–53.

32. Coustan-Smith E, Mullighan CG, Onciu M, et al. Early T-cell precursor leukaemia: a subtype of very high-risk acute lymphoblastic leukaemia. Lancet Oncol 2009; 10(2):147–56.

33. van den Ancker W, Westers TM, de Leeuw DC, et al. A threshold of 10% for myeloperoxidase by flow cytometry is valid to classify acute leukemia of ambiguous and myeloid origin. Cytometry B Clin Cytom 2013;84(2):114–8.

34. Guy J, Antony-Debré I, Benayoun E, et al. Flow cytometry thresholds of myeloperoxidase detection to discriminate between acute lymphoblastic or myeloblastic leukaemia. Br J Haematol 2013;161(4):551–5.

35. Bras AE, Osmani Z, de Haas V, et al. Standardised immunophenotypic analysis of myeloperoxidase in acute leukaemia. Br J Haematol 2021;193(5):922–7.

36. Borowitz MJ. Mixed phenotype acute leukemia. Cytometry B Clin Cytom 2014; 86(3):152–3.

37. Kovach AE, Raikar SS, Oberley MJ, et al. Standardization in the diagnosis of mixed phenotype acute leukemia (MPAL): semiquantitative, universally applicable flow cytometric criteria for immunophenotypic lineage assignment and isolated MPO. Blood 2021;138:4475.

38. Zhou M, Findley HW, Zaki SR, et al. Expression of myeloperoxidase mRNA by leukemic cells from childhood acute lymphoblastic leukemia. Leukemia 1993; 7(8):1180–3.

39. Kang H, Chen IM, Wilson CS, et al. Gene expression classifiers for relapse-free survival and minimal residual disease improve risk classification and outcome prediction in pediatric B-precursor acute lymphoblastic leukemia. Blood 2010; 115(7):1394–405.

40. Oberley MJ, Li S, Orgel E, et al. Clinical significance of isolated myeloperoxidase expression in pediatric B-lymphoblastic leukemia. Am J Clin Pathol 2017;147(4): 374–81.
41. Raikar SS, Park SI, Leong T, et al. Isolated myeloperoxidase expression in pediatric B/myeloid mixed phenotype acute leukemia is linked with better survival. Blood 2018;131(5):573–7.
42. McGinnis E, Yang D, Au N, et al. Clinical and laboratory features associated with myeloperoxidase expression in pediatric B-lymphoblastic leukemia. Cytometry B Clin Cytom 2021;100(4):446–53.
43. Weinberg OK, Dennis J, Zia H, et al. Adult mixed phenotype acute leukemia (MPAL): B/myeloid MPALisoMPO is distinct from other MPAL subtypes. Int J Lab Hematol 2022;45(2):170–8.
44. Campana D, Thompson JS, Amlot P, et al. The cytoplasmic expression of CD3 antigens in normal and malignant cells of the T lymphoid lineage. J Immunol 1987;138(2):648–55.
45. van Dongen JJ, Krissansen GW, Wolvers-Tettero IL, et al. Cytoplasmic expression of the CD3 antigen as a diagnostic marker for immature T-cell malignancies. Blood 1988;71(3):603–12.
46. Janossy G, Coustan-Smith E, Campana D. The reliability of cytoplasmic CD3 and CD22 antigen expression in the immunodiagnosis of acute leukemia: a study of 500 cases. Leukemia 1989;3(3):170–81.
47. Bradstock K, Matthews J, Benson E, et al. Prognostic value of immunophenotyping in acute myeloid leukemia. Australian Leukaemia Study Group. Blood 1994; 84(4):1220–5.
48. Vodinelich L, Tax W, Bai Y, et al. A monoclonal antibody (WT1) for detecting leukemias of T-cell precursors (T-ALL). Blood 1983;62(5):1108–13.
49. Haynes BF, Eisenbarth GS, Fauci AS. Human lymphocyte antigens: production of a monoclonal antibody that defines functional thymus-derived lymphocyte subsets. Proc Natl Acad Sci U S A 1979;76(11):5829–33.
50. Drexler HG, Thiel E, Ludwig WD. Acute myeloid leukemias expressing lymphoid-associated antigens: diagnostic incidence and prognostic significance. Leukemia 1993;7(4):489–98.
51. Legrand O, Perrot JY, Baudard M, et al. The immunophenotype of 177 adults with acute myeloid leukemia: proposal of a prognostic score. Blood 2000;96(3):870–7.
52. Lewis RE, Cruse JM, Sanders CM, et al. Aberrant expression of T-cell markers in acute myeloid leukemia. Exp Mol Pathol 2007;83(3):462–3.
53. Nadler LM, Anderson KC, Marti G, et al. B4, a human B lymphocyte-associated antigen expressed on normal, mitogen-activated, and malignant B lymphocytes. J Immunol 1983;131(1):244–50.
54. Anderson KC, Bates MP, Slaughenhoupt BL, et al. Expression of human B cell-associated antigens on leukemias and lymphomas: a model of human B cell differentiation. Blood 1984;63(6):1424–33.
55. Ball ED, Davis RB, Griffin JD, et al. Prognostic value of lymphocyte surface markers in acute myeloid leukemia [see comments]. Blood 1991;77(10):2242–50.
56. Weiss A, Littman DR. Signal transduction by lymphocyte antigen receptors. Cell 1994;76(2):263–74.
57. Patterson HC, Kraus M, Wang D, et al. Cytoplasmic Ig alpha serine/threonines fine-tune Ig alpha tyrosine phosphorylation and limit bone marrow plasma cell formation. J Immunol 2011;187(6):2853–8.
58. Leduc I, Preud'homme JL, Cogné M. Structure and expression of the mb-1 transcript in human lymphoid cells. Clin Exp Immunol 1992;90(1):141–6.

59. Hashimoto M, Yamashita Y, Mori N. Immunohistochemical detection of CD79a expression in precursor T cell lymphoblastic lymphoma/leukaemias. J Pathol 2002;197(3):341–7.

60. Pilozzi E, Pulford K, Jones M, et al. Co-expression of CD79a (JCB117) and CD3 by lymphoblastic lymphoma. J Pathol 1998;186(2):140–3.

61. Arber DA, Jenkins KA, Slovak ML. CD79 alpha expression in acute myeloid leukemia. High frequency of expression in acute promyelocytic leukemia. Am J Pathol 1996;149(4):1105–10.

62. Sato N, Kishi K, Toba K, et al. Simultaneous expression of CD13, CD22 and CD25 is related to the expression of Fc epsilon R1 in non-lymphoid leukemia. Leuk Res 2004;28(7):691–8.

63. Desiderio SV, Yancopoulos GD, Paskind M, et al. Insertion of N regions into heavy-chain genes is correlated with expression of terminal deoxytransferase in B cells. Nature 1984;311(5988):752–5.

64. Borowitz MJ, Lynn Guenther K, Shults KE, et al. Immunophenotyping of acute leukemia by flow cytometric analysis: use of CD45 and right-angle light scatter to gate on leukemic blasts in three-color analysis. Am J Clin Pathol 1993;100(5):534–40.

65. Paietta E, Racevskis J, Bennett JM, et al. Differential expression of terminal transferase (TdT) in acute lymphocytic leukaemia expressing myeloid antigens and TdT positive acute myeloid leukaemia as compared to myeloid antigen negative acute lymphocytic leukaemia. Br J Haematol 1993;84(3):416–22.

66. Zaliova M, Winkowska L, Stuchly J, et al. A novel class of ZNF384 aberrations in acute leukemia. Blood Adv 2021;5(21):4393–7.

67. Montefiori LE, Bendig S, Gu Z, et al. Enhancer hijacking drives oncogenic BCL11B expression in lineage-ambiguous stem cell leukemia. Cancer Discov 2021;11(11):2846–67.

68. Hulspas R, Dombkowski D, Preffer F, et al. Flow cytometry and the stability of phycoerythrin-tandem dye conjugates. Cytometry A 2009;75(11):966–72.

69. Maciorowski Z, Chattopadhyay PK, Jain P. Basic multicolor flow cytometry. Curr Protoc Immunol 2017;117(1):5.4.1–5.4.38.

70. Dongen JJM van, Lhermitte L, Böttcher S, et al. EuroFlow antibody panels for standardized n-dimensional flow cytometric immunophenotyping of normal, reactive and malignant leukocytes. Leukemia 2012;26(9):1908–75.

71. Van Gassen S, Callebaut B, Van Helden MJ, et al. FlowSOM: using self-organizing maps for visualization and interpretation of cytometry data. Cytometry 2015;87(7):636–45.

Clinical Flow Cytometry Analysis in the Setting of Chronic Myeloid Neoplasms and Clonal Hematopoiesis

Siba El Hussein, MD[a],*, Sanam Loghavi, MD[b],*

KEYWORDS

- Clonal hematopoiesis • Myelodysplastic neoplasms • Myeloproliferative neoplasms
- Flow cytometry analysis • CHIP • CCUS

KEY POINTS

- Flow cytometry analysis (FCA) is not currently incorporated in the diagnostic criteria for myelodysplastic neoplasms (MDS) in the World Health Organization classification of hematologic neoplasms.
- Increasing evidence supports the addition of FCA to the diagnostic workup during the evaluation of MDS as an adjunct diagnostic tool.
- FCA may provide additional helpful data to differentiate persistent clonal hematopoiesis from measurable residual disease following therapy in patients with acute myeloid leukemia.

INTRODUCTION

Chronic myeloid neoplasms including myelodysplastic neoplasms (MDS) and myeloproliferative neoplasms (MPNs) are clonal hematopoietic stem cell (HSC) disorders. Characterization of the molecular and genetic underpinning of these neoplasms had led to the development of targeted and nontargeted therapies with increasing investigative clinical trials rapidly developing for patients with these neoplasms. Chronic myeloid neoplasms have an inherent potential for clonal evolution and disease progression to acute myeloid leukemia (AML) sometimes years after the initial diagnosis. Therefore, detailed characterization of the bone marrow at baseline and during disease acceleration may prove invaluable in rendering an accurate assessment of patterns of disease progression with time. Characterization of bone marrow

[a] Department of Pathology, University of Rochester Medical Center, Rochester, NY, USA;
[b] Department of Hematopathology, The University of Texas MD Anderson Cancer Center, Houston, TX, USA
* Correspondence authors.
E-mail addresses: elhusseinsiba@gmail.com (S.E.H.); sloghavi@mdanderson.org (S.L.)

Clin Lab Med 43 (2023) 411–426
https://doi.org/10.1016/j.cll.2023.04.007
0272-2712/23/© 2023 Elsevier Inc. All rights reserved.

cellular compartments in the setting of chronic myeloid neoplasms has been historically performed using morphologic examination. However, within the last 2 decades, attention to the utility of flow cytometry analysis (FCA) as an adjunct diagnostic tool to study the maturation and immunophenotypic aberrancies of HSCs and other bone marrow subpopulations, has shed light on the invaluable role FCA in the evaluation of chronic myeloid neoplasms. Furthermore, recently, clonal hematopoiesis (CH) has been an emerging topic in clinical hematology-oncology, as its characterization as a precursor of myeloid neoplasms has underlined the importance of delving more into the intricacies of its biology, evolution and associated side effects on hematopoiesis and other organs (ie,: cardiovascular system). The emerging importance of characterizing CH is especially relevant in the setting of measurable residual disease (MRD) assessment for AML because some patients tend to have persistent CH following the treatment of their AML. In this article, we will provide a comprehensive account of the utility of FCA in the evaluation of bone marrow specimens for chronic myeloid neoplasms and related HSC abnormalities including persistent CH in the setting of AML, with emphasis on the evaluation of myeloid progenitors and maturing myelomonocytic cells, and a brief summary of the current FCA scoring systems pertaining to this topic.

EVALUATION OF BONE MARROW CELLULAR COMPARTMENTS USING FLOW CYTOMETRY ANALYSIS

FCA is used to detect aberrant expression of surface antigens on various cellular compartments of the bone marrow as well as phenotypic deviations from normal patterns of maturation in hematopoietic elements. The European LeukemiaNet (ELN) collaborative group has proposed minimal requirements for the standardization of FCA in the diagnostic workup of MDS.[1] These include a set of proposed core markers in a standardized panel designed for the evaluation of MDS as well as recurrent aberrancies identified in cases of MDS on different bone marrow cell lineages. **Fig. 1** summarizes the common aberrancies identified on these cell lineages in MDS and related myeloid stem cell neoplasms, **Fig. 2** provides a visual summary of the recommended markers for each cellular compartment.

Enumeration and Characterization of Myeloid Progenitors

CD34+ myeloid progenitors are enumerated by FCA based on their light scatter properties, dim CD45 expression and expression of CD34. Enumeration is subject to specimen quality and other technical factors but provides a relatively objective measure in the assessment of MDS. The highest number of CD34+ myeloid blasts have been reported in cases of MDS with increased blasts and MDS with isolated del(5q).[2] Abnormalities affecting myeloid progenitor cells include (1) increased numbers of blasts (>2%); (2) altered expression of CD45 (either increased or decreased), CD34 (increased or negative), CD13 (typically increased), CD117 (typically increased), CD123 (typically increased), CD38 (typically decreased), human leukocyte antigen – DR isotype (HLA-DR) (typically decreased), and increased side scatter; (3) abnormal expression patterns of CD13/CD33, CD38/CD117; (4) asynchronous expression of mature markers such as CD11b, CD15, CD10, or (5) lineage infidelity as shown by aberrant expression of lymphoid antigens such as CD2, CD5, CD7, CD19, CD22, and/or CD56[3–6] (see **Fig. 1**; **Figs. 3** and **4**). In addition, CD34+ myeloid progenitors in normal bone marrow include a heterogeneous population of cells composed of myeloid progenitors, plasmacytoid dendritic cell progenitors, and B cell progenitors also known as hematogones (see **Fig. 4**). This diversity is typically lost in cases of MDS. Of note, CD2, CD22, and

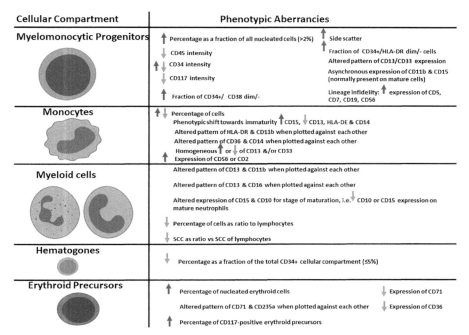

Cellular Compartment	Phenotypic Aberrancies	
Myelomonocytic Progenitors	↑ Percentage as a fraction of all nucleated cells (>2%) ↓ CD45 intensity ↑↓ CD34 intensity ↓ CD117 intensity ↑ Fraction of CD34+/ CD38 dim/-	↑ Side scatter ↑ Fraction of CD34+/HLA-DR dim/- cells Altered pattern of CD13/CD33 expression Asynchronous expression of CD11b & CD15 (normally present on mature cells) Lineage infidelity: ↑ expression of CD5, CD7, CD19, CD56
Monocytes	↑↓ Percentage of cells Phenotypic shift towards immaturity ↑CD15, ↓CD13, HLA-DE & CD14 Altered pattern of HLA-DR & CD11b when plotted against each other Altered pattern of CD36 & CD14 when plotted against each other Homogeneous ↑ or ↓ of CD13 &/or CD33 ↑ Expression of CD56 or CD2	
Myeloid cells	Altered pattern of CD13 & CD11b when plotted against each other Altered pattern of CD13 & CD16 when plotted against each other Altered expression of CD15 & CD10 for stage of maturation, i.e. ↓ CD10 or CD15 expression on mature neutrophils ↓ Percentage of cells as ratio to lymphocytes ↓ SCC as ratio vs SCC of lymphocytes	
Hematogones	↓ Percentage as a fraction of the total CD34+ cellular compartment (≤5%)	
Erythroid Precursors	↑ Percentage of nucleated erythroid cells Altered pattern of CD71 & CD235a when plotted against each other ↑ Percentage of CD117-positive erythroid precursors	↓ Expression of CD71 ↓ Expression of CD36

Fig. 1. Summary of the common aberrancies identified in cell lineages in myeloid stem neoplasms.

CD7 may be expressed on a small subset of CD34+ myeloid progenitors (typically on the CD38 bright compartment) in normal bone marrow specimens, and should not be over interpreted as evidence of MDS if other features assessed are within normal limits. Furthermore, aberrant myeloblasts should be distinguished from early regenerating myeloid stem cells, which show diminished CD38 expression; however, they

Progenitors	Maturing myeloids	Monocytes	Erythroids
CD45	CD45	CD45	CD45
CD34	CD34	CD34	CD71
CD117	CD117	CD117	CD235a
HLA-DR	HLA-DR	HLA-DR	CD117
CD11b	CD11b	CD11b	CD36
CD13	CD13	CD13	
CD7	CD16	CD16	
CD56	CD33	CD33	
CD19	CD14	CD14	
CD5	CD64	CD36	
CD15	CD56	CD64	
	CD15	CD56	
	CD10	CD2	

Fig. 2. Proposed core markers in the analysis of dysplasia in various bone marrow cellular elements by flow cytometry as recommended by the ELN collaborative group.

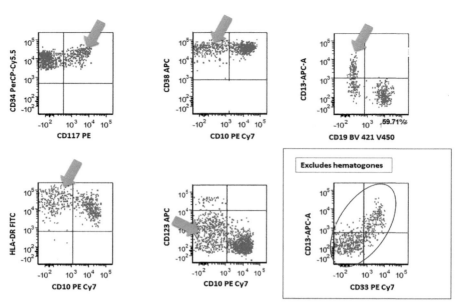

Fig. 3. Normal antigen expression intensity of CD34+ myeloid progenitors (*arrow*).

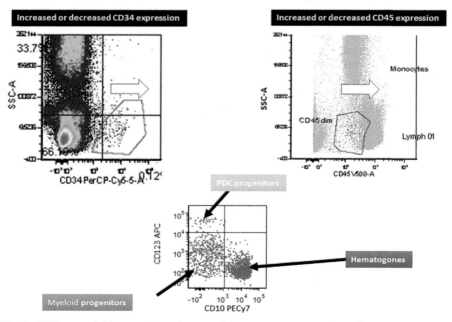

Fig. 4. CD34+ myeloid progenitors in normal bone marrow comprise a heterogenous population of cells composed of myeloid progenitors, plamacytoid dendritic cell (PDC) progenitors and hematogones, and CD123 moderate), PDCs (CD123 bright, HLA-DR, and CD2+). *Red arrow* indicated increased or decreased CD34/CD45 epression in CD34+ myeloid progenitors in the setting of MDS compared with normal.

characteristically have increased CD45 and CD34 expression and are dim for nearly all other antigens including CD13, CD33, CD117, CD123, and HLA-DR.

Enumeration of B-cell Progenitors/Hematogones

Decreased or absence of hematogones as assessed by CD19 and or CD10 is seen in the majority of MDS cases. To avoid the influence of hemodilution, the recommendation is to enumerate stage I hematogones as a fraction of CD34+ progenitors ($\leq$5% as reduced). Of note, a subset of MDS with ring sideroblasts/*SF3B1* mutation, or MDS with no detectable somatic mutations, can demonstrate the preservation of hematogones. These cases have been reported to show upregulated CD34, and decreased HLA-DR expression on myeloblasts, which can be a helpful clue.[7]

Assessment for Granulocytic and Monocytic Dysplasia Using Flow Cytometry Analysis

An ideal FCA assay designed for the evaluation of MDS should allow for the evaluation of maturing myelomonocytic cells. Maturing myelomonocytic cells in the bone marrow exhibit tightly regulated patterns of antigen expression for their stage of maturation.[8] **Fig. 5** provides an illustrative summary of these patterns. Deviation from these patterns may be seen in the setting MDS.

Typical alterations detected by FCA in the setting of MDS and related stem cell disorders include (1) decreased side scatter of mature granulocytes indicating cytoplasmic hypogranularity; (2) asynchronous expression of maturation markers (eg, CD11b vs CD16, and/or CD13 vs CD16); (3) aberrant expression of antigens as CD4 or CD56.[4,8] **Fig. 6** shows a comparison of normal granulocytes with those seen in the setting of MDS. The changes observed in maturing myeloid cells have been shown to be sensitive but not entirely specific. Similar changes can be seen

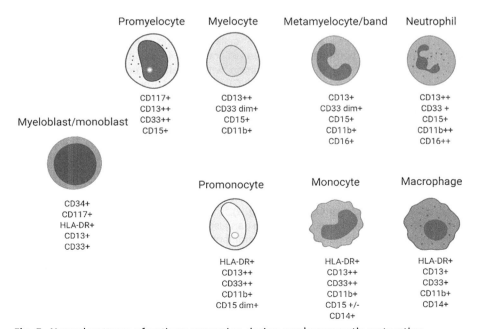

Fig. 5. Normal patterns of antigen expression during myelomonocytic maturation.

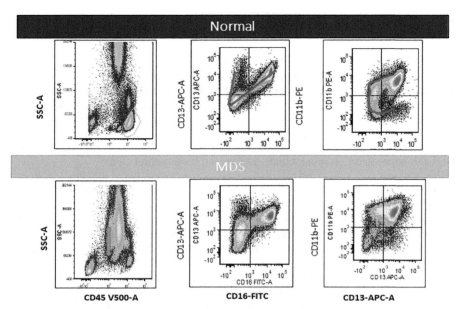

Fig. 6. Comparison of maturing myeloid cells in a normal bone marrow sample and a bone marrow sample involved by MDS. *Orange arrow* indicates decreased side scatter of maturing myeloid cells.

in patients with other nonneoplastic conditions and in the setting of chemotherapy, antibiotic exposure, growth factor administration and treatment with immunomodulatory agents.[9]

It should also be noted that immunophenotypic alterations of maturing myeloid cells may also be encountered in several other scenarios as well. Such examples include aged specimens (increased fraction of cells exhibiting decreased expression of CD11b and CD13), hemodilution (increased fraction of cells showing expression of CD10, CD11b, and CD16) and specimen with a left-shifted myeloid maturation (increased fraction of cells with CD13 low/CD16 low/CD10-negative cells).[3] Other aberrancies seen in granulocytes in the setting of an underlying MDS, include loss or decreased CD10, and aberrant expression of CD56 and HLA-DR[3,8] but these changes may also be observed in robustly regenerating/reactive bone marrow.

Alterations observed in the monocytic compartment include (1) an increased or decreased number of monocytes (compared with lymphocytes); (2) increased or decreased side scatter and decreased CD45; (3) decreased CD13, CD14, CD36, HLA-DR, and CD11b expression and increased CD15, CD123 which may also correspond to immaturity or left-shifted maturation of monocytes; and (4) substantial aberrant expression of CD2 and/or CD56 (see **Fig. 1**).[4,8] Many of the changes in monocytes as well as left-shifted monocytic maturation can also be observed in reactive and regenerative conditions and in nonneoplastic conditions. **Figs. 7** and **8** show a comparison of monocytes in a normal bone marrow sample and a sample involved by MDS.

Flow Cytometric Detection of Dyserythropoiesis

Aberrant antigen expression patterns in the granulocytic and monocytic cell lineages in the setting of MDS are well established; However, phenotypic aberrancies in the erythroid and megakaryocytic cell lineages are not as uniformly characterized, in

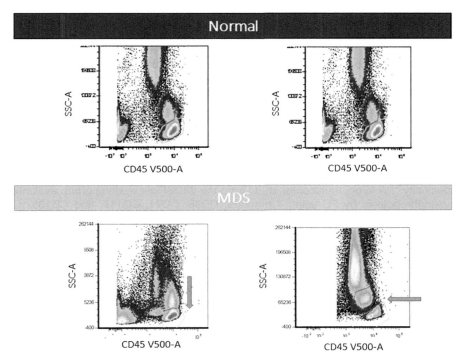

Fig. 7. Comparison of monocytes in a normal bone marrow sample and a bone marrow sample involved by MDS, with respect to side scatter (SCC) and CD45 expression. *Orange arrow* points at the monocytic population with decreased side scatter and decreased CD45 expression.

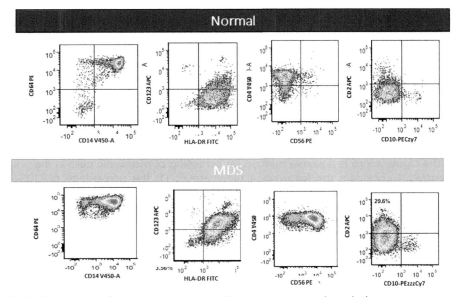

Fig. 8. Comparison of monocytes in a normal bone marrow sample and a bone marrow sample involved by MDS, with respect to CD2, CD4, CD10, CD14, CD56, CD64, CD123 and HLA-DR expression.

part due to a relative lack of relevant surface markers and partly because during sample preparation for routine FCA, red cell precursors are lysed together with red blood cells, and megakaryocytes are too scanty to harvest for analysis. Therefore, many FCA panels designed to assess MDS focus on the number and phenotype of myeloid blasts and the phenotype of maturing myeloid cells and monocytes.

Some common aberrancies in the erythroid series in MDS include increased percentage of nucleated red blood cells, altered patterns of CD71 and CD235a expression, decreased expression of CD71 and/or CD36, and increased percentage of CD117+ (immature) erythroid progenitors.[10,11] The addition of these 3 erythroid markers to the Ogata and Wells algorithms has been shown to increase their sensitivity from 74% to 86% and from 69% to 80%, respectively, without significant changes in specificity.[11] A large, multicenter study from the IMDSFlow working group evaluated dyserythropoiesis by FC using 4 markers: CD36, CD71, CD117, and CD105.[12] A weighted score was then calculated based on these 4 parameters and tested in 2 different cohorts, yielding a sensitivity of 24% to 33% and a specificity of 90% to 92%.[12] Furthermore, recently investigators have been able to successfully apply imaging flow cytometric techniques for quantification of morphometric changes in dysplastic erythroid precursors.[13]

The immunophenotypic features of pure erythroid leukemia (PEL), a myeloid stem cell neoplasm characterized by exuberant erythroid differentiation and biallelic *TP53* loss were recently described by Fang and colleagues.[14] These include decreased or negative CD38 expression, aberrant expression of CD7 (25%) and CD13 (29%), increased expression of CD4 (50%) or complete loss of CD4 (21%), and a complete absence of a CD34+ erythroid progenitor compartment. Although not increased in number, CD34-positive myeloblasts were frequently detected in PEL and demonstrated an aberrant immunophenotype in 90% of PEL cases.

FLOW CYTOMETRY-BASED SCORING SYSTEMS IN CHRONIC MYELOID NEOPLASMS

A plethora of FCA-based scoring systems have been developed throughout the last 2 decades to enhance the diagnostic workup of MDS/MPN, including: The "Ogata score,"[6,15] the "Wells algorithm,"[16,17] the "integrated flow cytometry (iFC)" score developed by the international consortium and the ELN Working Group,[1,18] and the newly conceptualized "Meyerson-Alayed scoring scheme (MASS)."[19]

The iFC score[5,18] includes a set of minimal requirements recommended to assess dysplasia, these include (1) detecting aberrant findings in at least 3 tested features comprising at least 2 cell compartments (see **Fig. 1**); (2) the documentation of these abnormalities for prognostic significance; and (3) integration in the diagnostic reports, together with morphologic, cytogenetic, and/or molecular findings.

The Ogata score is a simple method for screening of dysplastic cells in the bone marrow. It considers the following 4 parameters[6]: (1) the percentage of CD34+ myeloid progenitor cells in the bone marrow; (2) the frequency of hematogones within the CD34+ compartment; (3) CD45 expression on myeloid progenitors relative to CD45 expression on lymphocytes; and (4) neutrophil/lymphocyte side scatter (SSC) ratio (~6 is normal). **Fig. 9** shows a comparison of a normal bone marrow and a case of MDS demonstrating the parameters used in the Ogata score: The case of MDS shows increased CD34+ myeloid blasts, decreased granulocytic SSC indicative of cytoplasmic hypogranularity, and absent hematogones. The percentage of CD34+ cells by FCA is relevant for prognosis, and 2% or greater CD34+ cells has been reported to be significant. If the score is equal or greater than 2, the diagnostic sensitivity is 65% to 89% and specificity is 90% to 98%, and higher values are associated with

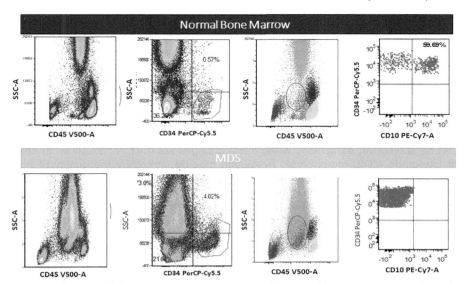

Fig. 9. Application of the Ogata score: Comparison of a normal bone marrow sample and a case of MDS demonstrating the parameters used in the Ogata score. The *red oval circle* highlights myeloblasts.

multilineage dysplasia, transfusion dependency, and high-risk karyotypes.[6,20] However, it is worth mentioning that the Ogata score is of limited applicability in low-risk MDS, hypocellular bone marrow samples (with <10% dysplastic granulocytes), hemodiluted specimens, and samples from pediatric patients.

The Wells algorithm has a scoring system ranging from 0 to 6, taking into consideration specific phenotypic aberrations in myeloblasts, granulocytes, and monocytes: if no abnormalities are identified on granulocytes, monocytes, or myeloblasts, 0 point is given; if granulocytes or monocytes demonstrate a single aberration, 1 point is given; if granulocytes or monocytes exhibit 2 abnormalities, or if both populations show one abnormality each, or if a CD34+ population is identified, 2 points are given. If one population (granulocytes or monocytes) demonstrates 4 abnormalities, or if a CD34+ population harbors 1 to 3 abnormalities, 3 points are given; And finally, if both 2 populations demonstrate 2 to 3 abnormalities each, 4 points are given. Additional points could be given either if myeloblasts demonstrate overt aberrancies or if the lymphoid-to-myeloid ratio was 1 or greater (ie, severe neutropenia).

MASS is a newly conceptualized scoring system, based on the presence of 2 of 5 criteria (CD177 expression ≤30% of granulocytes, low side-angle light scatter of granulocytes based on comparison with lymphocytes [SSC ratio <6], blast percentage >1%, B-cell progenitors as a percentage of CD34+ cells <5%, and abnormal blast CD45 expression compared with lymphocytes [CD45 mean fluorescent ratio <3.77 or >6.2]).[19] The modified MASS score excludes MASS-positive cases that demonstrate low B-cell progenitors and abnormal CD45 blast expression as the sole findings.[21] In summary, the MASS score shows many similarities to the Ogata score; however, it incorporates CD177 and a lower blast cutoff percentage (>1% vs >2%).

THE UTILITY OF FLOW CYTOMETRY ANALYSIS IN THE EVALUATION OF CHRONIC MYELOID NEOPLASMS

MDS are a heterogeneous group of clonal HSC disorders characterized by cytopenia(s) and morphologic dysplasia, recurrent molecular and/or cytogenetic aberrations, and an inherent risk for transformation to AML.[22] MPNs, however, are myeloid stem cell neoplasms that are characterized by an abnormal proliferation of one or more terminally differentiated myeloid cells in the peripheral blood. Flow cytometry immunophenotypic changes appreciated in MDS often overlap with MPN; However, these changes are typically less pronounced in cases of MPN compared with MDS.[23]

Establishing a diagnosis of MDS entails a comprehensive approach with focus on morphologic abnormalities of the various hematopoietic cell lineages as well as evaluation for evidence of clonality. However, the assessment of morphologic dysplasia can be subjective, particularly when these changes are mild, for example, in cases of low-grade MDS, morphologic evaluation may be limited by the quality of bone marrow biopsy and aspirate specimens in cases with suboptimal sampling. Furthermore, morphologic dysplasia is not specific and may be seen in nonneoplastic conditions.[24] It is therefore critical to use all tools at our disposal, such as FCA, when a diagnosis of MDS is in consideration. Although FCA findings are not currently incorporated as diagnostic criteria for MDS in the WHO Classification scheme,[25] increasing evidence supports the addition of FCA to the diagnostic workup when a patient is being evaluated for MDS.[4,6,20]

Although the diagnosis of MPN is typically more straightforward than MDS, the utility of FCA particularly in the "follow-up" of MPN cases has been recently highlighted: For example, using FCA, previously undiagnosed blastic plasmacytoid dendritic cell neoplasm (BPDCN) may be identified, in hypercellular bone marrows involved by MPN in evolution, in which the BPDCN component may be challenging to identify based on morphologic assessment alone.[26,27]

In line with identifying cellular components in the bone marrow that are otherwise not overtly detected morphologically, one group has studied the utility of assessing the percentage of physiologic plasmacytoid dendritic cells (PDCs) in the setting of AML-MRD assessment[28] and progression in low-grade MDS,[29] and has showed that the presence of high percentage of PDCs correlates with the absence of MRD,[28] and that decreased PDCs with time in low-grade MDS correlates with higher rates of disease progression into AML.[29] Furthermore, another study used FCA to demonstrate the presence of prominent bone marrow CH in elderly patients with BPDCN.[30] These findings highlight an emerging role for FCA in studying physiologic and aberrant, morphologically unappreciated bone marrow compartments, and their possible contribution to the biology of an associated underlying disease, providing further opportunities for more detailed characterization of myeloid neoplasms.

The majority of studies assessing the role of FCA in MDS and proposing scoring systems have focused on the aberrations involving leukocytes and their progenitors, mostly excluding the erythroid compartment, which commonly also shows immunophenotypic aberrancies. This exclusion limits the sensitivity of FCA for the identification of certain MDS cases, particularly those with erythroid predominance and *SF3B1* mutations,[7] highlighting the importance of a more comprehensive approach combining FCA with molecular analysis in the evaluation of patients with unexplained cytopenia(s).

THE UTILITY OF FLOW CYTOMETRY ANALYSIS IN EVALUATING CLONAL HEMATOPOIESIS WITHOUT OVERT MORPHOLOGIC DYSPLASIA

Clonal cytopenia of undetermined significance (CCUS) is now formerly recognized as a diagnostic entity in the fifth edition of the WHO classification.[22] A particular area of interest is the utility of FCA for distinguishing cases of MDS from idiopathic cytopenia(s) of undetermined significance (ICUS) and CCUS.[19,31,32] In their analysis of 79 patients with ICUS or CCUS, Dimopoulos and colleagues showed the FCA has limited value in distinguishing between these 2; However, phenotyping was able to reliably distinguish patients with higher mutational burden, suggesting these cases may represent early MDS that do not yet meet diagnostic criteria when using morphologic dysplasia alone, and identifying a group of patients who might require morphologic reassessment of dysplastic changes in their bone marrow.[31] Some of the most commonly observed FCA alterations in the myeloid and monocytic populations in the setting of CCUS included abnormal patterns of maturation and patterns of CD13, CD16, and CD11b expression similar to cases of bona fide MDS.

CH is thought to represent the precursor for many hematologic neoplasms. Somatic mosaicism is a direct product of aging and nearly universal after the age of 40 years. CH constitutes identifiable populations of blood/marrow cells originating from somatically mutated HSCs. In the absence of cytopenias or a history of a myeloid neoplasm, the presence of CH with a variant allele fraction (VAF) of at least 2% (ie, CH of indeterminate potential "CHIP") is associated with an increased risk of developing a hematologic malignancy at a rate of 0.5% to 1% per year.[33] However, the detection of CHIP in patients with cytopenia (ie, CCUS) with increased VAF (10%),[32,34–36] associated with a specific mutational pattern: that is, the presence of a splicing gene abnormality (*U2AF1*, *SF3B1*, *ZRZS2*, or *SRSF2*), or coalteration involving *ASXL1* or *TET2* with other genes,[34] may correlate with a particularly higher risk of transformation into an overt hematologic neoplasm.[34,37]

Currently complete remission (CR) following treatment of AML is defined as hematologic count recovery and bone marrow blast count of 5% or lesser. However, it is well known that the blast count may be increased (>5%) blasts in the setting of robust bone marrow regeneration following induction therapy, particularly in patients who receive growth factor therapy. FCA can serve as an invaluable tool in distinguishing regenerative myeloid precursors from AML blasts in the setting of postinduction therapy.[38] However, many patients who attain CR by morphologic evaluation may carry persistent low-level disease detectable by cytogenetic and fluorescence in situ hybridization (FISH) analysis, molecular analysis, or FCA.[39] Cytogenetic and FISH sensitivities in assessing CR seem to be similar (0.5×10^{-1}), whereas a sensitivity of at least 1×10^{-3} is recommended for the detection of MRD.[40] For these reasons, FCA or molecular methods are emerging as more valuable modalities for MRD assessment. In fact, the ELN[40,41] guidelines have recognized CR without MRD (CR MRD−) as a defined response endpoint in AML since 2017 and continues to do so.

A practical challenge in the interpretation of molecular results showing pathogenic mutations in the setting of posttherapy in AML is distinguishing true residual leukemia from preleukemic clones or CH or unrelated CH that emerged following therapy.[42–44] The presence of leukemia-related mutations such as *NPM1* mutation has been established as a harbinger of relapse in multiple studies,[45] whereas the significance of persistent CH is less understood.[30,43] For these reasons, the ELN also recommends the incorporation of FCA in the setting of MRD assessment because it studies aberrant populations from the immunophenotypic angle and may provide additional information pertaining to the nature of pathogenic clones detected by molecular analysis in the posttherapy setting (ie, CH vs residual leukemia).[40]

Background CH persists and emerges following the treatment of AML in many patients without a direct effect on the risk of relapse.[46] MRD serves is an important biomarker in patients with AML, dictating prognosis and treatment decisions because persistence of MRD is known to be associated with an increased risk of relapse. Patients with positive MRD may benefit either from more intensive consolidation therapy (including allogeneic HSC transplant)[44] or from other earlier interventional modalities.[41] Therefore, distinguishing residual AML from persistent CH is of paramount importance following induction therapy because CH may persist in the setting of disease remission, without increasing the patient's risk of AML relapse.[47] AML MRD assessment by FCA is generally performed using 2 well-established approaches, including the use of (1) leukemia-associated immunophenotype or (2) the deviation from normal (DFN) approach. The DFN approach is particularly important when the phenotype of the original leukemia is not available for comparison; however, this approach is limited by the fact that the residual CH may lead to mild immunophenotypic alterations of CD34+ myeloid stem cells when compared with normal.[43]

The immunophenotype of CH in the post-AML setting has been shown to demonstrate features akin to low-grade MDS. These phenotypic changes have been referred to as a "preleukemic" phenotype.[43] These changes are often observed in the CD34+ myeloid progenitor compartment and are characterized by an increased expression of CD13, an increased expression of CD117 and/or CD123, and a decreased expression CD38 and/or HLA-DR. A preleukemic phenotype typically does not manifest aberrant lymphoid markers or complete loss or gain of other antigens, and such changes should raise the possibility of AML MRD.[1,43,48,49] These preleukemic cells may be identifiable in a subset of cases at baseline diagnosis; however, they may be masked by the overabundance of large AML clones at the time of initial diagnosis.[43] The preleukemic phenotype has been shown to be associated with specific patterns of CH by molecular analysis, including high VAF of mutations and frequent *IDH2* and *SRSF2* mutations.[43] The presence of this preleukemic phenotype does not seem to correlate with risk of AML relapse.[43]

SUMMARY

In summary, FCA has proven to be an invaluable tool in the assessment of MDS and related myeloid stem cell neoplasms, particularly when morphologic dysplasia is not overt. In such cases, identification of immunophenotypic aberrancies typically associated with MDS could be the tipping point in making an accurate diagnosis. The most reliable cellular compartment for assessment in cases of suspected MDS is the CD34+ myeloid blast population as the maturing myeloid and monocytic cells may show immunophenotypic alterations in cases of reactive cytopenia or bone marrow regeneration. Furthermore, the utility of FCA has been shown in MPNs in progression, and/or with an underlying undiagnosed aberrant population. Finally, FCA may be helpful to distinguish CH or preleukemic populations from residual leukemia, which may have pertinent impact on patient management.

CLINICS CARE POINTS

- Flow cytometry is a useful ancillary tool in the diagnostic work up of chronic myeloid neoplasm, particularly myelodysplastic neoplasms and may aid in establishing a diagnosis in cases of myelodysplastic neoplasm (MDS) with subtle morphologic dysplasia.

KEY/ESSENTIAL HEADINGS

- FCA is a valuable diagnostic tool in the setting of myeloid neoplasms particularly in AML in morphologic remission, for distinguishing MDS from its mimics or precursors and identifying progression of MPNs.
- FCA is useful in distinguishing CH from MRD in the setting of AML, which impacts subsequent patient management.

CONFLICT OF INTEREST DISCLOSURE

None of the authors declares conflict of interest.

REFERENCES

1. Westers TM, Ireland R, Kern W, et al. Standardization of flow cytometry in myelo-dysplastic syndromes: a report from an international consortium and the European LeukemiaNet Working Group. Leukemia 2012;26:1730–41.
2. Davydova YO, Parovichnikova EN, Galtseva IV, et al. Diagnostic significance of flow cytometry scales in diagnostics of myelodysplastic syndromes. Cytometry B Clin Cytometry 2021;100(3):312–21.
3. Stachurski D, Smith BR, Pozdnyakova O, et al. Flow cytometric analysis of mye-lomonocytic cells by a pattern recognition approach is sensitive and specific in diagnosing myelodysplastic syndrome and related marrow diseases: emphasis on a global evaluation and recognition of diagnostic pitfalls. Leuk Res 2008;32: 215–24.
4. Loken MR, van de Loosdrecht A, Ogata K, et al. Flow cytometry in myelodysplas-tic syndromes: report from a working conference. Leuk Res 2008;32:5–17.
5. van de Loosdrecht AA, Alhan C, Bene MC, et al. Standardization of flow cytom-etry in myelodysplastic syndromes: report from the first European LeukemiaNet working conference on flow cytometry in myelodysplastic syndromes. Haemato-logica 2009;94:1124–34.
6. Ogata K, Kishikawa Y, Satoh C, et al. Diagnostic application of flow cytometric characteristics of CD34+ cells in low-grade myelodysplastic syndromes. Blood 2006;108:1037–44.
7. Chen Z, Ok CY, Wang W, et al. Low-grade myelodysplastic syndromes with pre-served CD34+ B-cell precursors (CD34+ hematogones). Cytometry B Clin Cy-tom 2020;98:36–42.
8. van Lochem EG, van der Velden VH, Wind HK, et al. Immunophenotypic differen-tiation patterns of normal hematopoiesis in human bone marrow: reference pat-terns for age-related changes and disease-induced shifts. Cytometry B Clin Cytometry 2004;60:1–13.
9. Truong F, Smith BR, Stachurski D, et al. The utility of flow cytometric immunophe-notyping in cytopenic patients with a non-diagnostic bone marrow: a prospective study. Leuk Res 2009;33:1039–46.
10. Mathis S, Chapuis N, Debord C, et al. Flow cytometric detection of dyserythropoi-esis: a sensitive and powerful diagnostic tool for myelodysplastic syndromes. Leukemia 2013;27:1981–7.
11. Cremers EM, Westers TM, Alhan C, et al. Implementation of erythroid lineage analysis by flow cytometry in diagnostic models for myelodysplastic syndromes. Haematologica 2017;102:320–6.
12. Westers TM, Cremers EM, Oelschlaegel U, et al. Immunophenotypic analysis of erythroid dysplasia in myelodysplastic syndromes. A report from the IMDSFlow working group. Haematologica 2017;102:308–19.
13. Rosenberg CA, Bill M, Rodrigues MA, et al. Exploring dyserythropoiesis in pa-tients with myelodysplastic syndrome by imaging flow cytometry and machine-learning assisted morphometrics. Cytometry B Clin Cytometry 2021;100(5): 554–67.
14. Fang H, Wang SA, You MJ, et al. Flow cytometry immunophenotypic features of pure erythroid leukemia and the distinction from reactive erythroid precursors. Cytometry B Clin Cytom 2022;102:440–7.

15. Ogata K, Della Porta MG, Malcovati L, et al. Diagnostic utility of flow cytometry in low-grade myelodysplastic syndromes: a prospective validation study. Haematologica 2009;94:1066–74.
16. Chu SC, Wang TF, Li CC, et al. Flow cytometric scoring system as a diagnostic and prognostic tool in myelodysplastic syndromes. Leuk Res 2011;35:868–73.
17. Wells DA, Benesch M, Loken MR, et al. Myeloid and monocytic dyspoiesis as determined by flow cytometric scoring in myelodysplastic syndrome correlates with the IPSS and with outcome after hematopoietic stem cell transplantation. Blood 2003;102:394–403.
18. Porwit A, van de Loosdrecht AA, Bettelheim P, et al. Revisiting guidelines for integration of flow cytometry results in the WHO classification of myelodysplastic syndromes-proposal from the International/European LeukemiaNet Working Group for Flow Cytometry in MDS. Leukemia 2014;28:1793–8.
19. Alayed K, Meyerson JB, Osei ES, et al. CD177 enhances the detection of myelodysplastic syndrome by flow cytometry. Am J Clin Pathol 2020;153:554–65.
20. Della Porta MG, Picone C, Pascutto C, et al. Multicenter validation of a reproducible flow cytometric score for the diagnosis of low-grade myelodysplastic syndromes: results of a European LeukemiaNET study. Haematologica 2012;97:1209–17.
21. Nirmalanantham P, Sakhi R, Beck R, et al. Flow cytometric findings in clonal cytopenia of undetermined significance. Am J Clin Pathol 2022;157:219–30.
22. Khoury JD, Solary E, Abla O, et al. The 5th edition of the world health organization classification of haematolymphoid tumours: myeloid and histiocytic/dendritic neoplasms. Leukemia 2022;36:1703–19.
23. Ouyang J, Zheng W, Shen Q, et al. Flow cytometry immunophenotypic analysis of Philadelphia-negative myeloproliferative neoplasms: correlation with histopathologic features. Cytometry B Clin Cytometry 2015;88:236–43.
24. Girard S, Genevieve F, Rault E, et al. When ring sideroblasts on bone marrow smears are inconsistent with the diagnosis of myelodysplastic neoplasms. Diagnostics 2022;12:1752.
25. Swerdlow SH, Campo E, Harris N, et al. WHO classification of tumours of haematopoietic and lymphoid tissues. Revised 4th edition. Lyon (France): IARC; 2017.
26. El Hussein S, Yabe M, Wang W, et al. Blastic plasmacytoid dendritic cell neoplasm (BPDCN) arising in the setting of polycythemia vera (PV): An illustration of the emerging role of flow cytometry analysis in monitoring progression of myeloproliferative neoplasms. EJHaem 2022;3(3):954–7.
27. Khan AM, Munir A, Raval M, et al. Blastic plasmacytoid dendritic cell neoplasm in the background of myeloproliferative disorder and chronic lymphocytic leukaemia. BMJ Case Rep 2019;12.
28. Xiao W, Goldberg AD, Famulare CA, et al. Loss of plasmacytoid dendritic cell differentiation is highly predictive for post-induction measurable residual disease and inferior outcomes in acute myeloid leukemia. Haematologica 2019;104:1378–87.
29. Chan A, Liu Y, Devlin S, et al. Reduced plasmacytoid dendritic cell output is associated with high risk in low-grade myelodysplastic syndrome. Hemasphere 2022;6:e685.
30. Khanlari M, Yin CC, Takahashi K, et al. Bone marrow clonal hematopoiesis is highly prevalent in blastic plasmacytoid dendritic cell neoplasm and frequently sharing a clonal origin in elderly patients. Leukemia 2022;36:1343–50.
31. Dimopoulos K, Hansen OK, Sjo LD, et al. The diagnostic and prognostic role of flow cytometry in idiopathic and clonal cytopenia of undetermined significance

(ICUS/CCUS): a single-center analysis of 79 patients. Cytometry B Clin Cytom 2020;98:250–8.

32. Gao L, Hyter S, Zhang D, et al. Morphologic, immunophenotypic, and molecular genetic comparison study in patients with clonal cytopenia of undetermined significance, myelodysplastic syndrome, and acute myeloid leukemia with myelodysplasia-related changes: a single institution experience. Int J Lab Hematol 2022;44:738–49.

33. Steensma DP, Bejar R, Jaiswal S, et al. Clonal hematopoiesis of indeterminate potential and its distinction from myelodysplastic syndromes. Blood 2015;126:9–16.

34. Malcovati L, Galli A, Travaglino E, et al. Clinical significance of somatic mutation in unexplained blood cytopenia. Blood 2017;129:3371–8.

35. Zheng G, Chen P, Pallavajjalla A, et al. The diagnostic utility of targeted gene panel sequencing in discriminating etiologies of cytopenia. Am J Hematol 2019;94:1141–8.

36. Warren JT, Link DC. Clonal hematopoiesis and risk for hematologic malignancy. Blood 2020;136:1599–605.

37. Cargo CA, Rowbotham N, Evans PA, et al. Targeted sequencing identifies patients with preclinical MDS at high risk of disease progression. Blood 2015;126:2362–5.

38. El Hussein S, Loghavi S. The impact of clonal hierarchy and heterogeneity on phenotypic manifestations of myelodysplastic neoplasms. Cancers 2022;14:5690.

39. Ouyang J, Goswami M, Tang G, et al. The clinical significance of negative flow cytometry immunophenotypic results in a morphologically scored positive bone marrow in patients following treatment for acute myeloid leukemia. Am J Hematol 2015;90:504–10.

40. Dohner H, Wei AH, Appelbaum FR, et al. Diagnosis and management of AML in adults: 2022 ELN recommendations from an international expert panel. Blood 2022;140(12):1345–77.

41. Schuurhuis GJ, Heuser M, Freeman S, et al. Minimal/measurable residual disease in AML: a consensus document from the European LeukemiaNet MRD Working Party. Blood 2018;131:1275–91.

42. Ravandi F. Is it time to routinely incorporate MRD into practice? Best Pract Res Clin Haematol 2018;31:396–400.

43. Loghavi S, DiNardo CD, Furudate K, et al. Flow cytometric immunophenotypic alterations of persistent clonal haematopoiesis in remission bone marrows of patients with NPM1-mutated acute myeloid leukaemia. Br J Haematol 2021;192:1054–63.

44. Hasserjian RP, Steensma DP, Graubert TA, et al. Clonal hematopoiesis and measurable residual disease assessment in acute myeloid leukemia. Blood 2020;135:1729–38.

45. Balsat M, Renneville A, Thomas X, et al. Postinduction minimal residual disease predicts outcome and benefit from allogeneic stem cell transplantation in acute myeloid leukemia with NPM1 mutation: a study by the acute leukemia French association group. J Clin Oncol 2017;35:185–93.

46. Tanaka T, Morita K, Loghavi S, et al. Clonal dynamics and clinical implications of postremission clonal hematopoiesis in acute myeloid leukemia. Blood 2021;138:1733–9.

47. Hourigan CS, Dillon LW, Gui G, et al. Impact of conditioning intensity of allogeneic transplantation for acute myeloid leukemia with genomic evidence of residual disease. J Clin Oncol 2020;38:1273–83.

48. Ogata K, Nakamura K, Yokose N, et al. Clinical significance of phenotypic features of blasts in patients with myelodysplastic syndrome. Blood 2002;100: 3887–96.

49. Tang G, Jorgensen LJ, Zhou Y, et al. Multi-color CD34(+) progenitor-focused flow cytometric assay in evaluation of myelodysplastic syndromes in patients with post cancer therapy cytopenia. Leuk Res 2012;36:974–81.

A Review of the Flow Cytometric Findings in Classic Hodgkin Lymphoma, Nodular Lymphocyte Predominant Hodgkin Lymphoma and T Cell/Histiocyte-Rich Large B Cell Lymphoma

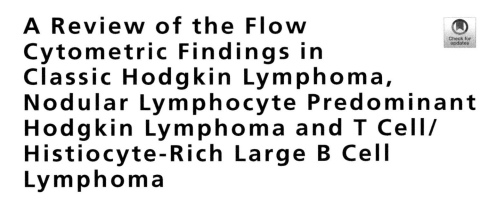

Feras Ally, MD[1], David Gajzer, MD[1], Jonathan R. Fromm, MD, PhD*

KEYWORDS

- T-cell/histiocyte-rich large B cell lymphoma • Classic Hodgkin lymphoma
- Nodular lymphocyte predominant Hodgkin lymphoma • Flow cytometry
- Antigen expression • Flow cytometric cell sorting

KEY POINTS

- Neoplastic cells from classic Hodgkin lymphoma (CHL), nodular lymphocyte predominant Hodgkin lymphoma (NLPHL), and T cell/histiocyte-rich large B cell lymphoma (THRLBCL) can be identified and immunophenotyped with high sensitivity by flow cytometry.
- The neoplastic cells of CHL and NLPHL directly interact with T cells and alter their microenvironment through these interactions.
- The reactive infiltrate in CHL, NLPHL, and THRLBCL predominates and immunophenotyping the reactive infiltrate can provide diagnostic information.

INTRODUCTION

Classic Hodgkin lymphoma (CHL), nodular lymphocyte predominant Hodgkin lymphoma (NLPHL), and T cell/histiocyte-rich large B cell lymphoma (THRLBCL) are B cell lymphomas of germinal center origin where the reactive infiltrate comprises the vast majority of cells in involved tissues, while neoplastic cells are rare. Recent studies suggest these neoplasms are pathobiologically related. CHL, NLPHL, and a subset of

Department of Laboratory Medicine and Pathology, University of Washington
[1] These 2 authors contributed equally.
* Corresponding author. Department of Laboratory Medicine, University of Washington, 825 Eastlake Avenue East, G-7800, Seattle, WA 98109.
E-mail address: jfromm@uw.edu

Clin Lab Med 43 (2023) 427–444
https://doi.org/10.1016/j.cll.2023.04.011
0272-2712/23/© 2023 Elsevier Inc. All rights reserved.
labmed.theclinics.com

THRLBCL cluster together on gene expression profiling suggesting similar pathobiology.[1] Morphologic, immunohistochemical, and clinical features demonstrate that THRLBCL and NLPHL are closely related. The two lymphomas can occur simultaneously in a given patient and NLPHL can transform into THRLBCL.[2-7] Additionally, the immunophenotypes of neoplastic cells as determined by immunohistochemistry are essentially identical, requiring architectural features to allow for their distinction.[4,6,8-10] Finally, genetic analysis of NLPHL and THRLBCL has demonstrated a similar cache of mutations[11] and consequently, THRLBCL and NLPHL have been postulated to belong on a biologic continuum.[11,12]

Traditionally, these lymphomas have not been amenable to immunophenotyping by flow cytometry, likely due to the lability and rarity of the neoplastic cells. However, over the last 15 years, flow cytometry combinations to immunophenotype the neoplastic cells of these 3 B cell lymphomas have been developed.[13-18] In addition, routine clinical flow cytometry assays for non-Hodgkin lymphomas can characterize the reactive infiltrates of these lymphomas to provide diagnostic information.[19-24] This review will summarize the findings of these flow cytometry studies that provide diagnostic information in the clinical hematopathology laboratory and insight into the pathobiology of these neoplasms.

Pathologic Features of Classic Hodgkin Lymphoma, Nodular Lymphocyte Predominant Hodgkin Lymphoma, and T Cell/Histiocyte-Rich Large B Cell Lymphoma

Classic Hodgkin lymphoma. CHL is a type of B cell lymphoma[25-29] characterized by neoplastic cells (Hodgkin and Reed-Sternberg [HRS] cells) in a special tumor microenvironment. HRS cells are infrequent,[30] often amounting to less than 1% of the white cells in an involved lymph node.[14,15] HRS cells have a distinct immunophenotype most commonly showing expression of CD30 and PAX-5, with variable CD15, without expression of CD3, CD20, and CD45 (by immunohistochemistry); these findings have been utilized to confirm the diagnosis in tissue sections.[8,30,31] HRS cells can have mononuclear or multilobated nuclei, often show T cells bound to their surface (the T cell-HRS cell rosette)[14,32-37] and are present in a mixed inflammatory, nonneoplastic background, composed of variable numbers of lymphocytes, histiocytes, plasma cells, and eosinophils. The interaction of the reactive infiltrate with HRS cells is critical in mediating the pathogenesis of CHL.[27,38,39] Studies have demonstrated that HRS cells are bound to T cells through the interaction of adhesion molecules; specifically, CD54 and CD58 on the HRS cells bind to the adhesion molecules lymphocyte function-associated antigen 1 (LFA-1) and CD2, respectively, on the T cells.[14,37,40]

Nodular lymphocyte predominant Hodgkin lymphoma. NLPHL is a rare B-cell lymphoma defined by the presence of rare, large neoplastic germinal center B-cell derived lymphocyte predominant (LP) cells present in a vaguely nodular, reactive background infiltrate composed of small, mature, nonneoplastic lymphocytes and histiocytes.[2,12,41,42] By immunohistochemistry performed on tissue sections, these LP cells express CD20, PAX-5, CD45, and BCL-6 but are negative for CD3, CD10, CD15, or CD30. The absence of CD15 and CD30 and the expression of CD20 and CD45 provide a reliable means of distinguishing LP cells from HRS cells of CHL. Reactive cell populations, including B-cells and follicular T cells (PD1/CD57+), are also present and frequently form rosettes around the LP cells.[29,30,41]

T cell/histiocyte-rich large B-cell lymphoma. THRLBCL is a type of B cell non-Hodgkin lymphoma where the neoplastic cells are rare, similar to what is observed with CHL and NLPHL. Nonneoplastic, reactive B cells are also few in number. The background tumor microenvironment of THRLBCL (as the entity's name would imply) is primarily composed of histocytes and T cells; this infiltrate is diffuse and lacks CD21-positive dendritic networks, a finding useful to help distinguish THRLBCL from NLPHL.[9,43,44] Neoplastic cells of THRLBCL are germinal center B cells with expression of BCL-6 but essentially no expression of CD10.[4,43,44] As with NLPHL, pan B-cell markers such as PAX-5, CD20, and CD79a are consistently expressed. Indeed, the immunophenotypes of the neoplastic cells of NLPHL and THRLBCL are nearly identical; this fact, coupled with the similarity of chromosomal alterations and gene expression of the neoplastic cells from the 2 lymphomas strongly suggest these neoplasms are pathobiologically related.[1,3,11] Because of the immunophenotypic overlap, distinguishing NLPHL and THRLBCL can, at times, be challenging for hematopathologists.

Technical considerationsfor evaluating CHL, NLPHL, and THRLBCL. Flow cytometry combinations used to characterize these lymphomas are shown in **Tables 1** and **2**. Because their neoplastic populations, unlike in B cell non-Hodgkin lymphomas (B-NHL), typically amount to less than 1% of the leukocytes in involved specimens, 500,000 and 1,000,000 cells should be collected with the assays. Relatively acellular specimens (from fine needle aspirations or small needle core biopsies) are still suitable for evaluation,[45] although our experience suggests that false-negative results are possible with specimens with less than 10,000 viable events. Procedures used to prepare specimens for analysis are identical to those used for B-NHL and are described elsewhere.[46,47]

Gating strategies to identify HRS cells from CHL. In contrast to the analysis of non-Hodgkin lymphoma, doublets are not excluded in the analysis of the CHL tube; HRS cells would be excluded by excluding doublets (HRS cells and T cells rosetting [see later discussion] results in doublet formation). After events are gated with a standard forward light scatter versus side light scatter viability gate, sequential gating strategies are used to identify HRS cells that require the expression of CD30, CD40, and CD95 and the absence of bright CD20 expression (**Fig. 1**; see "Flow cytometric studies of CHL, NLPHL and THRLBCL and their immunophenotypes" section). Of note, for many cases, an HRS population cannot be identified in any 2-dimensional plot and can only be identified after applying the gating strategy in **Fig. 1**.

Gating Strategies to Identify Neoplastic Cells from Nodular Lymphocyte Predominant Hodgkin Lymphoma and TCell/Histiocyte-RichLarge B Cell Lymphoma

We do not typically use defined gates to identify the neoplastic cells from these lymphomas, in contrast to the approach used for CHL (described above). Nevertheless, neoplastic cells from NLPHL and THRLBCL can be identified using a cache of informative antibodies. The neoplastic cells from these lymphomas will have increased forward and side light scatter compared with small lymphocytes. The neoplastic cells should show expression of CD20, CD40, and the germinal center markers (BCL-6 and CD75 positive); however, there is typically no expression of CD10. Finally, the neoplastic population will form a distinct cluster of events in multidimensional flow cytometric space.

Table 1
Combination used to immunophenotype neoplastic cells of classic Hodgkin lymphoma

Fluorochrome	PB	Fluorescein isothiocyanate	PE	ECD	PECY5.5	PECY7	APC	APC-A700	APC-H7
Antibody	CD95	CD64		CD30	CD5	CD40	CD20	CD15	CD71	CD45

| Table 2 Combinations used to immunophenotype the neoplastic cells of NLPHL and THRLBCL | | | | | | | | | | | |
Fluoro-chrome	V450	FITC/A488	PE	ECD	PECY5.5	PECY7	A594	APC	APC-A700	APC-H7
Tube 1	CD75	CD64 + CD10	CD32	CD5	CD40	CD20	CD38	CD54	CD71	CD45
Tube 2	DAPI	CD64	BCL-6	CD5	CD40	CD10	CD38	CD54	CD71	CD20

Flow Cytometric Studies of Classic Hodgkin Lymphoma, Nodular Lymphocyte Predominant Hodgkin Lymphoma, and T Cell/Histiocyte-Rich Large B Cell Lymphoma and Their Immunophenotypes

CHL

A large initial study of more than 400 samples using a combination similar to that shown in **Table 1** demonstrates that the neoplastic HRS cell population in CHL can be detected in approximately 89% of cases while the clinical specificity of the assay approaches 100%[15] (examples in **Fig. 2**). A more recent report from Chan and co-workers specifically focused on the evaluation of small biopsies using flow cytometry combinations for CHL; this group reports sensitivity and specificity of 95.4% and 98.2%, respectively, whereas positive and negative predictive values were 92.2% and 99.0%, respectively, for the detection of CHL.[45]

A detailed description of the immunophenotype of HRS cells was reported in our article from 2006,[14] evaluating 18 cases. All cases expressed CD30 and CD40 as expected because these antigens are required for a population to be considered an HRS population. CD15 expression was detected in 16 cases (89%). CD20 expression in 6 cases (35%), and CD19 expression in 5 cases (29%) was observed, typically present at low levels. In contrast to results in tissue sections,[30] some level of CD45 expression on HRS cells in was observed 73% of cases (where no T cell rosetting was present, see later discussion); of the positive cases, most (64%) showed dim to absent CD45. Occasional cases show HRS cells with CD45 expression at or only slightly below the level observed in the reactive lymphocytes. CD71 was expressed in all of

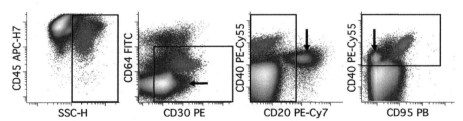

Fig. 1. Gating strategy to isolate HRS cells in CHL. A putative HRS population must fall in all 4 gates and be distinct in multidimensional flow cytometric space. The cells must have increased side scatter relative to the small reactive lymphocytes (*first dot plot*), be CD30-positive and have increased autofluorescence in the FITC channel compared with the immunoblasts and small lymphocytes (*second plot*), express no or low CD20 (*third plot*), and express CD40 at or greater intensity than reactive B cells (*fourth plot*). The B cells are identified by the vertical arrows (CD20+, CD40+) and immunoblasts are identified by the horizontal arrow. HRS cells are in red and are emphasized (highlighted); all other events are in blue. Flow cytometry dot plots were created using Woodlist version 3.1.3. (*Courtesy of* Dr Brent L. Wood.)

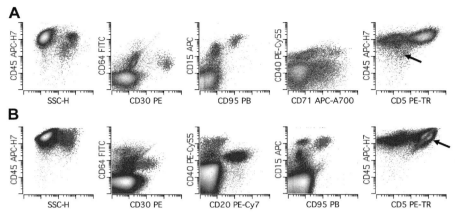

Fig. 2. Examples of flow cytometric characterization of CHL cases. (*A, B*). HRS cells (*red and emphasized*) are identified by their expression of CD30, CD40, CD95, absence of expression of CD64, and increased side light scatter (SSC-H) compared with normal lymphocytes; all remaining viable events are in blue. (*A*) HRS cells express CD15 (bright), CD30 (intermediate to bright), CD40 (intermediate), CD71 (intermediate), and CD95 (intermediate; data not shown), without expression of CD20 (data not shown) or CD64 (position of negative determined by isotype matched control experiment, data not shown). The HRS cells are essentially all unrosetted HRS cells (*single arrow*) having lower expression of CD45 relative to the lymphocytes and no expression of CD5. The neoplastic population comprises 0.97% of the white cells. (*B*) HRS cells express CD15 (bright), CD30 (low to intermediate), CD40 (intermediate to bright), CD71 (variable; data not shown), and CD95 (intermediate), without expression of CD20 or CD64. The entire HRS population shows expression of CD5 (overlaying the CD5-positive T cells, identified by an *arrow*), suggesting the population is rosetted without an unrosetted (CD5-negative) fraction. The neoplastic population comprises 0.3% of the white cells.

the CHL cases examined, often showing variable expression. Although not commonly used in our assays today, HRS cells from all cases examined showed some CD86 expression (often at an intermediate to bright-level). CD95 was expressed in all 14 cases evaluated (100%), with intermediate-level expression on at least a subset of the HRS cells in all cases. CD40, CD86, and CD95 expression on HRS cells was often greater than that on other cellular population in the lymph node.

Adhesion molecules and B7 family molecules. Subsequent studies evaluating the expression of adhesion molecules and PD-L1/PD-L2 were performed. The adhesion molecules CD54 (intercellular adhesion molecule 1 [ICAM-1]; binds LFA-1) and CD58 (LFA-3; binds CD2) were consistently and brightly expressed on HRS cells (measured in 6 cases of CHL). Evaluation of these antigens is relevant as CD54 and CD58 mediate the interaction of HRS cells with T cells (see "Identification of T Cell Rosettes by Flow Cytometry" section). All 6 CHL cases evaluated showed expression of CD273 (PD-L2), while 5 of 6 cases showed expression of CD274 (PD-L1) on the surface of HRS cells.

NLPHL
The flow cytometry 2-tube combination (see **Table 2**) has been shown to be sensitive (identified the neoplastic LP cells of NLPHL in 7 of 7 cases examined) and specific (only of 1 of 94 non-NLPHL cases misclassified) for the identification of LP cells in

NLPHL. The flow cytometry combination used to immunophenotype CHL (see **Table 1**) can also immunophenotype neoplastic LP cells in a minority of cases (**Fig. 3**).

B-cell–associated antigens. CD19 and CD20 were expressed in almost all cases (weak and moderate expression for CD19 and between moderate and bright expression for CD20). These antigens were expressed at, or above, the level of expression seen in normal small B cells. All 19 cases examined for CD40 showed moderately to bright expression on the LP cells, usually at a level higher than the small B cells. BCL-6 showed nuclear expression at a weak to moderate level; CD10 was consistently not expressed. CD75 (germinal center B-cell–associated marker)[48] was weakly to moderately expressed, typically in a variable pattern. Finally, CD32, an antigen that is not expressed at all or only weakly expressed on normal germinal centers and strongly expressed on reactive nongerminal center B cells, showed very-weak to absent expression, in keeping with the germinal center nature of LP cells. Ten cases were evaluated for surface light immunoglobulin chains on LP cells; 4 of 10 cases evaluated showed kappa surface light chain restriction and 6 showed the absence of surface light chains (consistent with prior observations in paraffin section that a subset of NLPHL cases show LP cells with kappa restriction[49,50]).

Miscellaneous antigens. CD71 (transferrin receptor, marker of activation) was moderately to brightly expressed, often at a level higher than all other cells in the lymph node suspension. As expected, CD45 was brightly expressed, consistently higher than that seen on the HRS cells of CHL. CD95 (FAS) was usually present on LP cells (94% positive in 16 cases tested using the tube described in **Table 1**), showing variable expression across cases.

Adhesion molecules. Expression of these macromolecules was evaluated on the LP cells due to their importance in facilitating the interaction of HRS cells with T cells (see later discussion).[14,40] CD54 was brightly expressed (and at a level higher expression than that observed on other cells in the lymph node suspension), whereas CD58 showed weak-to-moderate expression (LP cells of some cases showing lower and some cases showing higher expression compared with the small reactive B cells).

Expression of B7 family molecules. Expression of PD-L1 (CD274) and PD-L2 (CD273) was evaluated on LP cells in 5 cases, showing no-to-minimal expression on the LP cells from all cases tested.

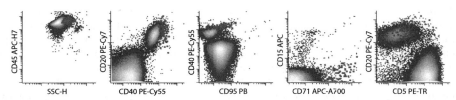

Fig. 3. An example of NLPHL characterized by CHL flow cytometry characterization tube. LP cells (*red* and emphasized) are identified by their bright expression of CD40 and CD71; all remaining viable events are in blue. LP cells express CD20 (intermediate), CD40 (bright), CD45, CD71 (bright), and CD95 (low) without expression of CD5, CD15, CD30, or CD64 (data not shown). The neoplastic population comprises 0.05% of the white cells. Note that LP cells have increased side scatter (SSC-H), relative to the small lymphocytes but the increase in side light scatter is not as high as that seen in CHL (see **Fig. 2**). CD40 expression on the LP cells is also increased relative to the small CD20+/CD40+ reactive B cells.

THRLBCL

Flow cytometry studies of the immunophenotype of neoplastic cells from THRLBCL have been uncommon due to the rarity of this lymphoma. Overall, in our studies, flow cytometry identified the neoplastic cells in 9 of the 11 THRLBCL involved lymph node biopsies (81.8%) using a combination to immunophenotype CHL (**Fig. 4**, see **Table 1**) and/or a combination of flow cytometry tubes designed to immunophenotype NLPHL (consensus tubes; **Fig. 5**, see **Table 2**). Consensus tubes were run in 8 THRLBCL cases, being positive in 75% (6 of 8 cases). The size of the neoplastic populations detected by flow cytometry was small (mean, 0.69% of white blood cells). Expression of various antigens on the neoplastic cells of THRLBCL is described below.

Expression of antigens on the neoplastic cells of T cell/histiocyte-rich large B cell lymphoma. *B-cell–associated antigens.* Expression of B-cell–associated antigens is similar to that expected from analogous immunohistochemistry studies. CD20 expression was observed at a moderate or bright level, at or greater than the intensity observed on normal reactive B cells. The germinal center maker BCL-6 demonstrated weak-to-moderate expression in the 5 cases in which the antigen was evaluated. CD75 (see discussion above)[48] was expressed in 83% of cases evaluated, often with variable expression. CD10 was rarely expressed and when present, expression was dim (similar to results seen in paraffin section), suggesting the somewhat uncommon germinal center immunophenotype of BCL-6+ and CD10−. CD40 is brightly expressed and like in NLPHL and CHL, the intensity of expression of this antigen is greater than that seen on associated reactive B cells. As noted above, CD32 is not expressed on normal germinal center B cells; in THRLBCL, expression of CD32 was somewhat inconsistent with no expression in some cases, whereas in other cases, the expression was similar to that of reactive B cells (total of 6 cases evaluated).

Adhesion molecules CD54 was overexpressed on the neoplastic cells of THRLBCL (and overexpressed relative to the other cells in the lymph node suspension). CD58 showed variable expression on the neoplastic cells of THRLBCL with 2 cases tested showing essentially no expression and 2 cases showing relatively strong expression. CD50 (ICAM-3) was expressed at a moderate level. In CHL, these interactions are in part responsible for shaping the tumor microenvironment, where both CD54 and CD58 are overexpressed. Whether the pattern of expression of CD54 and CD58 on the neoplastic cells of THRLBCL helps to define the microenvironment in this lymphoma is unknown.

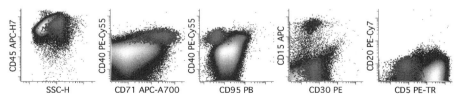

Fig. 4. An example of THRLBCL characterized by CHL flow cytometry characterization tube. Neoplastic cells (*red* and emphasized) are identified by their expression of CD40 and CD71 and lack of expression of CD64 and CD95; all remaining viable events are in blue. Neoplastic cells express CD40 (intermediate) CD45, CD71 (intermediate to bright), and CD95 (low to negative) without expression of CD5, CD15, CD20, significant CD30, or CD64 (data not shown). The lack of CD20 expression was also demonstrated by immunohistochemistry. The neoplastic population comprises 0.38% of the white cells. Note that neoplastic cells have increased side scatter (SSC-H) relative to the small lymphocytes and CD71 is expressed at a higher level than any other population in the tissue.

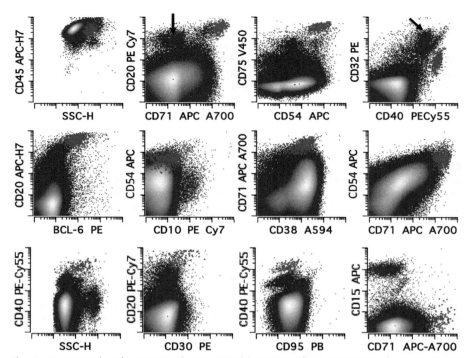

Fig. 5. An example of THRLBCL characterized by NLPHL flow cytometry characterization tubes. The large (as determined by increased forward and side light scatter compared with the small lymphocytes) neoplastic cells express CD20 (bright), CD32 (low to intermediate), CD38 (intermediate), CD40 (intermediate to bright), CD45 (bright), CD54 (intermediate to bright), CD71 (bright), CD75 (bright), and BCL-6 (low to intermediate) without CD5 (data not shown), CD10, or CD64 (data not shown). The neoplastic cells showed no expression of CD15 and less to no expression of CD30 in the CHL flow cytometry assay (data not shown). Normal small B cells are identified where appropriate with an arrow. (Modified with permission from Glynn and Fromm.[18])

Other (miscellaneous antigens) Little to no expression of CD15 was identified, whereas CD30 demonstrated low or very-low expression in 4 of 7 cases tested, differing significantly from what is observed in CHL and similar to the results seen in tissue sections of THRLBCL. Expression of CD71 (transferrin receptor, an activation antigen) varied across the evaluated cases, with low-to-intermediate expression on the neoplastic cells of some cases and intense expression in other cases. CD95 expression (uniformly expressed in CHL, see above) also varied across cases with some neoplastic cells showing very-low expression whereas other cases showed moderate expression that was brighter than that of the other cells in the lymph node. The pan-hematopoietic antigen CD45 was brightly expressed in all 9 cases tested, typically at the level of the small reactive lymphocytes.

Expression of B7 family molecules Four cases were evaluated for CD273 and CD274. CD273 was weakly expressed on the neoplastic cells in 3 cases and not expressed in the fourth. CD274 expression on the neoplastic cells varied (one case was negative, one case showed weak expression, one case showed moderate expression, and one case showed intermediate-to-bright expression).

CONCLUSIONS REGARDING UNIQUE ANTIGENS USED IN CHARACTERIZATION OF CHL, NLPHL, AND THRLBCL

Given the above flow cytometry-derived immunophenotypes, some conclusions about the unique antigens tested by these assays as well pathobiological insights provided by these studies are described below.

CD40. One common feature of these 3 lymphomas is the prominent expression of CD40. The antigen is uniformly expressed on the neoplastic populations of these lymphomas, at level equal to or greater than that of the background reactive B-cells. CD40 is expressed by antigen presenting cells such as macrophages, dendritic cells, and B cells and mediates the interaction with T cells (via CD40 L); these interactions ultimately result in the activation of the B cells or macrophages. Overexpression of CD40 in CHL likely contributes to the activation of NF-kappaB, which consequently promotes cell survival.[51] An increase in the NF-kappaB pathway has also been described in NLPHL.[1] A role for increased CD40 expression in the pathogenesis of THRLBCL has not been described but it seems reasonable to propose that high expression of the antigen might promote neoplastic cell survival.

CD75. CD75 is a germinal center associated marker that, in addition to expression on germinal center B cells, shows weak expression on mantle zone and extrafollicular B cells.[52] Less is known about its function. As noted above, CD75 expression was consistently seen in NLPHL and THRLBCL, an expected result given that the 2 lymphomas are of germinal center origin.

CD95 (FAS). When bound to its ligand (FAS ligand; CD95 L), CD95 (member of the tumor necrosis factor receptor family) initiates apoptosis. CD95 is expressed on the HRS cells of most CHL cases and interestingly CD95 L is also expressed. However, HRS cells seem to be resistant to CD95L-mediated cell death.[53,54] The microenvironment of Hodgkin lymphoma might be affected by these interactions because CD95 L on the HRS cells might induce apoptosis of CD8+/CD95+ T cells.[51] The flow cytometry studies presented here show that CD95 is also consistently expressed on neoplastic cells from NLPHL but not THRLBCL; how this affects the pathobiology of NLPHL and THRLBCL is unclear.

CD71 (transferrin receptor). Unpublished studies from our laboratory and others[55] have identified intermediate-to-bright expression of CD71 in normal proliferating cells such as germinal center B cells, immunoblasts, and in intermediate-grade and high-grade lymphomas (eg, DLBCL, NOS). CHL, NLPHL, and THRLBCL are composed of highly proliferating cells that uniformly express CD71, often at a significantly higher level than that seen in resting B-cells (see **Figs. 2, 3,** and **5**).

CD32. CD32 is an Fc receptor that has been implicated in resistance of B-cell lymphomas to anti-CD20 therapy. Work in other laboratories has demonstrated decreased expression on B cell lymphomas of germinal center origin (follicular lymphoma and diffuse large B-cell lymphoma of germinal center type).[56] Similarly, normal germinal center B-cells show decreased-to-absent expression of CD32 (unpublished data from our laboratory). As described above, while CHL, NLPHL, and TCHRLBCL are considered germinal center lymphomas, only NLPHL consistently showed lack of expression of the antigen. Some expression of CD32 was observed for both CHL and THRLBCL.

Adhesion molecules CD54 and CD58. Both CHL and NLPHL demonstrate the presence of T-cell neoplastic cell rosettes. As adhesion molecules facilitate the formation of rosettes, one might predict that the adhesion molecules might be overexpressed in lymphomas where rosettes have been described (CHL and NLPHL). Indeed, CD54 expression is increased on neoplastic cells of CHL, NLPHL, and THRLBCL (relative to background lymphocytes). We have previously shown that CD54 mediates the interaction of HRS cells with T cells in CHL.[14] One might thus speculate that increased CD54 expression on neoplastic cells of NLPHL and THRLBCL may play a role in the interaction of T cells. CD58 is consistently overexpressed in CHL and is also known

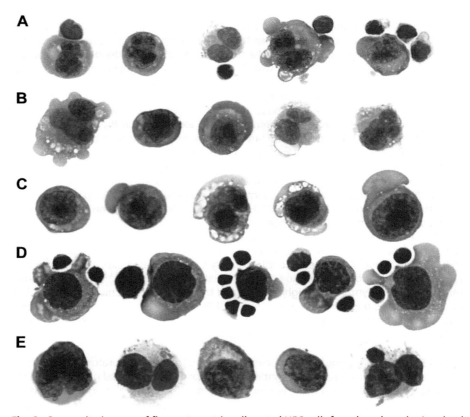

Fig. 6. Composite images of flow cytometric cell-sorted HRS cells from lymph nodes involved by CHL. The cells are purified using flow cytometric cell sorting with antibody combinations similar to those described in this article. Where noted bellow, specific cases were purified by flow cytometric cell sorting in the presence of unlabeled "blocking" antibodies to adhesion molecules (CD54, CD58, CD2, LFA-1) to disrupt interaction of HRS cells and T cells. (*A*) Case 1, purified without blocking antibodies; (*B*) same case as in "A," purified with the presence of blocking antibodies; (*C*) case 2 purified in the presence of blocking antibodies; (*D*) case 3, purified without blocking antibodies; and (*E*) case 4, without blocking antibodies. The details of combinations used for sorting are described elsewhere.[14]HRS cells bind T cells to varying degrees (compare case 3 and case 4). HRS cells from cases with numerous rosetted T cells demonstrate very bright expression of CD5 and CD45 due to the contribution of multiple T cells to the HRS-T cell rosette immunophenotype. Cases with few rosetted T cells (case 4) demonstrate no expression of CD5 and CD45 expression at a level lower than that of the reactive lymphocytes (typically).Cells stained with Wright-Geimsa. Images obtained with Olympus BH-2 microscope, Olympus (Waltham, MA) DP11 digital microscope camera, and processed with Adobe Photoshop (Adobe Photoshop-Adobe Inc, San Jose, CA) 7.0 to remove background; original magnification, X850. (© modified with permission from 2006 American Society for Clinical Pathology.[14].)

to play a role in the interaction of HRS cells and T cells[14,40]; however, CD58 is only weakly expressed in NLPHL and THRLBCL[18] (see later discussion). Insight into the phenomenon of T cell rosetting is described below.

CD273 (PD-L2) and CD274 (PD-L1). As described above, these 2 antigens are consistent expressed in CHL but essentially absent in NLPHL; THRLBCL showed variable expression. Some studies show that PD-L1/PD-L2 expression on neoplastic populations correlates with therapeutic efficacy of PD-1/PD-L1 blockade,[57,58] and CHL is responsive to PD-1/PD-L1 pathway blockade.[57] The studies presented here would predict THRLBCL to be more amenable to such immunotherapy than NLPHL. These conclusions supported by similar to studies in paraffin sections.[59]

Identification of T-Cell Rosettes by Flow Cytometry

In tissue sections morphology, CHL and NLPHL form T-cell neoplastic cell rosettes, that is, the neoplastic cells are surrounded by T cells.[32–37] Flow cytometric cell sorting experiments demonstrate neoplastic HRS cells bound to reactive T cells on flow cytometric cell sorting of neoplastic cells (**Fig. 6**).[14] Importantly, experiments in our laboratory show a correlation between the expression of T-cell antigens (such as CD3 and CD5) and the number of reactive T cells on the surface of the neoplastic cells. Frequently, we observe a diagonal relationship on a plot of CD45 versus CD5; all of the CD5 expression and most of the CD45 is contributed by the reactive rosetted T cells (see **Fig. 2**). Neoplastic LP cells of NLPHL show less rosetting of T cells by flow cytometry. Only 50% of NLPHL cases demonstrate the presence of rosettes by flow cytometry, whereas 90% of CHL cases demonstrate T-cell rosettes.[16] In addition, in NLPHL, flow cytometric cell sorting experiments only rarely demonstrate the presence of LP cell-T-cell rosettes.[16] Considered together, these studies suggest that HRS cells have greater avidity for T cells than do LP cells. We propose that differences in interaction with T cells are, in part, driven by differences in expression of adhesion molecules on the surface of these 2 neoplastic cell populations (see above). We have not observed rosettes for THRLBCL by flow cytometry, a result in accord with what has been observed in tissue sections. Studies in other laboratories have suggested that CD4+ T cells support the survival of HRS cells in CHL,[60] perhaps by direct interaction of HRS cells and T cells mediated by adhesion molecules. Given the lack of rosettes observed by flow cytometry, these mechanisms may be less important or not present in NLPHL and THRLBCL.

Table 3
Mean and standard error for measured reactive parameters

		Diagnosis		
	NLPHL	*T/HRLBCL*	*CHL*	*Reactive*
CD4/CD8	5.44 ± 0.41	9.99 ± 2.02	4.18 ± 0.62	3.94 ± 0.40
%dual CD4+/CD8+ T cells[a]	11.7 ± 1.84	3.70 ± 0.529	2.18 ± 0.257	2.67 ± 0.290
% CD4 T cells	50.8 ± 2.42	64.7 ± 5.45	42.8 ± 3.37	35.1 ± 1.92
% CD8 T cells	10.6 ± 0.856	18.0 ± 4.33	16.1 ± 1.77	13.8 ± 1.67
% T cells	69.0 ± 2.88	86.5 ± 3.10	62.1 ± 2.90	51.7 ± 2.16
% B cells	29.6 ± 2.91	5.02 ± 1.73	27.4 ± 2.86	42.4 ± 2.53

Data are mean ± standard error.
[a] Calculated as a percentage of all T cells.
Modified from Wu et al, 2016.[22]

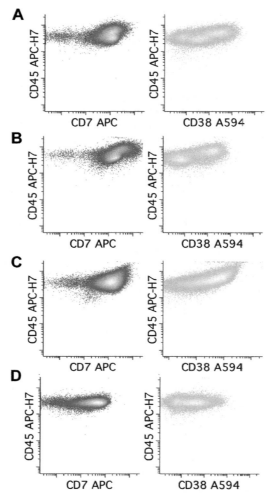

Fig. 7. Reactive lymphocytes in CHL, THRLBCL, and a reactive lymph node. (*A, B*) Reactive lymphocytes in 2 cases of CHL, (*C*) a case of THRLBCL, and (*D*) a reactive lymph node (for comparison). All 3 lymphoma cases demonstrate a CD4+ T cell population with increased CD45 and CD7 (first dot plot) and evidence of activation (subset with increased CD38; second dot plot). For the reactive lymph node, CD4+ T cells demonstrate uniform expression of CD45 across all levels of CD7 and no activated T cell subset (CD38+) is present. Red, CD4+ T cells; Green, all T cells.

Immunophenotyping the Reactive Infiltrate in Classic Hodgkin Lymphoma, Nodular Lymphocyte Predominant Hodgkin Lymphoma, and T Cell/Histiocyte-Rich Large B Cell Lymphoma

Given its prominence in tissue biopsies, our laboratory and others have evaluated whether immunophenotypic characterization of the reactive infiltrate of these lymphomas can provide diagnostic information. Others have proposed the identification of increased regulatory T cells[24] and increased CD7 expression on CD4+ T cells[21] (to suggest CHL) and increased CD4+/CD8+ T cells (to suggest NLPHL[20]).

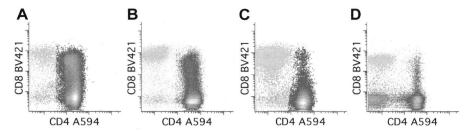

A   **B**   **C**   **D**

CD8 BV421   CD8 BV421   CD8 BV421   CD8 BV421

CD4 A594   CD4 A594   CD4 A594   CD4 A594

Fig. 8. Reactive T cells in NLPHL. Two NLPHL cases show prominent dual CD4+/CD8+ T cells, one shows a smaller population; a reactive lymph node case is shown for comparison. (*A*) NLPHL case; CD4+/CD8+ T cells represent 41.5% of T cells. (*B*) NLPHL case; CD4+/CD8+ T cells represent 20.1% of T cells. (*C*) NLPHL case; CD4+/CD8+ T cells represent 6.0% of T cells. (*D*) Reactive lymph node; CD4+/CD8+ T cells represent 2.6% of T cells. Population gated above background negative cells and calculated as a percentage of all CD3+ T cells. Red, CD4+ T cells; Green, CD8+ T cells.

In 2016, our group published a retrospective study examining reactive lymphocyte subsets in CHL, NLPHL, and THRLBCL.[22] T-cell subsets were examined in 34 cases of CHL, 27 cases of NLPHL, and 20 cases of THRLBCL. Forty-nine reactive lymph nodes composed the control group (summarized in **Table 3**; illustrative examples in **Figs. 7** and **8**). Reactive T cells were significantly increased in proportion for CHL, NLPHL, and

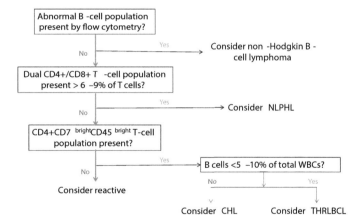

Fig. 9. Algorithm for using flow cytometry findings of reactive infiltrate as an adjunct in the diagnosis of CHL, THRLBCL, and NLPHL. The algorithm is used only if an abnormal light chain restricted B cell population is not identified by flow cytometry. If a T-cell population that coexpresses CD4 and CD8 is identified (population > ~6%–9% of the T cells), a diagnosis of NLPHL should be considered. If this CD4+CD8+ T cell population is absent, evaluate for the presence of a CD4+CD7^{bright}CD45^{bright} T-cell population. If the CD4+CD7^{bright} CD45^{bright} T-cell population is present and B cells comprise less than ~5 to 10% of the infiltrate, TCRLBCL should be considered. If the CD4+CD7^{bright}CD45^{bright} T-cell population is present but B cells comprise more than ~5 to 10% of the infiltrate, a diagnosis of CHL should be considered. Although the percentages described above are not absolute, as the percentage of the CD4+/CD8+ population increases, the probability of NLPHL increases. Similarly, in the presence of the CD4+CD7^{bright}CD45^{bright} T-cell population, as the percentage of reactive B cells decreases, the probability of THRLBCL increases. (Modified with permission from Wu et al.[22])

THRLBCL compared with reactive lymph node specimens, with THRLBCL showing the highest percentage. NLPHL had the highest percentage of reactive B cells (of the 3 lymphomas), although this percentage was still significantly decreased relative to reactive lymph nodes. As would be expect based on tissue immunohistochemistry, THRLBCL demonstrated a significantly decreased number of reactive B cells (relative to reactive lymph nodes and of lower percentage compared with NLPHL and CHL). THRLBCL also demonstrated a statistically significant increase in the mean percentage of CD4+ T cells (64.7%) when compared with NLPHL, CHL, and reactive lymph nodes. The mean percentage of CD4+/CD8+ T cells (evaluated as the percentage of T cells) was highest in NLPHL (see **Table 3**). CD8+ T cells showed no statistically significant differences of the mean percentages in this cohort.

As noted above, earlier studies have identified unique, reactive T-cell populations in both types of Hodgkin lymphoma that may be diagnostically useful.[19–21,24] In CHL, a population of CD4+ T cells has been identified in which there is concurrent bright/increased expression of CD7[21] or CD7 and CD45 (CD3+CD4+CD7[bright]CD45[bright] population) (76.5% of CHL cases; 26 of 34 cases evaluated).[19,22] In THRLBCL, 12 of 13 cases (92.3%) of T/HRLBCL contained the distinct CD3+CD4+CD7[bright] CD45[bright] population. This population is uncommon in NLPHL (8.3% of cases) or in reactive lymph nodes (4.1% of cases examined). In contrast, and as expected based on the studies by others, THRLBCL cases tend to not show the dual CD4+/CD8+ T cell (identified most prominently in NLPHL). Finally, our studies and those of others[23] have demonstrated increased CD4 to CD8 ratios of T cells in THRLBCL, in contrast to earlier studies by immunohistochemistry.[5,9,61] **Fig. 9** describes an algorithm utilizing the reactive populations described above to suggest a diagnosis of CHL, NLPHL, or THRLBCL.

SUMMARY

The flow cytometric assays described above have been designed to immunophenotype the neoplastic cells from CHL, NLPHL, and THRLBCL. Studies with these assays suggest that similarities in the immunophenotype on neoplastic cells likely contribute to the similar predominance of reactive cells in involved tissues in these lymphomas. Although not emphasized in this review, these combinations also allow for purification of neoplastic cells for downstream genetics studies. Finally, characterizing the reactive infiltrates can provide diagnostic information. Research to improve the diagnostic sensitivity of the flow cytometry assays is currently ongoing in our laboratory.

CLINICS CARE POINTS

- Flow cytometry assays for CHL, NLPHL, and THRLBCL can be a useful adjunct to morphology and immunohistochemistry.
- The flow cytometry assays are faster and usually cheaper way to provide immunophenotypic information when compared with immunohistochemistry.
- The flow cytometry assays are also useful research tools to study the pathologic condition of these lymphomas and improve diagnostics.

DISCLOSURE

The authors have no conflicts of interest to disclose.

REFERENCES

1. Brune V, Tiacci E, Pfeil I, et al. Origin and pathogenesis of nodular lymphocyte-predominant Hodgkin lymphoma as revealed by global gene expression analysis. J Exp Med 2008;205(10):2251–68.
2. Stein H, Swerdlow SH, Gascoyne RD, et al. Nodular lymphocyte predominant Hodgkin lymphoma. In: Swerdlow SH, Campos E, Harris NL, et al, editors. WHO classification of tumours of haematopoietic and lymphoid tissues. Lyon, France: IARC Press; 2017. p. 431–4.
3. Hartmann S, Doring C, Vucic E, et al. Array comparative genomic hybridization reveals similarities between nodular lymphocyte predominant Hodgkin lymphoma and T cell/histiocyte rich large B cell lymphoma. Br J Haematol 2015;169(3):415–22.
4. Abramson JS. T-cell/histiocyte-rich B-cell lymphoma: biology, diagnosis, and management. Oncol 2006;11(4):384–92. https://doi.org/10.1634/theoncologist.11-4-384.
5. Rudiger T, Gascoyne RD, Jaffe ES, et al. Workshop on the relationship between nodular lymphocyte predominant Hodgkin's lymphoma and T cell/histiocyte-rich B cell lymphoma. Review. Ann Oncol 2002;13(Suppl 1):44–51.
6. Pittaluga S, Jaffe ES. T-cell/histiocyte-rich large B-cell lymphoma. Haematologica 2010;95(3):352–6.
7. Lee AI, LaCasce AS. Nodular lymphocyte predominant Hodgkin lymphoma. Oncol 2009;14(7):739–51.
8. Stein H, Pileri SA, Weiss LM, et al. Hodgkin lymphomas: introduction. In: Swerdlow SH, Campos E, Harris NL, et al, editors. WHO classification of tumours of haematopoietic and lymphoid tissues. Lyon, France: IARC Press; 2017. p. 424–30. World Health Organization Classification of Tumors.
9. Tousseyn T, De Wolf-Peeters C. T cell/histiocyte-rich large B-cell lymphoma: an update on its biology and classification. Review. Virchows Arch 2011;459(6):557–63. https://doi.org/10.1007/s00428-011-1165-z.
10. Fraga M, Sanchez-Verde L, Forteza J, et al. T-cell/histiocyte-rich large B-cell lymphoma is a disseminated aggressive neoplasm: differential diagnosis from Hodgkin's lymphoma. Histopathology 2002;41(3):216–29.
11. Hartmann S, Doring C, Jakobus C, et al. Nodular lymphocyte predominant hodgkin lymphoma and T cell/histiocyte rich large B cell lymphoma–endpoints of a spectrum of one disease? PLoS One 2013;8(11):e78812.
12. Hartmann S, Eichenauer DA. Nodular lymphocyte predominant Hodgkin lymphoma: pathology, clinical course and relation to T-cell/histiocyte rich large B-cell lymphoma. Pathology 2020;52(1):142–53.
13. Cherian S, Fromm JR. Evaluation of primary mediastinal large B cell lymphoma by flow cytometry. Cytometry B Clin Cytom 2018;94(3):459–67.
14. Fromm JR, Kussick SJ, Wood BL. Identification and purification of classical Hodgkin cells from lymph nodes by flow cytometry and flow cytometric cell sorting. Am J Clin Pathol 2006;126(5):764–80.
15. Fromm JR, Thomas A, Wood BL. Flow cytometry can diagnose classical hodgkin lymphoma in lymph nodes with high sensitivity and specificity. Am J Clin Pathol 2009;131(3):322–32.
16. Fromm JR, Thomas A, Wood BL. Characterization and purification of neoplastic cells of nodular lymphocyte predominant hodgkin lymphoma from lymph nodes by flow cytometry and flow cytometric cell sorting. Am J Pathol 2017;187(2):304–17.

17. Fromm JR, Wood BL. A six-color flow cytometry assay for immunophenotyping classical Hodgkin lymphoma in lymph nodes. Am J Clin Pathol 2014;141(3): 388–96.

18. Glynn E, Fromm JR. Immunophenotypic characterization and purification of neoplastic cells from lymph nodes involved by T-cell/histiocyte-rich large B-cell lymphoma by flow cytometry and flow cytometric cell sorting. Cytometry B Clin Cytom 2020;98(1):88–98.

19. Fromm JR, Thomas A, Wood BL. Increased expression of T cell antigens on T cells in classical Hodgkin lymphoma. Cytometry B Clin Cytom 2010;78(6): 387–8.

20. Rahemtullah A, Reichard KK, Preffer FI, et al. A double-positive CD4+CD8+ T-cell population is commonly found in nodular lymphocyte predominant Hodgkin lymphoma. Am J Clin Pathol 2006;126(5):805–14.

21. Seegmiller AC, Karandikar NJ, Kroft SH, et al. Overexpression of CD7 in classical Hodgkin lymphoma-infiltrating T lymphocytes. Cytometry B Clin Cytom 2009; 76(3):169–74.

22. Wu D, Thomas A, Fromm JR. Reactive T cells by flow cytometry distinguish Hodgkin lymphomas from T cell/histiocyte-rich large B cell lymphoma. Cytometry B Clin Cytom 2016;90(5):424–32.

23. Kunder C, MJ C, Bakke A, et al. Predominance of CD4+ T cells in T-cell/histiocyte-rich large B-cell lymphoma and identification of a subset of patients with Peripheral B-cell Lymphopenia. Am J Clin Pathol 2017;147(6):596–603.

24. Bosler DS, Douglas-Nikitin VK, Harris VN, et al. Detection of T-regulatory cells has a potential role in the diagnosis of classical Hodgkin lymphoma. Cytometry B Clin Cytom 2008;74(4):227–35.

25. Stein H, Hummel M. Cellular origin and clonality of classic Hodgkin's lymphoma: immunophenotypic and molecular studies. Semin Hematol 1999;36(3):233–41.

26. Marafioti T, Hummel M, Foss HD, et al. Hodgkin and reed-sternberg cells represent an expansion of a single clone originating from a germinal center B-cell with functional immunoglobulin gene rearrangements but defective immunoglobulin transcription. Blood 2000;95(4):1443–50.

27. Mathas S, Hartmann S, Kuppers R. Hodgkin lymphoma: pathology and biology. Semin Hematol 2016;53(3):139–47.

28. Stein H, Pileri SA, MacLennan KA, et al. Classic hodgkin lymphoma. In: Swerdlow SH, Campos E, Harris NL, et al, editors. WHO classification of tumours of haematopoietic and lymphoid tissues. Lyon, France: IARC France; 2017. p. 435–42. World Health Organization Classification of Tumors.

29. Piris MA, Medeiros LJ, Chang KC. Hodgkin lymphoma: a review of pathological features and recent advances in pathogenesis. Pathology 2020;52(1):154–65.

30. Wang HW, Balakrishna JP, Pittaluga S, et al. Diagnosis of Hodgkin lymphoma in the modern era. Br J Haematol 2019;184(1):45–59.

31. Chan WC. The Reed-Sternberg cell in classical Hodgkin's disease. Hematol Oncol 2001;19(1):1–17.

32. Dorreen MS, Habeshaw JA, Stansfeld AG, et al. Characteristics of Sternberg-Reed, and related cells in Hodgkin's disease: an immunohistological study. Br J Cancer 1984;49(4):465–76.

33. Stuart AE, Williams AR, Habeshaw JA. Rosetting and other reactions of the Reed-Sternberg cell. J Pathol 1977;122(2):81–90.

34. Kadin ME, Newcom SR, Gold SB, et al. Letter: origin of Hodgkin's cell. Lancet 1974;2(7873):167–8.

35. Payne SV, Jones DB, Wright DH. Reed-Sternberg-cell/lymphocyte interaction. Lancet 1977;2(8041):768–9.
36. Payne SV, Newell DG, Jones DB, et al. The Reed-Sternberg cell/lymphocyte interaction: ultrastructure and characteristics of binding. Am J Pathol 1980; 100(1):7–24.
37. Veldman J, Visser L, Huberts-Kregel M, et al. Rosetting T cells in Hodgkin lymphoma are activated by immunological synapse components HLA class II and CD58. Blood 2020;136(21):2437–41.
38. Wein F, Kuppers R. The role of T cells in the microenvironment of Hodgkin lymphoma. J Leukoc Biol 2016;99(1):45–50.
39. Wein F, Weniger MA, Hoing B, et al. Complex immune Evasion strategies in classical hodgkin lymphoma. Cancer Immunol Res 2017;5(12):1122–32.
40. Sanders ME, Makgoba MW, Sussman EH, et al. Molecular pathways of adhesion in spontaneous rosetting of T-lymphocytes to the Hodgkin's cell line L428. Cancer Res 1988;48(1):37–40.
41. Schmitz R, Stanelle J, Hansmann ML, et al. Pathogenesis of classical and lymphocyte-predominant Hodgkin lymphoma. Annu Rev Pathol 2009;4:151–74.
42. Savage KJ, Mottok A, Fanale M. Nodular lymphocyte-predominant Hodgkin lymphoma. Semin Hematol 2016;53(3):190–202.
43. Ott G, Delabie J, Gascoyne RD, et al. T cell/histiocyte-rich large B-cell lymphoma. In: Swerdlow SH, Campos E, Harris NL, et al, editors. WHO classification of tumours of haematopoietic and lymphoid tissues. Lyon, France: IARC Press; 2017. p. 298–9. World Health Organization Classification of Tumors.
44. Cheng CL, O'Connor S. T cell-rich lymphoid infiltrates with large B cells: a review of key entities and diagnostic approach. J Clin Pathol 2017;70(3):187–201.
45. Chan A, Scarpa Carniello JV, Gao Q, et al. Role of flow cytometric immunophenotyping for classic hodgkin lymphoma in small biopsy and cytology specimens. Arch Pathol Lab Med 2022;146(4):462–8.
46. Fromm JR, Wood BL. Strategies for immunophenotyping and purifying classical Hodgkin lymphoma cells from lymph nodes by flow cytometry and flow cytometric cell sorting. Methods 2012;57(3):368–75.
47. Glynn E, Soma L, Wu D, et al. Flow cytometry for non-hodgkin and hodgkin lymphomas. Methods Mol Biol 2019;1956:35–60.
48. Carbone A, Gloghini A. CD75: a B-cell marker which should not be forgotten in lymphocyte predominant Hodgkin lymphoma. Am J Hematol 2014;89(4):449.
49. Schmid C, Sargent C, Isaacson PG. L and H cells of nodular lymphocyte predominant Hodgkin's disease show immunoglobulin light-chain restriction. Am J Pathol 1991;139(6):1281–9.
50. Stoler MH, Nichols GE, Symbula M, et al. Lymphocyte predominance Hodgkin's disease. Evidence for a kappa light chain-restricted monotypic B-cell neoplasm. Am J Pathol 1995;146(4):812–8.
51. Kuppers R. New insights in the biology of Hodgkin lymphoma. Hematology Am Soc Hematol Educ Program 2012;2012:328–34.
52. Arends JE, Bot FJ, Gisbertz IA, et al. Expression of CD10, CD75 and CD43 in MALT lymphoma and their usefulness in discriminating MALT lymphoma from follicular lymphoma and chronic gastritis. Histopathology 1999;35(3):209–15.
53. Kim LH, Eow GI, Peh SC, et al. The role of CD30, CD40 and CD95 in the regulation of proliferation and apoptosis in classical Hodgkin's lymphoma. Pathology 2003;35(5):428–35.
54. Verbeke CS, Wenthe U, Grobholz R, et al. Fas ligand expression in Hodgkin lymphoma. Am J Surg Pathol 2001;25(3):388–94.

55. Wu JM, Borowitz MJ, Weir EG. The usefulness of CD71 expression by flow cytometry for differentiating indolent from aggressive CD10+ B-cell lymphomas. Am J Clin Pathol 2006;126(1):39–46.

56. Lim SH, Vaughan AT, Ashton-Key M, et al. Fc gamma receptor IIb on target B cells promotes rituximab internalization and reduces clinical efficacy. Comparative Study. Blood 2011;118(9):2530–40.

57. Ansell SM, Lesokhin AM, Borrello I, et al. PD-1 blockade with nivolumab in relapsed or refractory Hodgkin's lymphoma. N Engl J Med 2015;372(4):311–9.

58. Taube JM, Klein A, Brahmer JR, et al. Association of PD-1, PD-1 ligands, and other features of the tumor immune microenvironment with response to anti-PD-1 therapy. Clin Cancer Res 2014;20(19):5064–74.

59. Chen BJ, Chapuy B, Ouyang J, et al. PD-L1 expression is characteristic of a subset of aggressive B-cell lymphomas and virus-associated malignancies. Clin Cancer Res 2013;19(13):3462–73.

60. Biggar R, Jaffe E, Goedert J, et al. Hodgkin lymphoma and immunodeficiency in persons with HIV/AIDS. Blood 2006;108(12):3786–91.

61. Felgar RE, Steward KR, Cousar JB, et al. T-cell-rich large-B-cell lymphomas contain non-activated CD8+ cytolytic T cells, show increased tumor cell apoptosis, and have lower Bcl-2 expression than diffuse large-B-cell lymphomas. Am J Pathol 1998;153(6):1707–15.

Clinical Cytometry for Platelets and Platelet Disorders

Andrew L. Frelinger III, PhD*, Benjamin E.J. Spurgeon, PhD

KEYWORDS

- Blood platelet disorders • Platelet function tests • Platelet activation
- Flow cytometry • Phenotyping • Thrombocytopenia

KEY POINTS

- Clinical flow cytometry is useful in the diagnosis of specific platelet disorders.
- Clinically important flow cytometric tests include tests for heparin-induced thrombocytopenia and vaccine-induced thrombotic thrombocytopenia.
- Studies are needed to evaluate the clinical utility of novel platelet subsets identified using large flow cytometry panels and high-dimensional immunophenotyping.

BACKGROUND

The critical role of platelets in hemostasis, aggregating to form hemostatic plugs, has been appreciated since at least 1910.[1] Platelets activated in hemostasis also participate in inflammatory processes. For example, P-selectin expressed on the surface of activated, but not resting platelets,[2] mediates platelet adhesion to monocytes and stimulation of cytokine synthesis and secretion.[3,4] More recently, it has been recognized that platelets are part of the first line of defense against infection, with Toll-like receptors and C-type lectin receptors mediating pathogen recognition.[5–8] In addition, platelets seem to function as immune cells, interacting with antigen-presenting cells[9] and themselves acting as antigen-presenting cells.[10,11] Thus, whereas clinical cytometry for platelets revolves mostly around their role in hemostasis, abnormalities in platelet number or function have the potential for a range of clinical consequences.

An important event in the development of flow cytometry for analysis of platelets was the use of PAC-1, a monoclonal IgM antibody specific for platelet glycoprotein (GP) IIb-IIIa (integrin αIIb/β3 or CD41/CD61), to identify activated platelets in whole

Center for Platelet Research Studies, Dana-Farber/Boston Children's Cancer and Blood Disorders Center, Harvard Medical School, Boston, MA 02115, USA
* Corresponding author. Division of Hematology/Oncology, Center for Platelet Research Studies, Boston Children's Hospital, 300 Longwood Avenue, Boston, MA 02115.
E-mail address: andrew.frelinger@childrens.harvard.edu

Clin Lab Med 43 (2023) 445–454
https://doi.org/10.1016/j.cll.2023.04.008
labmed.theclinics.com
0272-2712/23/© 2023 Elsevier Inc. All rights reserved.

blood.[12] Activation of platelets exposes fibrinogen binding sites on platelets[13] critical for aggregation and their role in hemostasis. GPIIb-IIIa was later identified as a platelet fibrinogen receptor, partly based on its absence in platelets from patients with Glanzmann thrombasthenia.[13,14] PAC-1 binds to activated but not resting platelets, blocks platelet aggregation, and fails to bind to Glanzmann thrombasthenia platelets.[15] Binding of a second antibody, S12 (against P-selectin), is also dependent on platelet activation, but requires stimulation sufficient to evoke secretion.[12] However, platelet secretion in response to strong activation with thrombin seems to be heterogeneous, with some platelets expressing less than 2000 and other platelets greater than 7500 S12 binding sites per platelet by flow cytometry.[16]

Michelson,[17] in 1987, used flow cytometry to evaluate whether distinct subpopulations of platelets exist in individual patients with chronic myeloid leukemia. Using antibodies directed to platelet surface GPIIb-IIIa and GPIb, platelets from patients with Glanzmann thrombasthenia were uniformly GPIIb-IIIa negative and GPIb positive, whereas those from patients with Bernard-Soulier syndrome were uniformly GPIIb-IIIa positive and GPIb negative. In contrast, children with chronic myeloid leukemia showed GPIIb-IIIa positive and negative platelet populations and GPIb positive and negative platelet populations. Taken together, these studies established flow cytometry as an important method to assess the degree of platelet activation and the efficacy of antiplatelet therapy in clinical disorders and to identify and investigate subpopulations of platelets in individual patients.

DISCUSSION

Inherited platelet function disorders are rare. Approaches to the diagnosis of an inherited platelet function disorder vary, but consensus guidelines from the International Society on Thrombosis and Haemostasis Subcommittee on Platelet Physiology[18] recommend flow cytometric analysis of granule release and the presence or absence of major platelet surface GPs as part of the first screen.

CURRENT CLINICAL APPLICATIONS

Clinical applications of flow cytometry and the relevant platelet biomarkers are summarized in **Table 1**. Although many clinical laboratories routinely perform complex flow cytometric tests ranging from CD4/CD8 immunodeficiency studies to leukemia and lymphoma phenotyping, few have established protocols for flow cytometric analysis of inherited platelet function disorders due to the relative rarity of these disorders. Consequently, tests for the presence or absence of major platelet surface GPs are often sent to specialized centers (eg, Versiti) or large reference laboratories (eg, Quest). This results in a delay in turnaround times, which impacts clinical utility and the ability to obtain a definitive diagnosis. In contrast, acquired platelet function disorders, such as heparin-induced thrombocytopenia, occur more frequently and several commercial flow cytometric tests with government agency clearance are available. Flow cytometry has enabled an important and timely tool, based on modifications of the heparin-induced thrombocytopenia assay, to identify vaccine-induced thrombotic thrombocytopenia related to COVID-19 vaccines.[19,20] Clinical flow cytometry of platelets may also be useful for characterization of drug-induced or immune thrombocytopenia. Tests have been reported that evaluate drug-dependent increases in platelet activation as measured by P-selectin expression, increased platelet surface immunoglobulin in patients with immune thrombocytopenia, and reactivity of sera from patients with immune thrombocytopenia with specific platelet surface GPs. Flow cytometry has also been used, mainly in clinical trials, to evaluate the

Table 1 Clinical applications of platelet flow cytometry	
Applications/Disorders	**Platelet Biomarkers**

Acute coronary syndromes[45,46]
Antiplatelet therapies[47–49]
Cystic fibrosis[50]
Diabetes[51,52]
Heart transplant vasculopathy[53]
Hemodialysis[54]
Heparin-induced thrombocytopenia[55,56]
Vaccine-induced thrombotic thrombocytopenia[19,20]
Ischemic stroke[57]
Myeloproliferative disorders[58,59]
Percutaneous coronary intervention[60]
Preeclampsia[61,62]
Systemic inflammation[63–65]
	Activation markers
	  CD62P
	  CD63
	  CD107a
	  PAC-1
	  PDMPs

Storage pool deficiency[66–68]	Dense granules
	  CD63
	  Mepacrine
	  Serotonin

Bernard-Soulier syndrome[17,69]	GPIb-IX-V complex
	  CD42a
	  CD42b
	  CD42d

Glanzmann thrombasthenia[17,70]	GPIIb/IIIa complex
	  CD41
	  CD61
	  PAC-1

P2Y12 antagonists[71,72]	Phosphoproteins *VASP*
Immune thrombocytopenia[73–76]	Platelet-associated immunoglobulin

Bone marrow function[77–79]	Platelet count
	  Immature platelet fraction
	  Reticulated platelets

Scott syndrome[80]	Procoagulant platelets *Annexin V*
Platelet-type von Willebrand disease[81]	von Willebrand factor

Abbreviations: PDMPs, platelet-derived microparticles; VASP, vasodilator-stimulated phosphoprotein.

pharmacodynamic efficacy of antiplatelet therapy with inhibitors of the platelet P2Y12 ADP receptor, including clopidogrel, prasugrel, and ticagrelor.

Platelet-derived microparticles (PDMPs) are elevated in many ischemic diseases and can be measured by flow cytometry. However, detection of PDMPs is variable and depends on instrument performance (PDMPs can be as small as 50 nm, which is lower than the limit of detection of many instruments). Modern machines, equipped with violet side scatter, allow the resolution of sub-100 nm particles and may be most advantageous for the sizing, counting, and characterization of PDMPs.[21] Sensitive PDMP assays may be useful in many pathologies, including arthritis, cancer, and thrombocytopenia.[22] However, because instruments vary widely in small-particle detection,[23] reference ranges must be established locally. Working groups are trying to standardize PDMP detection and have demonstrated the use of calibration beads to improve rigor and reproducibility.[23] Ongoing efforts are needed to facilitate multi-center studies for the validation and application of PDMPs as disease biomarkers, and (if successful) diagnostic assays could find their way into the clinic.

EMERGING APPLICATIONS AND FUTURE CHALLENGES

Novel platelet assays emerge intermittently, but their ability to act as clinical tools ultimately depends on their performance characteristics. Flow cytometry lacks definitive target standards for clinical and diagnostic use, so there is no clear roadmap to success, and validation strategies can differ among laboratories. Recent Clinical and Laboratory Standards Institute guidelines address the need for authoritative guidance for the validation of flow cytometry assays.[24] Development of new tests is hindered by the lack of platelet-based reference materials. Comparison with alternate methods is important for assay validation and has been performed for some platelet flow cytometric tests.[25–27]

Several conventional and spectral cytometers are approved for diagnostic use, as are many fluorescent reagents.[28] In contrast, mass cytometry is research use only but multicenter studies show it is able to generate robust and reproducible data across laboratories.[29,30] Whether mass cytometry is clinically useful or not, its discoveries can likely be replicated by conventional and spectral flow cytometry.[31,32] Because of its high-parameter capabilities, mass cytometry can be used to cast a wide net for biomarker discovery and results can be scaled down into smaller, more focused, multicolor flow cytometry panels. The advantage of high-parameter single-cell data, regardless of its source, is that the simultaneous measurement of multiple platelet biomarkers is likely to be more strongly associated with clinical outcomes than individual markers. Moreover, the combinatorial patterns of these markers can be used to identify specific subsets of platelets, whose relative abundance may have prognostic and/or diagnostic value in the same way, for example, that T-cell subsets are valuable for tracking HIV infection.[33]

Platelet phenotyping using biomarkers that span hemostasis, inflammation, and immunity is likely to identify subsets that are informative across a range of pathologies.[34] However, the use of platelet subsets as disease biomarkers requires a concerted validation effort. Perhaps the best-known flow cytometry validation (and commercialization) effort comes from the EuroFlow Consortium, who developed several tests for the classification and monitoring of hematologic malignancies.[35] These reputable tests may serve as a blueprint for the development of platelet-based assays and expedite the selection of stable fluorescent reagents. Liquid reagents containing polymer and tandem dyes may be unstable because of hydrolytic degradation. Lyophilization is a convenient solution that preserves the long-term stability of polymers and tandems,[36] and may preserve the stability of platelet agonists for assessment of in vitro platelet reactivity.

As panels increase in size and complexity, gating of platelet subtypes, as with gating of other cell types, becomes more challenging. Objective machine learning tools are preferred and may yield superior results over manual methods, which are tedious and introduce subjective bias. To date, we have demonstrated reproducible identification of platelet subtypes with manual and automated approaches.[34,37]

Prospective assay developers may wish to revisit the measurement of intraplatelet molecules. Phosphoproteins (eg, vasodilator-stimulated phosphoprotein) have already proven valuable for diagnostic use and their levels in response to endogenous inhibition are dysregulated in some pathologies.[38–40] Intraplatelet RNA is emerging as a novel biomarker in cancer diagnostics.[41] Megakaryocytes that take up tumor RNA and other tumor-derived factors are said to be "tumor-educated." Tumor-educated megakaryocytes give rise to platelets with an altered phenotype. Likewise, circulating platelets exposed to tumor RNA and other tumor-derived factors have altered RNA processing and an altered phenotype.[42] Resultant tumor-educated platelets represent a distinct subset of platelets with a molecular signature that ostensibly reflects that of the underlying cancer. Bulk sequencing of platelet RNA profiles can differentiate patients with cancer from healthy control subjects across various tumor types, although this approach is limited by low specificity and a high rate of false positives.[43] Ongoing studies of tumor-educated platelets using CITE-seq, a specialized form of flow cytometry that uses oligotagged antibodies to identify surface epitopes and single-cell sequencing, may allow users to filter out noise/irrelevant cells and provide significantly improved results.[44]

CLINICS CARE POINTS

- Use proper anticoagulant. EDTA prevents platelet-platelet aggregation and is suitable for evaluation of platelet surface GPIb but disrupts the GPIIb-IIIa complex and inhibits binding of some antibodies (eg, PAC-1). Sodium citrate (3.2%) is the preferred anticoagulant for platelet function tests.

- Careful blood collection is required for platelet function tests to avoid platelet activation. Use light tourniquets for short times, discard the first 1 to 3 mL of blood collected, and keep blood at room temperature (do not refrigerate or freeze).

- Platelets, because of their small size and potential overlap with debris, should be identified by forward and side light scatter and at least one platelet-identifying antibody.

- Evaluation of platelet activation requires fresh, unfixed samples. Fixation after staining allows samples to be stored until analysis. However, prolonged fixation may reduce the fluorescence of some probes and increase background for others.

DISCLOSURES

None.

REFERENCES

1. Duke WW. The relation of blood platelets to hemorrhagic disease. (re-publication of JAMA 1910;55:1185-1192). JAMA 1983;250(9):1201–9.
2. McEver RP, Martin MN. A monoclonal antibody to a membrane glycoprotein binds only to activated platelets. J Biol Chem 1984;259(15):9799–804.
3. Weyrich AS, McIntyre TM, McEver RP, et al. Monocyte tethering by P-selectin regulates monocyte chemotactic protein-1 and tumor necrosis factor-alpha secretion. Signal integration and NF-kappa B translocation. J Clin Invest 1995;95(5): 2297–303.
4. Weyrich AS, Elstad MR, McEver RP, et al. Activated platelets signal chemokine synthesis by human monocytes. J Clin Invest 1996;97(6):1525–34.
5. Brubaker SW, Bonham KS, Zanoni I, et al. Innate immune pattern recognition: a cell biological perspective. Annu Rev Immunol 2015;33:257–90.
6. Suzuki-Inoue K, Fuller GL, Garcia A, et al. A novel Syk-dependent mechanism of platelet activation by the C-type lectin receptor CLEC-2. Blood 2006;107(2): 542–9.

7. Sung PS, Huang TF, Hsieh SL. Extracellular vesicles from CLEC2-activated platelets enhance dengue virus-induced lethality via CLEC5A/TLR2. Nat Commun 2019;10(1):2402.

8. Kawai T, Akira S. Toll-like receptors and their crosstalk with other innate receptors in infection and immunity. Immunity 2011;34(5):637–50.

9. Han P, Hanlon D, Arshad N, et al. Platelet P-selectin initiates cross-presentation and dendritic cell differentiation in blood monocytes. Sci Adv 2020;6(11): eaaz1580.

10. Chapman LM, Aggrey AA, Field DJ, et al. Platelets present antigen in the context of MHC class I. J Immunol 2012;189(2):916–23.

11. Zufferey A, Speck ER, Machlus KR, et al. Mature murine megakaryocytes present antigen-MHC class I molecules to T cells and transfer them to platelets. Blood Adv 2017;1(20):1773–85.

12. Shattil SJ, Cunningham M, Hoxie JA. Detection of activated platelets in whole blood using activation-dependent monoclonal antibodies and flow cytometry. Blood 1987;70(1):307–15.

13. Bennett JS, Vilaire G. Exposure of platelet fibrinogen receptors by ADP and epinephrine. J Clin Invest 1979;64(5):1393–401.

14. Peerschke EI, Zucker MB, Grant RA, et al. Correlation between fibrinogen binding to human platelets and platelet aggregability. Blood 1980;55(5):841–7.

15. Shattil SJ, Hoxie JA, Cunningham M, et al. Changes in the platelet membrane glycoprotein IIb.IIIa complex during platelet activation. J Biol Chem 1985; 260(20):11107–14.

16. Johnston GI, Pickett EB, McEver RP, et al. Heterogeneity of platelet secretion in response to thrombin demonstrated by fluorescence flow cytometry. Blood 1987;69(5):1401–3.

17. Michelson AD. Flow cytometric analysis of platelet surface glycoproteins: phenotypically distinct subpopulations of platelets in children with chronic myeloid leukemia. J Lab Clin Med 1987;110(3):346–54.

18. Gresele P. Subcommittee on platelet Physiology of the International Society on thrombosis and hemostasis. Diagnosis of inherited platelet function disorders: guidance from the SSC of the ISTH. J Thromb Haemost 2015;13(2):314–22.

19. Handtke S, Wolff M, Zaninetti C, et al. A flow cytometric assay to detect platelet activating antibodies in VITT after ChAdOx1 nCov-19 vaccination. Blood 2021; 137(26):3656–9.

20. Cesari F, Sorrentino S, Gori AM, et al. Detection of platelet-activating antibodies associated with vaccine-induced thrombotic thrombocytopenia by flow cytometry: an Italian experience. Viruses 2022;14(6).

21. McVey MJ, Spring CM, Kuebler WM. Improved resolution in extracellular vesicle populations using 405 instead of 488 nm side scatter. J Extracell Vesicles 2018; 7(1):1454776.

22. Italiano JEJ, Mairuhu AT, Flaumenhaft R. Clinical relevance of microparticles from platelets and megakaryocytes. Curr Opin Hematol 2010;17(6):578–84.

23. Cointe S, Judicone C, Robert S, et al. Standardization of microparticle enumeration across different flow cytometry platforms: results of a multicenter collaborative workshop. J Thromb Haemostasis 2017;15(1):187–93.

24. CLSI. Validation of assays performed by flow cytometry. 1st edition. Clinical and Laboratory Standards Institute; 2021.

25. Dovlatova N, Lordkipanidze M, Lowe GC, et al. Evaluation of a whole blood remote platelet function test for the diagnosis of mild bleeding disorders. J Thromb Haemost 2014;12(5):660–5.

26. van Asten I, Schutgens REG, Baaij M, et al. Validation of flow cytometric analysis of platelet function in patients with a suspected platelet function defect. J Thromb Haemost 2018;16(4):689–98.
27. Gremmel T, Koppensteiner R, Panzer S. Comparison of aggregometry with flow cytometry for the assessment of agonists-induced platelet reactivity in patients on dual antiplatelet therapy. PLoS One 2015;10(6):e0129666.
28. Novakova M, Glier H, Brdičková N, et al. How to make usage of the standardized EuroFlow 8-color protocols possible for instruments of different manufacturers. J Immunol Methods 2019;475:112388.
29. Bagwell CB, Hunsberger B, Hill B, et al. Multi-site reproducibility of a human immunophenotyping assay in whole blood and peripheral blood mononuclear cells preparations using CyTOF technology coupled with Maxpar Pathsetter, an automated data analysis system. Cytometry B Clin Cytometry 2020;98(2):146–60.
30. Sahaf B, Pichavant M, Lee BH, et al. Immune profiling mass cytometry assay harmonization: multicenter experience from CIMAC-CIDC. Clin Cancer Res 2021;27(18):5062–71.
31. Gadalla R, Noamani B, MacLeod BL, et al. Validation of CyTOF against flow cytometry for immunological studies and monitoring of human cancer clinical trials. Front Oncol 2019;9:415.
32. Jaimes MC, Leipold M, Kraker G, et al. Full spectrum flow cytometry and mass cytometry: a 32-marker panel comparison. Cytometry 2022;101(11):942–59.
33. Chattopadhyay PK, Roederer M. Good cell, bad cell: flow cytometry reveals T-cell subsets important in HIV disease. Cytometry 2010;77(7):614–22.
34. Spurgeon BEJ, Frelinger AL 3rd. Comprehensive phenotyping of human platelets by single-cell cytometry. Cytometry 2022;101(4):290–7.
35. van Dongen JJM, Lhermitte L, Böttcher S, et al. EuroFlow antibody panels for standardized n-dimensional flow cytometric immunophenotyping of normal, reactive and malignant leukocytes. Leukemia 2012;26(9):1908–75.
36. Chan RCF, Kotner JS, Chuang CMH, et al. Stabilization of pre-optimized multicolor antibody cocktails for flow cytometry applications. Cytometry B Clin Cytometry 2017;92(6):508–24.
37. Spurgeon BEJ, Frelinger AL III. Platelet phenotyping by full spectrum flow cytometry. Current Protocols 2023;3:e687.
38. Aye MM, Kilpatrick ES, Aburima A, et al. Acute hypertriglyceridemia induces platelet hyperactivity that is not attenuated by insulin in polycystic ovary syndrome. J Am Heart Assoc 2014;3(1):e000706.
39. Berger M, Raslan Z, Aburima A, et al. Atherogenic lipid stress induces platelet hyperactivity through CD36-mediated hyposensitivity to prostacyclin: the role of phosphodiesterase 3A. Haematologica 2020;105(3):808–19.
40. Kahal H, Aburima A, Spurgeon B, et al. Platelet function following induced hypoglycaemia in type 2 diabetes. Diabetes & Metabolism 2018;44(5):431–6.
41. Wurdinger T, Veld SGJG, Best MG. Platelet RNA as pan-tumor biomarker for cancer detection. Cancer Res 2020;80(7):1371–3.
42. Roweth HG, Battinelli EM. Lessons to learn from tumor-educated platelets. Blood 2021;137(23):3174–80.
43. t Veld SGJG, Arkani M, Post E, et al. Detection and localization of early- and late-stage cancers using platelet RNA. Cancer Cell 2022;40(9):999–1009.
44. Stoeckius M, Hafemeister C, Stephenson W, et al. Simultaneous epitope and transcriptome measurement in single cells. Nat Methods 2017;14(9):865–8.
45. Coulter SA, Cannon CP, Ault KA, et al. High levels of platelet inhibition with abciximab despite heightened platelet activation and aggregation during thrombolysis

for acute myocardial infarction: results from TIMI (thrombolysis in myocardial infarction) 14. Circulation 2000;101(23):2690–5.

46. Stellos K, Bigalke B, Stakos D, et al. Platelet-bound P-selectin expression in patients with coronary artery disease: impact on clinical presentation and myocardial necrosis, and effect of diabetes mellitus and anti-platelet medication. J Thromb Haemost 2010;8(1):205–7.

47. Ault KA, Cannon CP, Mitchell J, et al. Platelet activation in patients after an acute coronary syndrome: results from the TIMI-12 trial. Thrombolysis in Myocardial Infarction. J Am Coll Cardiol 1999;33(3):634–9.

48. Gawaz M, Ruf A, Neumann FJ, et al. Effect of glycoprotein IIb-IIIa receptor antagonism on platelet membrane glycoproteins after coronary stent placement. Thromb Haemost 1998;80(6):994–1001.

49. Peter K, Kohler B, Straub A, et al. Flow cytometric monitoring of glycoprotein IIb/IIIa blockade and platelet function in patients with acute myocardial infarction receiving reteplase, abciximab, and ticlopidine: continuous platelet inhibition by the combination of abciximab and ticlopidine. Circulation 2000;102(13):1490–6.

50. O'Sullivan BP, Linden MD, Frelinger AL 3rd, et al. Platelet activation in cystic fibrosis. Blood 2005;105(12):4635–41.

51. Serebruany VL, Malinin A, Ong S, et al. Patients with metabolic syndrome exhibit higher platelet activity than those with conventional risk factors for vascular disease. J Thromb Thrombolysis 2008;25(2):207–13.

52. Israels SJ, McNicol A, Dean HJ, et al. Markers of platelet activation are increased in adolescents with type 2 diabetes. Diabetes Care 2014 37(8):2400–3.

53. Fateh-Moghadam S, Bocksch W, Ruf A, et al. Changes in surface expression of platelet membrane glycoproteins and progression of heart transplant vasculopathy. Circulation 2000;102(8):890–7.

54. Kawabata K, Nakai S, Miwa M, et al. Platelet GPIIb/IIIa is activated and platelet-leukocyte coaggregates formed in vivo during hemodialysis. Nephron 2002;90(4):391–400.

55. Althaus K, Pelzl L, Hidiatov O, et al. Evaluation of a flow cytometer-based functional assay using platelet-rich plasma in the diagnosis of heparin-induced thrombocytopenia. Thromb Res 2019;180:55–61.

56. Runser A, Schaning C, Allemand F, et al. An optimized and standardized rapid flow cytometry functional method for heparin-induced thrombocytopenia. Biomedicines 2021;9(3).

57. Grau AJ, Ruf A, Vogt A, et al. Increased fraction of circulating activated platelets in acute and previous cerebrovascular ischemia. Thromb Haemost 1998;80(2):298–301.

58. Villmow T, Kemkes-Matthes B, Matzdorff AC. Markers of platelet activation and platelet-leukocyte interaction in patients with myeloproliferative syndromes. Thromb Res 2002;108(2–3):139–45.

59. Jensen MK, de Nully Brown P, Lund BV, et al. Increased circulating platelet-leukocyte aggregates in myeloproliferative disorders is correlated to previous thrombosis, platelet activation and platelet count. Eur J Haematol 2001;66(3):143–51.

60. Gawaz M, Neumann FJ, Ott I, et al. Platelet activation and coronary stent implantation. Effect of antithrombotic therapy. Circulation 1996;94(3):279–85.

61. Janes SL, Goodall AH. Flow cytometric detection of circulating activated platelets and platelet hyper-responsiveness in pre-eclampsia and pregnancy. Clin Sci (Lond) 1994;86(6):731–9.

62. Konijnenberg A, van der Post JA, Mol BW, et al. Can flow cytometric detection of platelet activation early in pregnancy predict the occurrence of preeclampsia? A prospective study. Am J Obstet Gynecol 1997;177(2):434–42.

63. Gawaz M, Dickfeld T, Bogner C, et al. Platelet function in septic multiple organ dysfunction syndrome. Intensive Care Med 1997;23(4):379–85.

64. Joseph JE, Harrison P, Mackie IJ, et al. Increased circulating platelet-leucocyte complexes and platelet activation in patients with antiphospholipid syndrome, systemic lupus erythematosus and rheumatoid arthritis. Br J Haematol 2001; 115(2):451–9.

65. Russwurm S, Vickers J, Meier-Hellmann A, et al. Platelet and leukocyte activation correlate with the severity of septic organ dysfunction. Shock 2002;17(4):263–8.

66. Gordon N, Thom J, Cole C, et al. Rapid detection of hereditary and acquired platelet storage pool deficiency by flow cytometry. Br J Haematol 1995;89(1): 117–23.

67. Maurer-Spurej E, Pittendreigh C, Wu JK. Diagnosing platelet delta-storage pool disease in children by flow cytometry. Am J Clin Pathol 2007;127(4):626–32.

68. Cai H, Mullier F, Frotscher B, et al. Usefulness of flow cytometric mepacrine up-take/release combined with CD63 assay in diagnosis of patients with suspected platelet dense granule disorder. Semin Thromb Hemost 2016;42(3): 282–91.

69. Cohn RJ, Sherman GG, Glencross DK. Flow cytometric analysis of platelet surface glycoproteins in the diagnosis of Bernard-Soulier syndrome. Pediatr Hematol Oncol 1997;14(1):43–50.

70. Jennings LK, Ashmun RA, Wang WC, et al. Analysis of human platelet glycoproteins IIb-IIIa and Glanzmann's thrombasthenia in whole blood by flow cytometry. Blood 1986;68(1):173–9.

71. Schwarz UR, Geiger J, Walter U, et al. Flow cytometry analysis of intracellular VASP phosphorylation for the assessment of activating and inhibitory signal transduction pathways in human platelets: definition and detection of ticlopidine/clopidogrel effects. Thromb Haemost 1999;82(3):1145–52.

72. Aleil B, Ravanat C, Cazenave JP, et al. Flow cytometric analysis of intraplatelet VASP phosphorylation for the detection of clopidogrel resistance in patients with ischemic cardiovascular diseases. J Thromb Haemost 2005;3(1):85–92.

73. Lazarchick J, Genco PV, Hall SA, et al. Detection of platelet antibodies by flow cytometric analysis. Diagn Immunol 1984;2(4):238–41.

74. Huh HJ, Park CJ, Kim SW, et al. Flow cytometric detection of platelet-associated immunoglobulin in patients with immune thrombocytopenic purpura and nonimmune thrombocytopenia. Ann Clin Lab Sci 2009;39(3):283–8.

75. Hagenstrom H, Schlenke P, Hennig H, et al. Quantification of platelet-associated IgG for differential diagnosis of patients with thrombocytopenia. Thromb Haemost 2000;84(5):779–83.

76. Tomer A, Koziol J, McMillan R. Autoimmune thrombocytopenia: flow cytometric determination of platelet-associated autoantibodies against platelet-specific receptors. J Thromb Haemost 2005;3(1):74–8.

77. Briggs C, Kunka S, Hart D, et al. Assessment of an immature platelet fraction (IPF) in peripheral thrombocytopenia. Br J Haematol 2004;126(1):93–9.

78. Schoorl M, Schoorl M, Oomes J, et al. New fluorescent method (PLT-F) on Sysmex XN2000 hematology analyzer achieved higher accuracy in low platelet counting. Am J Clin Pathol 2013;140(4):495–9.

79. Romp KG, Peters WP, Hoffman M. Reticulated platelet counts in patients undergoing autologous bone marrow transplantation: an aid in assessing marrow recovery. Am J Hematol 1994;46(4):319–24.
80. Halliez M, Fouassier M, Robillard N, et al. Detection of phosphatidyl serine on activated platelets' surface by flow cytometry in whole blood: a simpler test for the diagnosis of Scott syndrome. Br J Haematol 2015;171(2):290–2.
81. Giannini S, Cecchetti L, Mezzasoma AM, et al. Diagnosis of platelet-type von Willebrand disease by flow cytometry. Haematologica 2010;95(6):1021–4.

Utility of Flow Cytometry Analysis in the Detection of Nonhematologic Neoplasms

An Overview

Hibbah Nabeel, MD[a], Bachir Alobeid, MD[b],*

KEYWORDS

- Flow cytometry • Nonhematopoietic • Nonhematologic • Neoplasm • Carcinoma
- Effusion • Pediatric • Solid tumor

KEY POINTS

- Flow cytometry analysis has tremendously evolved over the past decades and has stood the test of time as a powerful tool in the assessment of hematologic neoplasms.
- The role of flow cytometry analysis has also expanded beyond assessment of hematologic neoplasms to immunophenotypically evaluate various adult and pediatric nonhematologic neoplasms encountered in different body sites.
- Specially designed multicolor antibody panels and even routine hematologic panels have been used in the assessment of nonhematologic neoplasms.
- Despite all the advances, flow cytometry analysis is still infrequently applied in the routine daily diagnostic workup of nonhematologic neoplasms due to certain limitations and diagnostic pitfalls.

INTRODUCTION AND BACKGROUND

Flow cytometry analysis (FCM) is a well-established multiparameter powerful diagnostic modality widely used for the assessment of hematologic neoplasms (HN). Although the main current applications of FCM remain the diagnosis and follow-up of HN, it has also been used to detect nonhematologic neoplasms (non-HN). Indeed, one of the earliest diagnostic applications of FCM in the 1980s of last century was in the detection of urinary bladder carcinoma. At that time FCM was established as a valuable adjunct to cytology in the diagnosis, management, and follow-up of patients

[a] Department of Pathology and Cell Biology, Columbia University Irving Medical Center, 630 West 168th street, VC14-236 New York, NY 10032, USA; [b] Department of Pathology and Cell Biology, Columbia University Irving Medical Center, 630 West 168th street, VC14-229 New York, NY 10032, USA
* Corresponding author. 630 West 168th street, VC14-229 New York, NY 10032.
E-mail address: ba2024@cumc.columbia.edu

Clin Lab Med 43 (2023) 455–465
https://doi.org/10.1016/j.cll.2023.05.001
0272-2712/23/© 2023 Elsevier Inc. All rights reserved.
labmed.theclinics.com

with suspected or known urinary bladder carcinoma.[1] Urinary bladder irrigation specimens, containing suspensions of single exfoliated urothelial carcinoma cells, readily lending themselves to FCM, were examined using simultaneous nonimmunophenotypic multiparameter FCM measurements of aneuploidy and nuclear size. Carcinoma cells were distinguished from normal cells by an increase in the proportion of urinary bladder epithelial cells with more than diploid (polyploid) DNA and aneuploid cell peaks.

FCM has tremendously evolved over the past decades. It is currently considered a powerful, versatile tool used widely for cellular immunophenotypic analysis of HN. The role of FCM has also expanded to immunophenotypically evaluate various non-HN encountered in body cavity malignant effusions, lymph nodes, and other body sites, using specially designed multicolor antibody panels for non-HN and even routine antibody panels otherwise typically used for assessment of HN.

This review focuses on the more recently published literature on evolution and advances in the utility of FCM in the detection and evaluation of non-HN, its limitations and pitfalls, as well as future directions and promising applications.

Utility of Flow Cytometry in the Analysis of Nonhematologic Neoplasms in Body Cavity Malignant Effusions

Body cavity (pleural, peritoneal, and pericardial) malignant effusions are common complications of advanced non-HN. The effusions are often drained for diagnostic and therapeutic purposes by minimally invasive procedures. Cytology, aided by immunohistochemical analysis (IHC), remains the main method of evaluation of effusion samples. Because neoplastic cells are naturally dispersed and suspended as single cells in the effusion fluid and washing samples, they are amenable to FCM. Although FCM is a rapid, powerful modality for multiparameter immunophenotypic evaluation, it is still infrequently applied in the characterization of malignant effusions secondary to non-HN in the routine daily diagnostic setting. Over the past 3 decades, several studies have been published exploring the diagnostic utility of FCM in malignant effusion specimens secondary to non-HN, either by using DNA ploidy to detect malignant aneuploid cells or by using various panels of immunophenotypic epithelial and nonepithelial cell markers.

Earlier studies extensively explored the role of DNA ploidy by FCM. The studies were based on the proposition that detection of cells demonstrating abnormal DNA content strongly supported the diagnosis of malignancy.[2-7] These studies reported varying sensitivity and specificity by FCM.[3,4,6,7] However, there is conflicting data on the use of DNA ploidy as a sole marker of malignancy, as reactive mesothelial cells can demonstrate hyperploidy as well,[4,7] which was demonstrated by FISH analysis in one study.[8] Despite this, the studies overall suggest that DNA ploidy analysis by FCM is a useful adjunct to cytology.[2-7]

Several epithelial markers, such as Ber-EP4, B72.3, CD15, CD138, CK18, antipancytokeratin, antiepithelial membrane antigen (EMA), and integrin, have been used to establish the efficacy of FCM in the analysis of carcinomas.[9-16] Sigstad and colleagues used FCM to perform quantitative analysis of integrin expression and showed FCM to be an efficient tool for quantitative analysis of adhesion molecules in effusions. The group ascertained that the characterization of adhesion molecule expression can be achieved using FCM and that it is an effective tool for the study of cancer-related expression patterns, as well as for comparative analysis of different malignancies, such as adenocarcinoma and malignant mesothelioma using intensity of expression of an integrin subunit (αv) as a parameter to differentiate between tumor types.[11] Pillai and colleagues used a combination of quantitative and qualitative criteria to infer the presence of malignancy. The group studied the expression of Ber-EP4 as a marker for all carcinomas and reported that the sensitivity and specificity of FCM was 88.15% and 97.64%, respectively, compared with 73.68% and 100% of cytology alone for the presence of a malignant effusion. A caveat is that Ber-EP4 can possibly be downregulated in various carcinomas, potentially resulting in false-negative results. Alternatively, Ber-EP4–positive cells are frequently seen in peritoneal washings, and the likely origin for such cells is exfoliation of ovarian, tubal, or uterine epithelium or even recent surgery. However, such cells have low-level expression of Ber-EP4 and occur in much lower numbers compared with malignant epithelial cells in effusions. Quantitative parameters can thus be used to differentiate between benign and malignant effusions.[12] Kentrou and colleagues reported EMA and Ber-EP4 as the most sensitive markers for malignancy in effusions, whereas the detection of desmin-33–negative/cytokeratin-positive cells had the simultaneous highest positive and negative predictive values.[4]

These studies not only established FCM as a useful adjunct to cytology for the diagnosis of malignant effusions, especially in the setting of atypical or suspicious cytologic findings, or when cytologic preparations were paucicellular or hemorrhagic, but also elucidated the role of FCM as a tool to quantitate expression of various markers and follow-up of patients after chemotherapy, providing helpful information to aid accurate diagnosis.

The utility of FCM for prognostication in body cavity non-HN was also explored. Tamai and colleagues used FCM to detect and quantify the expression of carcinoembryonic antigen (CEA) by tumor cells from freshly excised human gastric cancer specimens including ascites fluid specimens. The study demonstrated that FCM detected CEA in both the cell membrane and cytoplasm, with the additional benefit of quantifying CEA expression, not achievable by IHC alone. They reported a significant correlation between CEA expression by FCM and the postoperative survival in patients with gastric cancer with poorly differentiated adenocarcinoma, highlighting another use of this dynamic tool.[17]

In summary, these studies demonstrate that multicolor FCM with its superior qualitative and quantitative properties can play an important adjunct role to cytology and IHC in the rapid diagnosis of malignant effusions, especially in paucicellular or hemorrhagic cytology specimens or when cytologic diagnosis is equivocal (atypical/suspicious). The combined use of FCM and cytology has higher sensitivity and specificity and helps triage cases efficiently.

Utility of Flow Cytometry in the Assessment of Nonhematologic Neoplasms in Lymph Nodes and Other Solid Tissues

FCM is routinely performed in the workup of lymph nodes and other solid organ biopsy specimens for the assessment of HN. Lymph nodes also are the most frequent site of involvement by metastatic non-HN and sometimes the first manifestation of the disease. FCM has been used to detect metastatic epithelial malignancies in various specimen types including lymph nodes and solid organs. Ravoet and colleagues used 3 antibody panels: CD45/Glycophorin-A/EMA, CD45/CD138/EMA, and CD45/Glycophorin-A/Cytokeratin. This approach was able to not only detect but also quantify metastatic involvement. Among the 116 histologically assessable samples, agreement between FCM and histology was found in 102 samples (87.9%; 95% confidence interval = 81–93). For the diagnosis of carcinoma, the agreement between FCM and histology was 100%. Moreover, FCM detected significant infiltration by carcinoma cells in one case when morphology failed, which is not surprising because FCM can detect an exceptionally low level of abnormal cells (possibly micrometastasis in this case). However, sampling issues should also be considered, with metastatic infiltration being limited to the part of the specimen submitted for FCM or less likely contamination of the FCM sample by epithelial cells from normal tissues (eg, skin).[13] Hartana and colleagues demonstrated that FCM was effective in detecting micrometastases to sentinel lymph nodes in patients with renal tumors using cytokeratin-18 (as intracellular marker) with carbonic anhydrase and cadherin-6 (as surface markers). Stability of the assay was established by low intra-assay and inter-assay variability.[14]

A retrospective study we performed at our institution evaluated the utility of FCM in detecting non-HN by using routine antibody panels, designed and validated for the detection of HN.[15] The analysis focused on the CD45-negative, viable populations in various samples. The study revealed that most of the non-HN cases detected by the routine panels were neuroendocrine carcinomas (33/57), primarily small cell carcinoma. Other types of carcinomas such as squamous cell carcinoma and adenocarcinoma (**Fig. 1**), as well as other neoplasms were also detected. In addition to lacking CD45 expression, a defining feature of non-HN, the neoplasms commonly expressed CD56, as reported in other studies as well, followed by CD117 and CD138.[15,16,18–28] In most cases, at least one marker included in the routine panels was detected on the neoplastic cells. CD56 expression was seen in nearly all cases of neuroendocrine tumors (**Fig. 2**), whereas CD138 expression (**Fig. 3**) was more common in squamous cell carcinoma and adenocarcinoma. Other expressed markers included CD38, HLA-DR, CD13, CD34, and CD10. The presence of non-HN was confirmed in all samples by morphologic evaluation. This study highlighted the importance of analyzing CD45 negative events and demonstrated the utility of FCM in detecting non-HN even when applying routine antibody panels. Of note, CD10 was positive in an ascitic fluid sample from a patient with colonic carcinoma. CD10 is an understudied/unexplored discriminant marker by FCM, useful for the diagnosis of clear cell variant of renal cell carcinoma, hepatocellular carcinoma, and gynecologic tumors such as endometrial stromal sarcoma.[15]

A similar study reported by Stacchini and colleagues evaluated 9422 specimens submitted for routine flow cytometric investigation; 47 of the samples were suspected to harbor non-HN based on detection of CD45-negative events. The group designed a panel of monoclonal antibodies to characterize the CD45-negative populations suspected to represent non-HN. The panel included CD45 for leukocyte identification, CD326 to mark epithelial cells, CD33 to identify myeloid cells, CD138 to trace plasma cells, and CD56 for the identification of neuroendocrine tumors. FCM detected CD326-positive epithelial cells in 34 of 36 specimens, whereas altered scatter characteristics and variable reactivity to the other antigens tested allowed the detection of non-HN in the remaining 9 specimens. No CD326-positive events were detected in

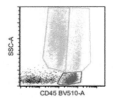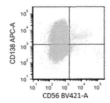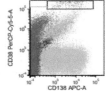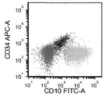

Fig. 1. FCM of a peritoneal fluid sample. The gated CD45-negative, intermediate to high side scatter events (*green dots*) show partial CD138 expression and more uniform expression of CD10, and negativity for CD34, CD38, and CD56. The concurrent cytology evaluation demonstrated involvement of the peritoneal fluid by adenocarcinoma.

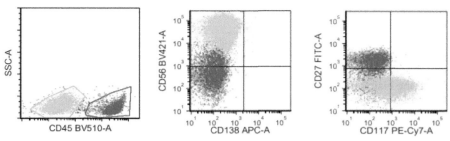

Fig. 2. FCM of a lymph node sample. The CD45-negative, low side scatter population of events (*green dots*) shows uniform expression of CD56, partial positivity for CD117, and no expression of CD138. The concurrent histology evaluation demonstrated involvement of the lymph node by Merkel cell carcinoma.

melanoma or sarcoma cases. The presence of non-HN was confirmed subsequently by histology in every case. Elaborating on the technique, the group recommended carefully analyzing CD45-negative events; because epithelial elements are variable in size and cytoplasmic complexity, they can be found in all areas of scatter plot including areas potentially considered as "cell debris". Scatter parameters and back gating on CD326-, CD56-, and/or CD138-positive events was fundamental in detecting non-HN. In diagnosis of CD56-positive neuroendocrine neoplasms, caution should be practiced to avoid misclassification of CD56-positive/CD45-negative events as natural killer cell neoplasms, especially if nonspecific staining/autofluorescence is misinterpreted as weak CD45 expression[19]; this can be avoided by careful evaluation and establishing clear cut-offs of CD56-positive/CD45-negative populations. The group concluded that the clue to the presence of non-HN was in analysis of CD45-negative cells with altered scatter parameters,[18] a conclusion supported by other studies.[12,15]

These studies demonstrated that FCM of lymph node samples is a valuable ancillary tool for detection of non-HN. It could help triage cases in a timely efficient manner, guiding immunohistochemical stains, particularly when HN have been excluded.

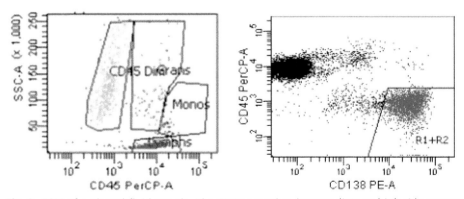

Fig. 3. FCM of a pleural fluid sample. The CD45-negative, intermediate to high side scatter population of events (*green dots*) shows uniform expression of CD138 (*red dots*). The concurrent cytology showed poorly differentiated adenocarcinoma of mammary origin in the pleural fluid.

Utility of Flow Cytometry in the Assessment of Pediatric Nonhematologic Neoplasms

Pediatric non-HN, also referred to as "small round blue cell tumors," are derived from embryonic mesenchymal and neuroectodermal precursors. They are usually evaluated using comprehensive IHC, as the tumors show overlapping morphologic features on routine histology. Pediatric non-HN include neuroblastoma, Ewing sarcoma/primitive neuroectodermal tumor (PNET), rhabdomyosarcoma, Wilms tumor, retinoblastoma, and desmoplastic small round cell tumor. Several studies have investigated the role of FCM in the detection of pediatric non-HN, particularly neuroblastoma, as it has propensity to involve the bone marrow (BM), as well as for its morphologic resemblance to HN.[16,18–36] Many studies have reported FCM as an effective modality in detecting neuroblastoma involving various specimen types including BM, body cavity effusions, and peripheral blood.[16,29–35] Various markers have been evaluated to establish the phenotype of different pediatric small blue cell tumors, including CD56, CD81, GD2, CD271, CD57, vimentin, CD99, and myogenin.[16,18–26,29–31,33,35]

FCM is established as a useful ancillary study that aids in diagnosis of neuroblastoma. A study by Furlanetto and colleagues demonstrated that FCM achieved a sensitivity of 100%, a specificity of 86%, a positive predictive value of 67%, and a negative predictive value of 100% in detection of neuroblastoma in the BM.[30] Ferreira and colleagues systematically applied FCM analysis for diagnostic screening and further classification of pediatric solid tumors. They proposed a strategy that aimed at differential diagnosis between tumoral versus nontumoral samples, HN versus non-HN, and the subclassification of pediatric non-HN. Apart from achieving high concordance between FCM and conventional diagnostic methods, they reported that different pediatric non-HN subtypes displayed distinct antigen expression profiles. Neuroblastoma uniformly expressed CD56, CD9, CD81 (high), and GD2 (high) with heterogeneous expression of CD57 and CD58. Strong GD2 expression was limited to neuroblastoma. PNET displayed a phenotype similar to neuroblastoma cells, except that they were negative for GD2 and showed stronger expression of CD99 and CD271. Nuclear expression of MYOD1 and myogenin was restricted to rhabdomyosarcoma. Hemangiopericytoma demonstrated CD45-negative and CD34-positive phenotype. Furthermore, GD2 and CD271 were considered as the 2 most helpful markers to differentiate between neuroblastoma and PNET. They also used FCM to characterize pediatric carcinomas, which are rare entities. They demonstrated expression of EpCAM in adrenal carcinoma and nasopharyngeal carcinoma, whereas all noncarcinoma tumor cell samples were negative for EpCAM.[22]

The same group designed and validated a single panel of antibodies for fast and accurate screening, orientation, and classification of pediatric non-HN. The design of this panel relied on a total of 42 different markers selected from a larger set of markers reported in the literature, which were tested in a large series of pediatric samples suspicious for infiltration by non-HN. In its final version, the "solid tumor orientation tube" (STOT) consisted of a single 8-color/12-antibody combination (CD99-CD8/myogenin/CD4-EpCAM/CD56/GD2/CD3-CD19/cyCD3-CD271/CD45). Prospective validation of STOT in 149 samples showed concordant results in 138/149 cases (92.6%) with the diagnosis according to WHO/ICCC-3 classification. The group not only established the ability of this tube to distinguish between benign and malignant cells, HN, and non-HN but also allowed accurate discrimination among CD45-negative/CD56-positive non-HN.[26]

Apart from aiding in fast and accurate diagnosis of pediatric non-HN, FCM has been studied as a tool for prognostication in patients with neuroblastoma cells detected in the BM, which has significantly worse prognosis compared with children with negative BM by FCM. This suggestion was supported by a pilot study that evaluated the role of FCM in detecting measurable residual disease and predicting the outcome of patients with advanced neuroblastoma.[27] In contrast, another study has suggested that BM mesenchymal cells, which are also CD45-negative and CD56-positive, might pose an obstacle to accurate neuroblastoma disease assessment by FCM.[28]

In a multivariate analysis, immunophenotyping by FCM proved to be an independent prognostic factor when analyzed jointly with other neuroblastoma risk factors, more so than molecular polymerase chain reaction (PCR) analysis of PHOX2B and TH gene expression, which was conducted in a subgroup of patient samples.[32] Consequently, FCM has been recommended as a useful adjunct to molecular studies given the high false-positive results seen with PCR.[32,34] Of note, Nagai and colleagues used FCM analysis to detect neuroblastoma cells in the peripheral blood to guide stem cell transplantation through peripheral blood in patients with advanced neuroblastoma.[31]

The aforementioned studies have widely explored and clearly established the role of FCM as a valuable ancillary modality useful to aid in the fast and accurate diagnosis of pediatric non-HN, especially neuroblastoma, as well as a useful adjunct tool for prognostication of disease.

DISCUSSION AND SUMMARY

FCM is a versatile diagnostic modality widely used in routine immunophenotypic evaluation of HN. However, this body of literature review reveals that the role of FCM in the detection and evaluation of non-HN has been extensively explored as well (**Table 1**). Although cytology specimens and most solid tissue samples are amenable to FCM, this diagnostic modality is still not widely used in the routine workup or follow-up of non-HN. FCM can be especially helpful in the analysis of body cavity malignant effusions and limited fine-needle aspiration or cerebrospinal fluid samples.[9–12,15,17,20,21,23,33,35,37] FCM provides more rapid immunophenotyping than conventional IHC, can identify rare malignant cells that could be missed on routine cytology alone, and can be used to evaluate limited paucicellular samples. Given the short turnaround time of FCM assays and

Table 1
Immunophenotypic markers applied in the evaluation of nonhematologic neoplasms by flow cytometry analysis

Immunophenotypic Markers	Utility and Application in FCM Analysis of Non-HN	References
NCAM (CD56), CD117	Neuroendocrine tumors	9,10,15,16,18–23,35
EPCAM (Ber-EP4, MOC-31, CD326) CD138, CD15, CK18, integrin, EMA, claudin 4, B-72.3	Epithelial tumors	9–12,15,16,18,37
GD2, CD81, CD56, CD90, CD57	Neuroblastoma	16,18–35
CD99, CD271, CD57, CD56	Ewing sarcoma/PNET	16,22,26
MYOD1, myogenin, CD56	Rhabdomyosarcoma	16,22,24,26
CD56, NG2, CD10	Germ cell tumors	22,26
N-cadherin, EMA	Mesothelial origin	10,11
CD34	Hemangiopericytoma	22,26
CD56, CD58, EPCAM	Wilms tumor	26

the accuracy with which it can characterize neoplastic cells by using comprehensive multicolor panels of antibodies, it can be a useful tool for the detection of non-HN, especially when making a timely diagnosis is of the essence; this can help expedite further downstream immunophenotypic analysis of specimens and triage samples for appropriate genetic and molecular studies. In addition, FCM cell sorting and potential subsequent targeted molecular analysis can be helpful in obtaining additional diagnostic information from clinical samples of low-level disease or limited fine needle aspiration or body fluid samples. It is also further useful when cytologic diagnosis is equivocal (atypical/suspicious) or if the cytologic preparations are paucicellular or hemorrhagic. Most studies have reported good sensitivity of FCM to identify neoplastic cells in cytology specimens.

However, in many situations other methods of pathology evaluation including immunomorphology may be required to overcome certain limitations of FCM. As mentioned earlier, despite the great body of published literature on the efficacy of FCM in detection of non-HN, its use for diagnostic purposes is relatively limited and mostly used in research settings.

The need for preparation of single-cell suspensions of neoplastic cells from solid tissue samples is one limiting factor of FCM. The required physical disaggregation and extraction of neoplastic cells from solid tissue samples might affect antigen preservation and viability of neoplastic cells. Enzymatic digestion has been proposed to improve the cellular yield, but it can also alter surface antigens of target.[36] Most studies have designed and applied various specialized antibody panels targeting non-HN cells; however, there is lack of reliable, standardized, and validated antibody panels, as well as lack of standardized approach for the diagnostic application of FCM to non-HN.[18,23,26] Another limitation of FCM analysis is that it does not provide information on the architecture of the tumor, although it provides additional valuable information on cell lineage and stage of differentiation, along with patterns of antigenic expression, which helps in guiding additional IHC.[26] FCM is unable to distinguish with certainty between benign or malignant epithelial cells,[13,26] and this may represent a pitfall in specimens contaminated by benign epithelial cells, especially those obtained by endoscopy. The transit of the endoscope across the alimentary canal or respiratory tree potentially causes sample contamination by normal epithelial cells of the mucosa. Similarly, percutaneous fine-needle aspiration samples of salivary gland tumors may be affected by nonneoplastic glandular tissue contamination.[18] Furthermore, poorly differentiated non-HN may downregulate markers included in FCM panels, making FCM unhelpful in detecting poorly differentiated non-HN, although such cases account for a small number of neoplasms.[12,37] Sampling errors can also result in false negatives.

Finally, to maximize the benefits and efficacy of FCM in the detection of non-HN, and to increase its diagnostic utility, further future studies are necessary to design and evaluate antibody panels, as well as establish standardized sample preparation protocols and gating strategies that contribute to improving the yield of this powerful versatile assay in assessing non-HN.

CLINICS CARE POINTS

- The role of FCM has been widely explored and established as a useful adjunct in the detection of non-HN using various antibody panels.
- FCM is still infrequently applied in the routine daily workup of non-HN, and its use is mostly restricted to investigative settings due to certain limitations and diagnostic pitfalls.

> - To maximize the utility of FCM in the detection of non-HN, more studies are needed to design and evaluate standardized antibody panels and establish sample preparation protocols and gating strategies that contribute to improving the yield of FCM in assessing non-HN.

DISCLOSURE

The authors have no financial or nonfinancial conflict of interests.

REFERENCES

1. Hermansen DK, Badalament RA, Fair WR, et al. Detection of bladder carcinoma in females by flow cytometry and cytology. Cytometry 1989;10:739–42.
2. Chen LM, Lazcano O, Katzmann JA, et al. The role of conventional cytology, immunocytochemistry, and flow cytometric DNA ploidy in the evaluation of body cavity fluids: a prospective study of 52 patients. Am J Clin Pathol 1998; 109:712–21.
3. Saha I, Dey P, Vhora H, et al. Role of DNA flow cytometry and image cytometry on effusion fluid. Diagn Cytopathol 2000;22:81–5.
4. Kentrou NA, Tsagarakis NJ, Tzanetou K, et al. An improved flow cytometric assay for detection and discrimination between malignant cells and atypical mesothelial cells, in serous cavity effusions. Cytometry B 2011;80B:324–34.
5. Friedman MT, Gentile P, Tarectecan A, et al. Malignant mesothelioma: immunohistochemistry and DNA ploidy analysis as methods to differentiate mesothelioma from benign reactive mesothelial cell proliferation and adenocarcinoma in pleural and peritoneal effusions. Arch Pathol Lab Med 1996;120:959–66.
6. Arjen Rijken MD, Andrew Dekker MD, Suzanne Taylor MD, et al. Diagnostic value of DNA analysis in effusions by flow cytometry and image analysis: a prospective study on 102 patients as compared with cytologic examination. Am J Clin Pathol 1991;95(1):6–12.
7. Lazcano O, Chen LM, Tsai C, et al. Image analysis and flow cytometric DNA studies of benign and malignant body cavity fluids: reappraisal of the role of current methods in the differential diagnosis of reactive *versus* malignant conditions. Mod Pathol 2000;13:788–96.
8. Fiegl M, Zojer N, Kaufmann H, et al. Hyperdiploidy and apparent aneusomy in mesothelial cells from non-malignant effusions as detected by fluorescence in situ hybridization (FISH). Cytometry 1999;38:15–23.
9. Risberg B, Davidson B, Dong HP, et al. Flow cytometric immunophenotyping of serous effusions and peritoneal washings: comparison with immunocytochemistry and morphological findings. J Clin Pathol 2000;53(7):513–7.
10. Davidson B, Dong HP, Holth A, et al. Flow cytometric immunophenotyping of cancer cells in effusion specimens: diagnostic and research applications. Diagn Cytopathol 2007;35:568–78.
11. Sigstad E, Dong HP, Nielsen S, et al. Quantitative analysis of integrin expression in effusions using flow cytometric immunophenotyping. Diagn Cytopathol 2005; 33(5):325–31.
12. Pillai V, Dorfman DM. Flow cytometry of nonhematopoietic neoplasms. Acta Cytol 2016;60:336–43.
13. Ravoet C, Demartin S, Gerard R, et al. Contribution of flow cytometry to the diagnosis of malignant and non malignant conditions in lymph node biopsies. Leuk Lymphoma 2004;45(8):1587–93.

14. Hartana C, Kinn J, Rosenblatt R, et al. Detection of micrometastases by flow cytometry in sentinel lymph nodes from patients with renal tumours. Br J Cancer 2016;115:957–66.
15. Annunziata J, Miller ML, Park DC, et al. Detection of nonhematologic neoplasms by routine flow cytometry analysis. Am J Clin Pathol 2020;153(1):99–104.
16. Chang A, Benda PM, Wood BL, et al. Lineage-specific identification of nonhematopoietic neoplasms by flow cytometry. Am J Clin Pathol 2003;119(5):643–55.
17. Tamai M, Tanimura H, Yamaue H, et al. Expression of carcinoembryonic antigen in fresh human gastric cancer cells assessed by flow cytometry. J Surg Oncol 1993; 52(3):176–80.
18. Stacchini A, Aliberti S, Demurtas A, et al. Flow cytometry dentification of nonhemopoietic neoplasms during routine immunophenotyping. Int J Lab Hematol 2019;41(2):208–17.
19. Bryson GJ, Lear D, Williamson R, et al. Detection of the CD56+/CD45- immunophenotype by flow cytometry in neuroendocrine malignancies. J Clin Pathol 2002; 55(7):535–7.
20. Farinola MA, Weir EG, Ali SZ. CD56 expression of neuroendocrine neoplasms on immunophenotyping by flow cytometry: a novel diagnostic approach to fine-needle aspiration biopsy. Cancer 2003;99:240–6.
21. Leon ME, Hou JS, Galindo LM, et al. Fine-needle aspiration of adult small-round-cell tumors studied with flow cytometry. Diagn Cytopathol 2004;31:147–54.
22. Ferreira-Facio CS, Milito C, Botafogo V, et al. Contribution of multiparameter flow cytometry immunophenotyping to the diagnostic screening and classification of pediatric cancer. PLoS One 2013;8(3):e55534.
23. Gautam U, Srinivasan R, Rajwanshi A, et al. Comparative evaluation of flow-cytometric immunophenotyping and immunocytochemistry in the categorization of malignant small round cell tumors in fine-needle aspiration cytologic specimens. Cancer 2008;114(6):494–503.
24. Bozzi F, Collini P, Aiello A, et al. Flow cytometric phenotype of rhabdomyosarcoma bone marrow metastatic cells and its implication in differential diagnosis with neuroblastoma. Anticancer Res 2008;28(3A):1565–9.
25. Swerts K, De Moerloose B, Dhooge C, et al. Detection of residual neuroblastoma cells in bone marrow: comparison of flow cytometry with immunocytochemistry. Cytometry 2004;61B:9–19.
26. Ferreira-Facio CS, Botafogo V, Ferrão PM, et al. Flow cytometry immunophenotyping for diagnostic orientation and classification of pediatric cancer based on the EuroFlow solid tumor orientation tube (STOT). Cancers (Basel) 2021;13(19): 4945.
27. Cai J-Y, Pan Ci, Tang Y-J, et al. Minimal residual disease is a prognostic marker for neuroblastoma with bone marrow infiltration. Am J Clin Oncol 2012;35(3): 275–8.
28. Theodorakos I, Paterakis G, Papadakis V, et al. Interference of bone marrow CD56+ mesenchymal stromal cells in minimal residual disease investigation of neuroblastoma and other CD45-/CD56+ pediatric malignancies using flow cytometry. Pediatr Blood Cancer 2019;66:e27799.
29. Okcu MF, Wang RY, Bueso-Ramos C, et al. Flow cytometry and fluorescence in situ hybridization to detect residual neuroblastoma cells in bone marrow. Pediatr Blood Cancer 2005;45(6):787–95.
30. Furlanetto G, Spagnol F, Alegretti AP, et al. Flow cytometry as a diagnostic tool in neuroblastoma. J Immunol Methods 2021;498:113135.

31. Nagai J, Ishida Y, Koga N, et al. A new sensitive and specific combination of CD81/CD56/CD45 monoclonal antibodies for detecting circulating neuroblastoma cells in peripheral blood using flow cytometry. J Pediatr Hematol Oncol 2000;22(1):20–6.
32. Popov A, Druy A, Shorikov E, et al. Prognostic value of initial bone marrow disease detection by multiparameter flow cytometry in children with neuroblastoma. J Cancer Res Clin Oncol 2019;145:535–42.
33. Shen H, Tang Y, Xu X, et al. Rapid detection of neoplastic cells in serous cavity effusions in children with flow cytometry immunophenotyping. Leuk Lymphoma 2012;53(8):1509–14.
34. Esser R, Glienke W, Bochennek K, et al. Detection of neuroblastoma cells during clinical follow up: advanced flow cytometry and rt-PCR for tyrosine hydroxylase using both conventional and real-time PCR. Klin Pädiatr 2011;223(6):326–31.
35. Quiros-Caso C, Arias Fernández T, Fonseca-Mourelle A, et al. Routine flow cytometry approach for the evaluation of solid tumor neoplasms and immune cells in minimally invasive samples. Cytometry B Clin Cytometry 2022;102(4):272–82.
36. Corver WE, Cornelisse CJ. Flow Cytometry of human solid tumours: clinical and research applications. Curr Diagn Pathol 2002;8:249–67.
37. Pillai V, Cibas ES, Dorfman DM. A simplified flow cytometric immunophenotyping procedure for the diagnosis of effusions caused by epithelial malignancies. Am J Clin Pathol 2013;139(5):672–81.

Evolving Approach to Clinical Cytometry for Immunodeficiencies and Other Immune Disorders

Amir A. Sadighi Akha, MD, DPhil[a], Krisztián Csomós, PhD[b],
Boglárka Ujházi, MSc[b], Jolán E. Walter, MD, PhD[b],
Attila Kumánovics, MD[a],*

KEYWORDS

- Primary immunodeficiency • Inborn errors of immunity • Autoimmunity
- Flow cytometry • T-bet[+] B cells

KEY POINTS

- Our understanding of immune cells has been mainly due to our ability to identify them by flow cytometric methods.
- Improvements in existing flow cytometers, invention of spectral and mass cytometry, the surge in the variety and number of available fluorochromes, and increase in the computational power and sophistication of analytic approaches have increased the ability and scope of immunophenotyping and can be used to discover novel subsets.
- The significant progress in our understanding of primary immunodeficiencies has led to a conceptual shift, which questions the traditional boundaries between these diseases and other categories of immune-mediated disease.
- T-bet[+] B cells display a high degree of heterogeneity, plasticity, and sex-specific regulation and have distinct trafficking and tissue distribution characteristics.
- T-bet[+] B cells can be identified in all of the traditional B cell subsets except transitional B cells.

FLOW CYTOMETRY: NOVEL METHODS DRIVE THE DISCOVERY OF NOVEL SUBSETS

Our current understanding of immune cells and their respective subsets has been mainly due to our ability to identify and quantify them by flow cytometric methods. This achievement has hinged on the availability of antibodies specific for the numerous

[a] Department of Laboratory Medicine and Pathology, Mayo Clinic, Rochester, MN, USA;
[b] Division of Pediatric Allergy/Immunology, University of South Florida, Johns Hopkins All Children's Hospital, St. Petersburg, FL, USA
* Corresponding author.
E-mail address: kumanovics.attila@mayo.edu

Clin Lab Med 43 (2023) 467–483
https://doi.org/10.1016/j.cll.2023.05.002   labmed.theclinics.com
0272-2712/23/© 2023 Elsevier Inc. All rights reserved.

markers expressed by different immune cells and of instruments with the necessary sensitivity and resolution to detect them. The first requisite was addressed by Kohler and Milstein's development of monoclonal antibodies[1] and complemented by the availability and use of an increasing number of fluorochrome conjugates.[2] The second was made possible by inventing fluorescent flow cytometers, which required advances in physics, chemistry, instrumentation manufacturing, and computation. The first flow cytometers that could detect signals from fluorescently labeled antibodies, and were fundamentally the same as the current ones, were introduced in the early 1970s.[3] These instruments had a single laser as the light source and could identify cells based on fluorescein-labeled antibodies. This allowed the identification and sorting of lymphocytes into two subsets: T and B lymphocytes.[4] With further development, the number of markers increased to three by the 1980s and to five in the 1990s.[2] Currently, a single laser can excite five to six dyes and commercial equipment may contain four or five different lasers. This has culminated in the description of dozens of subsets for both B and T cells in human peripheral blood, which have to be considered during the evaluation of immunodeficiencies and other immune disorders.[5–10]

In conventional (polychromatic) flow cytometry, the emitted light is measured at certain (selected) wavelengths. One of the main impediments to increasing the number of fluorophores that can be used in the same assay is the increasing spectral overlap between the emitted light and the various fluorescent dyes. Accounting for these fluorescence spill-over emissions into nondetection (secondary) channels (wavelengths) requires additional controls, such as single stain controls, and a mathematical correction process called compensation. Currently, the two main approaches used to overcome this impediment are spectral fluorescent flow cytometry and mass cytometry.

In spectral flow cytometry,[11] the light is dispersed using gratings or prisms and the whole spectrum is measured, not just selected wavelengths. In this type of flow cytometry, the spectral signature is the most significant parameter. The individual signals are identified by spectral unmixing. This increases the individual resolution of fluorophores with similar emission spectra and allows the development of multicolor panels with up to 30-40 markers. Spectral flow cytometry allows subtraction of cellular autofluorescence, which increases signal-to-noise ratios and the detection of dim samples.

Mass cytometry is another successful method to avoid the limitations of fluorescence. The use of transition element (lanthanide) isotopes not normally found in biological systems as labels, instead of fluorescent tags, is an elegant solution for practically eliminating spectral interference.[12] In mass cytometry, the elemental ions (metal-isotope-tagged antibodies) are measured by a time-of-flight inductively coupled plasma mass spectrometer (also known as cytometry by time-of-flight). This approach allows the routine use of 40-50 markers per cell. The lack of background ("autofluorescence" in traditional flow cytometry) and compensation issues without losing sensitivity is an additional advantage of this method. The lower sampling efficiency (cell loss) and increased acquisition time are the main disadvantages of mass cytometry. The data are recorded in the same way as in fluorescent flow cytometry, allowing analysis using the same flow cytometry software. Although the quantitative and qualitative results obtained by fluorescent and mass cytometry methods are closely matched and largely interchangeable,[13] allowing its incorporation into clinical testing, for now mass cytometry mostly remains in the confines of research.

Traditional manual analysis mainly uses one-parameter histograms and two-parameter (two-dimensional, bivariate, or biaxial) data plots. Clinical flow cytometry still largely relies on manual gating and looks for predetermined phenotypes based on prior knowledge and experience. Although automated tools exist for sequential gating around cell populations in two-parameter plots, the markers analyzed are still defined by the operator relying on a priori knowledge.

In discovery research, where 20-50 markers are measured, gating of one (histograms) or two (bivariant plots) markers at a time is no longer practical and useful for viewing and interpreting the data. This has prompted the introduction of novel analysis methods, including multivariate approaches and the replacement of user-guided gating/clustering. **Figs. 1** and **2** compare the traditional and high-dimensional gating approaches for identifying particular B cell subsets and illustrate the advantages of a high-dimensional gating strategy. Most markers used for B-cell subset phenotyping show a continuous expression (nonbinary) and are individually non-discriminatory (eg, CD24 and CD38), necessitating the use of marker combinations to identify a particular subset. Although a clear discrimination of transitional B cells from mature naive B cells is difficult with conventional manual gating (see **Fig. 1**), high-dimensional analysis can clearly separate transitional B cells (Cluster 1; light blue) from mature naive B cells (Cluster 2; dark blue), as shown in **Fig. 2**A and C.

Fully automated methods most often used are based on dimensionality reduction and clustering.[14–17] Dimensionality reduction projects high-dimensional data into a lower dimensional space by losing as little information as possible. Overall, principal component analysis (PCA) is probably the best-known approach. PCA is a linear reduction method used to understand the global structure of the data set. Currently, the nonlinear *t*-distributed stochastic neighbor embedding (t-SNE) algorithm is probably the most used approach for dimensionality reduction in flow cytometry. The advantage is that t-SNE algorithm preserves local structures. Clustering-based approaches place cells with similar marker profiles into cell clusters in the original high-dimensional space. Clustering is an unsupervised machine learning approach used for pattern discovery. Clustering approaches are classified according to the algorithm used for identifying the similarities between cells, such as hierarchical and

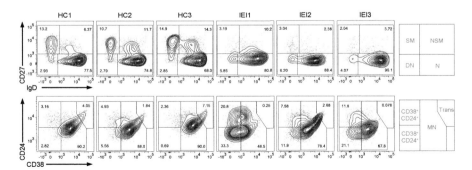

Fig. 1. *B-cell subset analysis by conventional biaxial gating using traditional surface B-cell markers.* Frozen PBMC samples were stained for viability and conventional B-cell markers (CD19, CD27, IgD, CD24, and CD38). Total B cells are defined as CD19$^+$ from single cells/lymphocytes (not shown). Representative biaxial contour plots of three healthy controls (HC) and three patients with inborn errors of immunity (IEI). Total naive (*N*), non-switched memory (NSM), switched memory (SM), and IgD CD27 double-negative (DN) B cells are defined as IgD$^+$ CD27$^-$, IgD$^+$ CD27$^+$, IgD$^-$ CD27$^+$, IgD$^-$ CD27$^-$ cells, respectively (upper plots). Transitional (Trans), mature naive (MN), and two CD38$^-$ subsets are identified from total naive B cells (CD19$^+$ IgD$^+$ CD27$^-$) as CD38^{high}CD24^{high}, CD38^{int}CD24^{int}, CD38$^-$CD24$^+$, and CD38$^-$CD24$^-$ cells, respectively (lower plots).

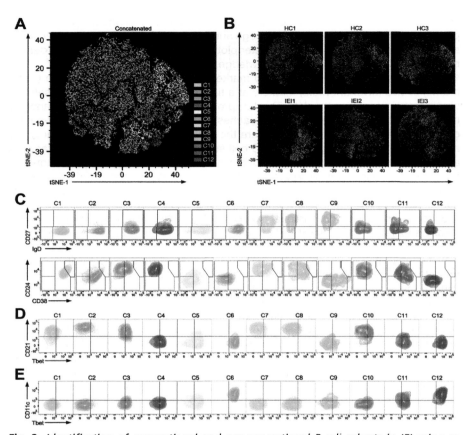

Fig. 2. *Identification of conventional and nonconventional B-cell subsets in IEI using an extended B cell staining panel with automated unsupervised clustering.* Concatenated live B cells from the same data set as shown in **Fig. 1** were subjected to unsupervised high-dimensional analysis using FlowSOM. CD11c, CD21, CD24, CD27, CD38, IgD, and T-bet parameters were simultaneously used to assign live CD19⁺ B cells from each subject by a self-organizing map (SOM) in a 10×10 grid resulting in 100 different nodes. Then, nodes were classified into 12 metaclusters, each representing a unique B-cell subset. To visualize B-cell subset composition, t-SNE analysis was performed on the concatenated data set using default settings. (*A*) t-SNE analysis of concatenated CD19⁺ B cells from three HCs and three IEI patients. Each color represents a B-cell subset. (*B*) Subset distribution by subjects defined by t-SNE analysis. (*C–E*) Projection of each t-SNE-defined subset of concatenated data set into conventional biaxial contour plots. (*C*) Upper row: IgD versus CD27, lower row: CD38 versus CD24. (*D*) T-bet versus CD21. (*E*) T-bet versus CD11c. Colors in (*A–E*) depict the same subsets. t-SNE-defined subsets (C1–12) allow the identification of both conventional (see **Fig. 1**) and nonconventional subsets. High-dimensional gating allows the resolution of conventional subsets, such as the mature naive subset, into multiple subdivisions. For example, the resolution of the mature naive subset (C2–C6) by the decrease of CD38 in C3–C6, the decrease of CD24 in C5–C6 and decrease of CD21 in C4–C6, whereas T-bet is gradually increasing in C3–C6, and CD11c is high in C6. The DN clusters (C10, C11, and C12) are resolved with decreasing CD21, and increasing T-bet and CD11c expression into DN1 (C10) and DN2 (C11–C12) subsets.

density-based clustering. Clustering has its limitations in understanding biology, as a continuum of transitional cell states often exists. Additional methods, such as trajectory inference (or pseudo-time/pseudo-temporal ordering), can be used to order single-cell data along developmental trajectories and arrange cells based on marker expression gradients.[18] These can, for example, be used to recapitulate the development of naive B cells from hematopoietic stem cells.[19] Fortunately, most of the computational algorithmic methods used for high-dimensional flow cytometry can also be used for other single-cell data, such as single-cell RNA-seq and others which are increasingly used in discovery research.[20]

Flow cytometry using either traditional operator-based or algorithmic approaches allows for the discovery of new cell types by using novel and often unexpected combinations of markers. High-dimensional flow cytometry or not, different research groups may use different sets of markers and analyze them using different definitions, gating approaches and algorithms. This necessitates additional studies to establish that various prior descriptions in fact identify the same cell type and to determine the best way to define the novel population for clinical practice. The multiple independent approaches that culminated in the discovery of T-bet$^+$ B cells are a good example of this process.

CONCEPTUAL EVOLUTION IN OUR UNDERSTANDING OF PRIMARY IMMUNODEFICIENCIES

In tandem with advances in immunophenotyping, there has been a significant progress in our understanding of primary immunodeficiencies (PIDs). PIDs are caused by germline mutations that affect the development and/or function of immune cells. The point of departure for the current understanding of this group of diseases is arguably the discovery of X-linked agammaglobulinemia by Ogden Bruton,[21] and the early independent description of what is now known as severe combined immunodeficiency (SCID) by Glanzmann and Riniker[22] and Hitzig and colleagues[23] The first attempt to classify PIDs in 1968 included only 11 entities.[24] In the intervening period, advances in molecular genetics and cellular immunology have substantially increased the number of identified conditions and their phenotypic and biological definition,[25,26] with the most recent report of the International Union of Immunological Societies (IUIS) Committee including a total of 485 entities.[27] The field's progress is multilayered in nature and goes beyond a simple exponential increase in the number of identified entities. The broadening of clinical phenotypes, description of PIDs with narrow phenotype, discovery of PID phenocopies, and a conceptual shift from PIDs to inborn errors of immunity (IEIs) are among the most important advances in this respect:

The increase in the number of documented patients with different IEIs has coincided with the broadening of the clinical phenotypes in comparison to the initial reports for each entity. This is at least in part due to the distinct mechanistic effects of different mutations in a gene, including loss of function (LOF), gain of function (GOF), haploinsufficiency, and dominant-negative effects; see Refs[28–31] as examples of these mechanisms. The most telling example is observed with mutations in recombinase-activating genes 1 and 2 (*RAG1* and *RAG2*), where a continuum of changes in the catalytic activity of the RAG complex can manifest as T$^-$ B$^-$ NK$^+$ SCID; Omenn syndrome with immunodeficiency, generalized erythroderma, and tissue damage due to infiltration with autologous oligoclonal T cells; leaky SCID; and combined immunodeficiency with granulomas and/or autoimmunity.[32] Immune dysregulation is a cardinal feature of the latter 3, with extensive evidence of impairments in both central and peripheral tolerance.

In classical immunodeficiencies such as SCID and X-linked agammaglobulinemia, it is appreciated that the patient would be subject to recurrent infections and that the affected arm of the immune system would determine the nature of the pathogens involved, that is, bacteria, viruses, parasites, or fungi.[25] The discovery of entities such as Mendelian susceptibility to mycobacterial disease, where more than a dozen genetic etiologies impair interferon (IFN)-γ-mediated immunity and predispose the patient to infection with a narrow group of organisms, and inherited defects in the toll-like receptor (TLR)-3 signaling pathway that underlie herpes simplex encephalitis of childhood, form the biologic basis for the concept of PIDs with narrow phenotype.[33–35]

In tandem with the growing understanding of the genetic basis of PIDs, it has become clear that somatic mutations in genes involved in PIDs and autoantibodies to cytokines and/or other proteins of the immune system can manifest as phenocopies of specific PIDs in the absence of the underlying germline mutations for the particular PID. The most recent IUIS classification includes 10 separate categories, of which 9 tabulate genetically identified categories of PIDs, whereas the 10th one is devoted to known phenocopies of these diseases.[27,36]

Since their inception, PIDs had been viewed as entities that substantially increase the risk of infection in affected individuals. It is now realized that based on the nature of the affliction, the patients may present with allergy, autoimmunity, autoinflammation, or malignancy as component(s) or main feature(s) of their disease.[37] This has led to the adoption of the term "Inborn Errors of Immunity", instead of PID in the IUIS classification as a more inclusive description for this group of diseases.[27,36]

This change in terminology is not an arcane nosological exercise. It argues against categorical boundaries between immunodeficiencies and other immune-mediated diseases and has important implications in both clinical and laboratory practice. At the clinical level, it would translate into searching and/or expecting a broader set of signs, symptoms, and pathologic consequences than originally envisaged in patients with PIDs. At the laboratory level, it could necessitate the use of additional markers for evaluating the spectrum of the patient's condition and/or modify the utility and interpretive scope of existing laboratory tests. In the context of flow cytometry, this is relevant to assays evaluating immune cells. In this article, we focus on T-bet⁺ B cells as an example for exploring the implications of this change on the scope and interpretation of clinical cytometry tests.

T-BET⁺ B CELLS

In humans, under normal conditions, the peripheral blood B-cell compartment mainly consists of transitional B cells, naive B cells, memory B cells, and a small subset of antibody secreting cells, which can be effectively distinguished by a combination of cluster of differentiation (CD)19, CD24, CD27, CD38, and immunoglobulin D (IgD) (see Fig. 1).[38,39] For years, in diagnostic immunophenotyping, CD27 expression has been widely used as the defining marker of human memory B cells.[40,41] However, a broad base of basic and clinical research has identified a number of functionally significant memory B-cell subsets that are CD27⁻,[42] underscoring the limitations of using CD27 as a universal marker for the study of human memory B cells. Currently placed under the rubric of double-negative (DN) memory B cells, characterized by the absence of both CD27 and IgD expression, the CD27⁻ memory B cells themselves comprise diverse subsets with distinct phenotypes, functions, and anatomic locations.

T-bet⁺ B cells, a predominantly CD27⁻ memory B-cell subset, have been the focus of increasing interest over the past decade. Their characterization is the result of extensive independent studies in mice and humans on an overlapping group of B cell subsets variously called DN B cells, DN2, CD21[low] B cells, tissue-based, atypical, exhausted, and age-associated B cells (ABCs),[42] henceforth solely referred to as T-bet[+] B cells. While not the first studies on the subject, the companion papers published by the Cancro[43] and Marrack[44] laboratories have had a pivotal role in defining this population. The two groups used different criteria to identify these cells, with the Cancro group defining them as B220[+] CD19[+] CD21[-] CD23[-] CD95[-] CD43[-] splenic cells,[43] whereas the Marrack laboratory relied on CD11c expression on B220[+] CD19[+] splenic cells for this purpose.[44] Because of the expansion of this population with age, both groups named them ABCs.

ABCs display particular signaling characteristics. They do not divide in response to B-cell receptor (BCR) cross-linking alone but do so when stimulated through TLR7 or TLR9.[43] Gene expression profiling showed high expression levels of T-bet (T-box transcription factor TBX21, also called *T-box expressed in T cells*) in ABCs,[44] a finding subsequently replicated in numerous laboratories, hence the moniker T-bet[+] B cells. T-bet was originally identified in mice as a critical factor for T helper (Th)1 differentiation and IFN-γ expression.[45] Subsequent studies have shown that it is expressed widely and functions in most major immune cell types.[46] T-bet[+] B cells can produce antibodies, with their isotype switching skewed toward immunoglobulin G (IgG)1 in humans and IgG2a/c in mice.[47] They can also produce pro-inflammatory and anti-inflammatory cytokines such as IFN-γ, tumor necrosis factor (TNF)-α, interleukin (IL)-17, and IL-10.[43,48,49] Owing to their high level of major histocompatibility complex (MHC) class II expression, they are also good antigen-presenting cells.[43,44,50]

In terms of ontogeny, initial adoptive transfer studies had established that follicular B cells may serve as the precursors for T-bet[+] cells.[44] Subsequent studies in mice showed that T-bet[+] B cells display somatic hypermutation, require cell-intrinsic MHC class II and CD40 expression and do not develop in the absence of CD154,[51] implying that these cells are the product of an antigen-driven process. In order for a follicular B cell to differentiate to a T-bet[+] B cell, the antigens encountered by the B cell must include TLR7 or TLR9 agonists. Subsequent exposure to either IFN-γ or IL-21 would enable the emergence of T-bet[+] cells through this pathway. IL-4 can inhibit the IL-21-mediated differentiation but will not affect the IFN-γ-driven process.[52] Nonetheless, it has been suggested that follicular B cells may not be the sole precursor for T-bet[+] B cells[50,53,54] and that transitional B cells, marginal zone B cells, and B1 B cells and extrafollicular differentiation may also contribute to T-bet[+] B cell pools or that the T-bet[+] phenotype may be established through homeostatic proliferation in a manner analogous to normal T-cell homeostasis.[55]

Collectively, mouse and human studies have confirmed the role of these cells in a broad set of contexts including humoral antimicrobial immunity, autoimmune and autoinflammatory disorders, particular IEIs, and the immunobiology of aging.[42,55-58]

Identifying CD21[low] B cells in patients with high human immunodeficiency virus (HIV) loads is one of the first examples of studying B cells with T-bet[+]-like features in human infections.[59] These cells were later described as FcRL4[+] memory B cells.[60] They are distinctively large lymphocytes that preferentially reside near epithelial surfaces, plausibly due to their heightened expression of CCR1 and CCR5 chemokine receptors.[61,62] Expression of Fc (Fragment crystallizable) Receptor Like 4 (FcRL4) dampens BCR-mediated signaling by recruiting Src homology 2 domain-containing protein tyrosine phosphatase (SHP)-1 and/or SHP-2 to its immunoreceptor tyrosine-based inhibitory motifs[63] while enhancing TLR9-mediated signaling by concentrating in endosomes after exposure to TLR9 agonists.[64] They show similar levels of somatic hypermutation and isotype switching with the CD27[+] memory B cells and can secrete high levels of antibodies on stimulation with T-cell cytokines.[61] Subsequent work has confirmed that these cells are in fact T-bet+.[65,66]

HIV is not unique in this respect, as increases in T-bet+ B cells can be seen in a number of viral, bacterial, and parasitic infections, including hepatitis C virus,[67] tuberculosis,[68] malaria[69–71] and severe acute respiratory syndrome coronavirus 2 (SARS-COV-2)[72–74] infections, and also after vaccination.[75,76] The human studies have been paralleled by animal models, including the study of gamma herpesvirus 68, lymphocytic choriomeningitis virus, murine cytomegalovirus and vaccinia infections,[77,78] Ehrlichia muris, a mouse obligate intracellular tick-borne pathogen,[79–81] and other bacterial infections.[82]

Based on the clearance or persistence of the infection, the increased frequency of T-bet+ B cells in the peripheral blood may be transient or sustained. By contrast, during steady-state conditions, these cells mainly reside in the spleen and do not circulate systemically,[47] leading to the assertion that the peripheral blood and splenic pools of T-bet+ B cells are not in equilibrium.[55]

In addition to microbe-specific humoral responses, T-bet+ B cells arise in the context of autoimmunity. This was first reported by the Marrack group in mouse models of autoimmunity and the peripheral blood of patients with rheumatoid arthritis and scleroderma.[44] Subsequent studies have confirmed and expanded these initial findings. There is now compelling evidence for the association of T-bet+ B cells with systemic lupus erythematosus (SLE)[53,83] and their similarity with the T-bet+ B cells in mouse models of the disease.[44,84] The presence of these cells in the peripheral blood strongly correlates with SLE disease activity,[83] a finding reminiscent of the relationship between the frequency of T-bet+ B cells with viral, bacterial, or parasitic load during infection. In addition to SLE, T-bet+ B cells are a common feature of other autoimmune and autoinflammatory disorders including rheumatoid arthritis,[44,85] multiple sclerosis,[86,87] Sjogren's syndrome,[88] Crohn's disease,[89] axial spondyloarthritis,[90] and Down's syndrome.[91] Producing autoantibodies, making cytokines particularly those associated with a Th1 signature, and activating inflammatory T cells are among the suggested mechanisms for the contribution of T-bet+ B cells to autoimmunity.[57]

T-bet+ B cells have also been identified in certain IEIs. It has been shown that a subgroup of patients with common variable immunodeficiency, who in addition to infections are prone to autoimmunity and present with conditions such as autoimmune cytopenia and interstitial lung disease, have an increased frequency of T-bet+ B cells.[92–95] More recently, the study of B-cell development in humans with partial RAG deficiency has shown defective humoral tolerance with a shift toward increased frequency of T-bet+ B cells.[10] Investigating other IEIs has helped to further delineate the requirements for the development of T-bet+ B cells.[96] The study of a patient with T-bet deficiency has shown that T-bet is required for the in vivo and in vitro development of CD11c^hi CD21^low B cells,[96] thereby helping to resolve the controversy surrounding the role of T-bet in the generation of these cells.[97–99] It has also been shown that patients with complete autosomal recessive STAT1 deficiency or with IFN-γ receptor 1 (IFN-γR1) deficiency have reduced frequencies of CD11c^hi CD21^low T-bet+ B cells and that IFN-γ and IL-27 in part compensate for one another in the generation of these cells.[96] In addition, B cells from patients with impaired BCR-mediated nuclear factor kappa-light-chain-enhancer of activated B cells (NF-κB) signaling due to LOF CARD1 and MALT1 mutations have a limited ability to develop into T-bet+ B cells.[100]

The contribution of T-bet+ B cells to both antimicrobial immunity and self-reactive responses has been the focus of detailed investigation. Earlier studies showed that the engagement of TLR7/TLR9 is required, but not sufficient, for the development of

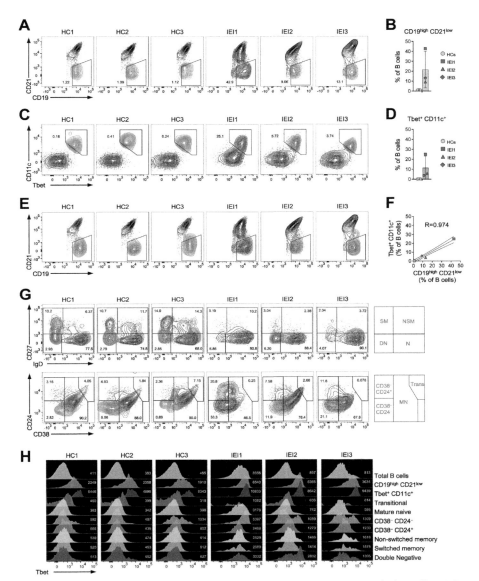

Fig. 3. *Detection of nonconventional B-cell subsets in IEI using an extended B cell staining panel and conventional biaxial gating.* Frozen PBMC samples were stained for viability and surface stained for CD19, CD27, IgD, CD24, CD38, CD21, CD11c, and then fixed, permeabilized and stained for T-bet intracellularly. Contour plots and graphs show indicated B-cell subsets from the same HCs (*n* = 3) and IEI patients (*n* = 3) as in **Figs. 1** and **2**. Proportions of specific B-cell subsets are indicated as percentage of total B cells in each contour plot. Graphs show the proportions of specific B-cell subsets in HCs (gray symbols) and IEI patients (red symbols). (*A*) Contour plots depict CD19^{high} CD21^{low} B cells (blue) from total B cells. (*B*) Graph shows the proportion of CD19^{high} CD21^{low} cells. (*C*) Contour plots depict T-bet^{+} CD11c^{+} B cells (red) from total B cells. (*D*) Graph shows the proportion of T-bet^{+} CD11c^{+}. (*E*) Contour plots show the distribution of T-bet^{+} CD11c^{+} cells (red) among total B cells (black) (T-bet^{+} CD11c^{+} cells are overlayed on total B cells). (*F*) Correlation between the

T-bet$^+$ B cells.[52] Subsequent studies have revealed the divergent roles of these molecules in B-cell tolerance and autoimmunity: TLR7 deficiency diminishes autoimmune manifestations, whereas TLR7 duplication,[101,102] or TLR7 GOF mutations[103] exacerbate it, with high TLR7 dosage causing acute inflammatory pathology and profound dendritic cell dysregulation.[101,102] By contrast, TLR9 deficiency would lead to more pronounced autoimmunity.[104,105] This has led to the hypothesis that in addition to established central and peripheral mechanisms of B-cell tolerance that are based on BCR epitope specificity, molecular pattern recognition systems can play a role in establishing peripheral B-cell tolerance.[106]

T-bet$^+$ B cells significantly increase with age in both humans and mice,[43,44] hence the name ABCs. Aging leads to a set of functional and structural alterations in the immune system that can manifest as a decreased ability to fight infection, diminished response to vaccination, increased incidence of cancer, higher prevalence of autoimmunity, and constitutive low-grade inflammation (also known as inflammaging). These are broadly referred to as immunosenescence,[107,108] which should not be conflated with cellular senescence as defined by Hayflick.[109] B cell changes with aging include a significant decrease in B-cell precursors, a progressive shift towards homeostatic expansion of antigen-experienced cells and B-cell intrinsic defects including, but not limited to, impaired induction of E47 with a consequent decrease in activation-induced cytidine deaminase and its downstream effects.[110,111]

The contribution of T-bet$^+$ B cells to B-cell immunosenescence has to be viewed in this broader context. T-bet$^+$ B cells produce TNF-α, which interferes with B-cell maturation by inducing pro-B-cell apoptosis and exerting an overall inflammatory effect on the bone marrow microenvironment.[49,112] T-bet$^+$ B cells express B-cell activating factor receptor (BAFF-R) and transmembrane activator and calcium-modulator and cyclophilin ligand (CAML) interactor (TACI) receptors but are independent of BAFF-R for their survival.[43] As BAFF and its receptors mediate peripheral B-cell homeostasis,[113] this would allow T-bet$^+$ B cells to sequester BAFF at the expense of the follicular and marginal zone B cells and to gradually displace them with advancing age. This shift in the peripheral B-cell pool can have a number of functional corollaries: One of them is that the response to antigenic challenges would increasingly depend on recruiting T-bet$^+$ B cells instead of naive follicular B cells,[114] thereby augmenting the role of the already existing repertoire in both primary and recall responses.[55] The other is that with their predilection to produce pro-inflammatory cytokines, they may contribute to the constitutive low-grade inflammation observed with age.

It is worth noting that the contribution of T-bet$^+$ B cells to antimicrobial immunity, autoimmunity, IEIs, and aging should not be viewed as discrete phenomena, but as interrelated components of a broader picture. An example of this is the discovery of shared transcriptional profiles of these cells in the context of malaria, HIV, and autoimmunity.[48]

---

fraction of CD19^{high} CD21^{low} (x-axis) and T-bet$^+$ CD11c$^+$ (y-axis) in HCs and IEI patients. Linear regression line is shown with 95% confidence intervals, Pearson R value is indicated. (G) Contour plots show the distribution of T-bet$^+$ CD11c$^+$ cells (red) among N, NSM, SM, and DN B cells (black) in upper panels and the naive T-bet$^+$ CD11c$^+$ cells (red) among Tran, MN, CD38$^-$CD24$^+$, and CD38$^-$CD24$^-$ total naive B cells (IgD$^+$ CD27$^-$) (black) in lower panels. Total naive (N), non-switched memory (NSM), switched memory (SM) and IgD CD27 double-negative (DN) B cells. (H) Histograms show the expression level of T-bet in total B cells, CD19^{high} CD21^{low}, T-bet$^+$ CD11c$^+$, Tran, MN, CD38$^-$CD24$^-$, CD38$^-$CD24$^+$, NSM, SM, and DN B cells. Geometric mean fluorescent intensity (gMFI) of T-bet for each population is indicated.

In summary, the cells we have discussed under the name T-bet$^+$ B cells can trace their origin to many different studies in experimental animal models and clinical medicine. Although all these studies included flow cytometry, the markers used varied broadly. This variation in the mode of discovery has led to a variety of names and definitions for these cells, thereby delaying their clinical use. To determine the best approach to identifying these cells, we added CD21, CD11c and T-bet to the conventional panel of CD19, CD24, CD27, CD38 and IgD that is routinely used in clinical B-cell flow cytometry and evaluated peripheral blood mononuclear cells (PBMCs) from three healthy controls and three patients with IEIs. In addition to detecting a number of conventional and nonconventional B-cell subsets (**Fig. 2**C), **Fig. 3** shows that gating CD21^{low} B cells based on CD19 and CD21 expression (**Fig. 3**A), and T-bet$^+$ B cells based on CD11c and T-bet expression (see **Fig. 3**C), result in largely overlapping populations (see **Fig. 3**E) that show good correlation with each other (see **Fig. 3**F). However, the two populations are not identical, and the numerical results are different (see **Fig. 3**B, D, and F). T-bet$^+$ B cells are known to display a high degree of heterogeneity, plasticity and sex-specific regulation, and to have distinct trafficking and tissue distribution characteristics. The current assessment shows that T-bet$^+$ B cells can be detected in all of the traditional B-cell subsets identified using CD19, CD27, IgD, CD24 and CD38, except for transitional B cells (see **Figs. 2**D, E and **3**G, and H), strongly suggesting that the best approach to identifying these cells is the detection of T-bet itself.

SUMMARY

Improvements in existing flow cytometers, invention of spectral and mass cytometry, the surge in the variety and number of available fluorochromes, and an increase in the computational power and sophistication of analytic approaches have increased the abilities and scope of immunophenotyping. In tandem, the significant progress in our understanding of PIDs has led to a conceptual shift which questions the traditional boundaries between these diseases and other categories of immune-mediated disease. Together, these provide an opportunity and a need to use additional markers for evaluating the spectrum of the patient's condition, and/or modify the utility and interpretive scope of existing laboratory tests.

Laboratory immunologists have routinely exercised context-dependent interpretation of flow cytometric findings; a concurrent decrease in class-switched memory B cells and increase in transitional B cells is an important case in point.[39] The current premise goes beyond the current conventional limits. Here, we have focused on T-bet$^+$ B cells as an example to explore this possibility. The discovery of these cells has relied on the use of overlapping but not identical sets of markers, leading to a variety of names and definitions. To determine the best approach to identifying these cells, we added CD21, CD11c, and T-bet to the conventional combination of CD19, CD24, CD27, CD38 and IgD used for B-cell flow cytometry and found that CD19^{hi} CD21^{low} and CD11c$^+$ T-bet$^+$ populations show good correlation but are not identical.

We contend that the best way to detect this population is by directly testing for T-bet expression. The development and clinical implementation of this test will be a valuable tool in the context of infection, autoimmunity, IEIs and aging.

CLINICS CARE POINTS

- Recent medical and technological advances have blurred the traditional boundaries between various immune diseases in flow cytometry testing.

- A novel B-cell subset, variably known as CD21^{low} B cells, age-associated B cells, and T-bet$^+$ B cells, has been independently discovered by using different marker combinations in the contexts of infection, immunodeficiency, autoimmunity, malignancy and aging.
- Direct testing for T-bet expression is our recommended approach for evaluating this population in clinical cytometry.

REFERENCES

1. Kohler G, Milstein C. Continuous cultures of fused cells secreting antibody of predefined specificity. Nature 1975;256:495–7.
2. Chattopadhyay PK, Hogerkorp CM, Roederer M. A chromatic explosion: the development and future of multiparameter flow cytometry. Immunology 2008; 125:441–9.
3. Hulett HR, Bonner WA, Barrett J, et al. Cell sorting: automated separation of mammalian cells as a function of intracellular fluorescence. Science 1969; 166:747–9.
4. Kreth HW, Herzenberg LA. Fluorescence-activated cell sorting of human T and B lymphocytes. I. Direct evidence that lymphocytes with a high density of membrane-bound immunoglobulin are precursors of plasmacytes. Cell Immunol 1974;12:396–406.
5. Spitzer MH, Gherardini PF, Fragiadakis GK, et al. An interactive reference framework for modeling a dynamic immune system. Science 2015;349:1259425.
6. Cheng Y, Newell EW. Deep profiling human T cell heterogeneity by mass cytometry. Adv Immunol 2016;131:101–34.
7. Hsieh EW, Hernandez JD. Novel tools for primary immunodeficiency diagnosis: making a case for deep profiling. Curr Opin Allergy Clin Immunol 2016;16: 549–56.
8. Winkler F, Bengsch B. Use of mass cytometry to profile human T cell exhaustion. Front Immunol 2019;10:3039.
9. Glass DR, Tsai AG, Oliveria JP, et al. An Integrated multi-omic single-cell Atlas of human B cell identity. Immunity 2020;53:217–232 e5.
10. Csomos K, Ujhazi B, Blazso P, et al. Partial RAG deficiency in humans induces dysregulated peripheral lymphocyte development and humoral tolerance defect with accumulation of T-bet(+) B cells. Nat Immunol 2022;23:1256–72.
11. Nolan JP. The evolution of spectral flow cytometry. Cytometry 2022;101:812–7.
12. Bandura DR, Baranov VI, Ornatsky OI, et al. Mass cytometry: technique for real time single cell multitarget immunoassay based on inductively coupled plasma time-of-flight mass spectrometry. Anal Chem 2009;81:6813–22.
13. Ravkov EV, Charlton CM, Barker AP, et al. Evaluation of mass cytometry in the clinical laboratory. Cytometry B Clin Cytom 2019;96:266–74.
14. Saeys Y, Van Gassen S, Lambrecht BN. Computational flow cytometry: helping to make sense of high-dimensional immunology data. Nat Rev Immunol 2016; 16:449–62.
15. Saeys Y, Van Gassen S, Lambrecht B. Response to Orlova et al. "Science not art: statistically sound methods for identifying subsets in multi-dimensional flow and mass cytometry data sets". Nat Rev Immunol 2017;18:78.
16. Hu Z, Bhattacharya S, Butte AJ. Application of machine learning for cytometry data. Front Immunol 2021;12:787574.
17. Chester C, Maecker HT. Algorithmic tools for Mining high-dimensional cytometry data. J Immunol 2015;195:773–9.

18. Saelens W, Cannoodt R, Todorov H, et al. A comparison of single-cell trajectory inference methods. Nat Biotechnol 2019;37:547–54.
19. Bendall SC, Davis KL, Amir el AD, et al. Single-cell trajectory detection uncovers progression and regulatory coordination in human B cell development. Cell 2014;157:714–25.
20. Gao X, Cockburn IA. The development and function of CD11c(+) atypical B cells - insights from single cell analysis. Front Immunol 2022;13:979060.
21. Bruton OC. Agammaglobulinemia. Pediatrics 1952;9:722–8.
22. Glanzmann E, Riniker P. Essential lymphocytophthisis; new clinical aspect of infant pathology. Ann Paediatr 1950;175:1–32.
23. Hitzig WH, Biro Z, Bosch H, et al. Agammaglobulinemia & alymphocytosis with atrophy of lymphatic tissue. Helv Paediatr Acta 1958;13:551–85.
24. Seligmann M, Fudenberg HH, Good RA. A proposed classification of primary immunologic deficiencies. Am J Med 1968;45:817–25.
25. Notarangelo LD, Bacchetta R, Casanova JL, et al. Human inborn errors of immunity: an expanding universe. Sci Immunol 2020;5:eabb1662.
26. Schmitt EG, Cooper MA. Genetics of Pediatric immune-mediated diseases and human immunity. Annu Rev Immunol 2021;39:227–49.
27. Tangye SG, Al-Herz W, Bousfiha A, et al. Human inborn errors of immunity: 2022 Update on the classification from the International union of immunological Societies Expert Committee. J Clin Immunol 2022;42:1473–507.
28. Minegishi Y, Saito M, Tsuchiya S, et al. Dominant-negative mutations in the DNA-binding domain of STAT3 cause hyper-IgE syndrome. Nature 2007;448:1058–62.
29. Flanagan SE, Haapaniemi E, Russell MA, et al. Activating germline mutations in STAT3 cause early-onset multi-organ autoimmune disease. Nat Genet 2014;46:812–4.
30. Hsu AP, Sampaio EP, Khan J, et al. Mutations in GATA2 are associated with the autosomal dominant and sporadic monocytopenia and mycobacterial infection (MonoMAC) syndrome. Blood 2011;118:2653–5.
31. Kuehn HS, Ouyang W, Lo B, et al. Immune dysregulation in human subjects with heterozygous germline mutations in CTLA4. Science 2014;345:1623–7.
32. Villa A, Notarangelo LD. RAG gene defects at the verge of immunodeficiency and immune dysregulation. Immunol Rev 2019;287:73–90.
33. Casanova JL. Human genetic basis of interindividual variability in the course of infection. Proc Natl Acad Sci U S A 2015;112:E7118–27.
34. Casanova JL. Severe infectious diseases of childhood as monogenic inborn errors of immunity. Proc Natl Acad Sci U S A 2015;112:E7128–37.
35. Casanova JL, Abel L. Human genetics of infectious diseases: unique insights into immunological redundancy. Semin Immunol 2018;36:1–12.
36. Bousfiha A, Moundir A, Tangye SG, et al. The 2022 Update of IUIS phenotypical classification for human inborn errors of immunity. J Clin Immunol 2022;42:1508–20.
37. Fischer A, Provot J, Jais JP, et al, members of the CFPIDsg. Autoimmune and inflammatory manifestations occur frequently in patients with primary immunodeficiencies. J Allergy Clin Immunol 2017;140:1388–13893 e8.
38. Sanz I, Wei C, Jenks SA, et al. Challenges and Opportunities for consistent classification of human B cell and plasma cell populations. Front Immunol 2019;10:2458.
39. Kumanovics A, Sadighi Akha AA. Flow cytometry for B-cell subset analysis in immunodeficiencies. J Immunol Methods 2022;509:113327.

40. Klein U, Rajewsky K, Kuppers R. Human immunoglobulin (Ig)M+IgD+ peripheral blood B cells expressing the CD27 cell surface antigen carry somatically mutated variable region genes: CD27 as a general marker for somatically mutated (memory) B cells. J Exp Med 1998;188:1679-89.
41. Tangye SG, Liu YJ, Aversa G, et al. Identification of functional human splenic memory B cells by expression of CD148 and CD27. J Exp Med 1998;188: 1691-703.
42. Cancro MP, Tomayko MM. Memory B cells and plasma cells: the differentiative continuum of humoral immunity. Immunol Rev 2021;303:72-82.
43. Hao Y, O'Neill P, Naradikian MS, et al. A B-cell subset uniquely responsive to innate stimuli accumulates in aged mice. Blood 2011;118:1294-304.
44. Rubtsov AV, Rubtsova K, Fischer A, et al. Toll-like receptor 7 (TLR7)-driven accumulation of a novel CD11c(+) B-cell population is important for the development of autoimmunity. Blood 2011;118:1305-15.
45. Szabo SJ, Kim ST, Costa GL, et al. A novel transcription factor, T-bet, directs Th1 lineage commitment. Cell 2000;100:655-69.
46. Lazarevic V, Glimcher LH, Lord GM. T-bet: a bridge between innate and adaptive immunity. Nat Rev Immunol 2013;13:777-89.
47. Johnson JL, Rosenthal RL, Knox JJ, et al. The transcription factor T-bet resolves memory B cell subsets with distinct tissue distributions and antibody Specificities in mice and humans. Immunity 2020;52:842-855 e6.
48. Holla P, Dizon B, Ambegaonkar AA, et al. Shared transcriptional profiles of atypical B cells suggest common drivers of expansion and function in malaria, HIV, and autoimmunity. Sci Adv 2021;7:eabg8384.
49. Ratliff M, Alter S, Frasca D, et al. In senescence, age-associated B cells secrete TNFalpha and inhibit survival of B-cell precursors. Aging Cell 2013;12:303-11.
50. Rubtsov AV, Rubtsova K, Kappler JW, et al. CD11c-Expressing B cells are located at the T cell/B cell Border in spleen and are Potent APCs. J Immunol 2015;195:71-9.
51. Russell Knode LM, Naradikian MS, Myles A, et al. Age-associated B cells express a diverse repertoire of V(H) and Vkappa genes with somatic hypermutation. J Immunol 2017;198:1921-7.
52. Naradikian MS, Myles A, Beiting DP, et al. Cutting Edge: IL-4, IL-21, and IFN-gamma Interact to Govern T-bet and CD11c expression in TLR-activated B cells. J Immunol 2016;197:1023-8.
53. Jenks SA, Cashman KS, Zumaquero E, et al. Distinct effector B cells induced by Unregulated toll-like receptor 7 contribute to pathogenic responses in systemic lupus erythematosus. Immunity 2018;49:725-739 e6.
54. Woodruff MC, Ramonell RP, Nguyen DC, et al. Extrafollicular B cell responses correlate with neutralizing antibodies and morbidity in COVID-19. Nat Immunol 2020;21:1506-16.
55. Cancro MP. Age-associated B cells. Annu Rev Immunol 2020;38:315-40.
56. Mouat IC, Horwitz MS. Age-associated B cells in viral infection. PLoS Pathog 2022;18:e1010297.
57. Mouat IC, Goldberg E, Horwitz MS. Age-associated B cells in autoimmune diseases. Cell Mol Life Sci 2022;79:402.
58. Phalke S, Rivera-Correa J, Jenkins D, et al. Molecular mechanisms controlling age-associated B cells in autoimmunity. Immunol Rev 2022;307:79-100.
59. Moir S, Malaspina A, Ogwaro KM, et al. HIV-1 induces phenotypic and functional perturbations of B cells in chronically infected individuals. Proc Natl Acad Sci U S A 2001;98:10362-7.

60. Moir S, Ho J, Malaspina A, et al. Evidence for HIV-associated B cell exhaustion in a dysfunctional memory B cell compartment in HIV-infected viremic individuals. J Exp Med 2008;205:1797–805.
61. Ehrhardt GR, Hsu JT, Gartland L, et al. Expression of the immunoregulatory molecule FcRH4 defines a distinctive tissue-based population of memory B cells. J Exp Med 2005;202:783–91.
62. Ehrhardt GR, Hijikata A, Kitamura H, et al. Discriminating gene expression profiles of memory B cell subpopulations. J Exp Med 2008;205:1807–17.
63. Ehrhardt GR, Davis RS, Hsu JT, et al. The inhibitory potential of Fc receptor homolog 4 on memory B cells. Proc Natl Acad Sci U S A 2003;100:13489–94.
64. Sohn HW, Krueger PD, Davis RS, et al. FcRL4 acts as an adaptive to innate molecular switch dampening BCR signaling and enhancing TLR signaling. Blood 2011;118:6332–41.
65. Knox JJ, Buggert M, Kardava L, et al. T-bet+ B cells are induced by human viral infections and dominate the HIV gp140 response. JCI Insight 2017;2:e92943.
66. Austin JW, Buckner CM, Kardava L, et al. Overexpression of T-bet in HIV infection is associated with accumulation of B cells outside germinal centers and poor affinity maturation. Sci Transl Med 2019;11:eaax0904.
67. Chang LY, Li Y, Kaplan DE. Hepatitis C viraemia reversibly maintains subset of antigen-specific T-bet+ tissue-like memory B cells. J Viral Hepat 2017;24:389–96.
68. Joosten SA, van Meijgaarden KE, Del Nonno F, et al. Patients with tuberculosis have a dysfunctional circulating B-cell compartment, which Normalizes following successful Treatment. PLoS Pathog 2016;12:e1005687.
69. Weiss GE, Crompton PD, Li S, et al. Atypical memory B cells are greatly expanded in individuals living in a malaria-endemic area. J Immunol 2009;183:2176–82.
70. Zinocker S, Schindler CE, Skinner J, et al. The V gene repertoires of classical and atypical memory B cells in malaria-susceptible West African children. J Immunol 2015;194:929–39.
71. Obeng-Adjei N, Portugal S, Holla P, et al. Malaria-induced interferon-gamma drives the expansion of Tbethi atypical memory B cells. PLoS Pathog 2017;13:e1006576.
72. Notarbartolo S, Ranzani V, Bandera A, et al. Integrated longitudinal immunophenotypic, transcriptional and repertoire analyses delineate immune responses in COVID-19 patients. Sci Immunol 2021;6:eabg5021.
73. Cervantes-Diaz R, Sosa-Hernandez VA, Torres-Ruiz J, et al. Severity of SARS-CoV-2 infection is linked to double-negative (CD27(-) IgD(-)) B cell subset numbers. Inflamm Res 2022;71:131–40.
74. Castleman MJ, Stumpf MM, Therrien NR, et al. Autoantibodies elicited with SARS-CoV-2 infection are linked to alterations in double negative B cells. Front Immunol 2022;13:988125.
75. Lau D, Lan LY, Andrews SF, et al. Low CD21 expression defines a population of recent germinal center graduates primed for plasma cell differentiation. Sci Immunol 2017;2. eaai8153.
76. Andrews SF, Chambers MJ, Schramm CA, et al. Activation Dynamics and immunoglobulin evolution of Pre-existing and newly generated human memory B cell responses to Influenza Hemagglutinin. Immunity 2019;51:398–410 e5.
77. Rubtsova K, Rubtsov AV, van Dyk LF, et al. T-box transcription factor T-bet, a key player in a unique type of B-cell activation essential for effective viral clearance. Proc Natl Acad Sci U S A 2013;110:E3216–24.

78. Barnett BE, Staupe RP, Odorizzi PM, et al. Cutting Edge: B cell-intrinsic T-bet expression is required to control Chronic viral infection. J Immunol 2016;197: 1017–22.

79. Racine R, Chatterjee M, Winslow GM. CD11c expression identifies a population of extrafollicular antigen-specific splenic plasmablasts responsible for CD4 T-independent antibody responses during intracellular bacterial infection. J Immunol 2008;181:1375–85.

80. Kenderes KJ, Levack RC, Papillion AM, et al. T-Bet(+) IgM memory cells generate multi-lineage effector B cells. Cell Rep 2018;24:824–837 e3.

81. Yates JL, Racine R, McBride KM, et al. T cell-dependent IgM memory B cells generated during bacterial infection are required for IgG responses to antigen challenge. J Immunol 2013;191:1240–9.

82. Newell KL, Cox J, Waickman AT, et al. T-bet(+) B cells dominate the Peritoneal Cavity B cell response during murine intracellular bacterial infection. J Immunol 2022;208:2749–60.

83. Wang S, Wang J, Kumar V, et al. IL-21 drives expansion and plasma cell differentiation of autoreactive CD11c(hi)T-bet(+) B cells in SLE. Nat Commun 2018;9: 1758.

84. Manni M, Ricker E, Pernis AB. Regulation of systemic autoimmunity and CD11c(+) Tbet(+) B cells by SWEF proteins. Cell Immunol 2017;321:46–51.

85. Adlowitz DG, Barnard J, Biear JN, et al. Expansion of activated peripheral blood memory B cells in rheumatoid arthritis, Impact of B cell Depletion Therapy, and Biomarkers of response. PLoS One 2015;10:e0128269.

86. Claes N, Fraussen J, Vanheusden M, et al. Age-associated B cells with Proinflammatory characteristics are expanded in a proportion of multiple sclerosis patients. J Immunol 2016;197:4576–83.

87. Couloume L, Ferrant J, Le Gallou S, et al. Mass cytometry identifies expansion of T-bet(+) B cells and CD206(+) Monocytes in early multiple sclerosis. Front Immunol 2021;12:653577.

88. Saadoun D, Terrier B, Bannock J, et al. Expansion of autoreactive unresponsive CD21-/low B cells in Sjogren's syndrome-associated lymphoproliferation. Arthritis Rheum 2013;65:1085–96.

89. Wang Z, Wang Z, Wang J, et al. T-bet-Expressing B cells are Positively associated with Crohn's disease activity and Support Th1 inflammation. DNA Cell Biol 2016;35:628–35.

90. Wilbrink R, Spoorenberg A, Arends S, et al. CD27(-)CD38(low)CD21(low) B-cells are increased in axial spondyloarthritis. Front Immunol 2021;12:686273.

91. Malle L, Patel RS, Martin-Fernandez M, et al. Autoimmunity in Down's syndrome via cytokines, CD4 T cells and CD11c(+) B cells. Nature 2023;1–10.

92. Warnatz K, Wehr C, Drager R, et al. Expansion of CD19(hi)CD21(lo/neg) B cells in common variable immunodeficiency (CVID) patients with autoimmune cytopenia. Immunobiology 2002;206:502–13.

93. Rakhmanov M, Keller B, Gutenberger S, et al. Circulating CD21low B cells in common variable immunodeficiency resemble tissue homing, innate-like B cells. Proc Natl Acad Sci U S A 2009;106:13451–6.

94. Isnardi I, Ng YS, Menard L, et al. Complement receptor 2/CD21- human naive B cells contain mostly autoreactive unresponsive clones. Blood 2010;115: 5026–36.

95. Unger S, Seidl M, van Schouwenburg P, et al. The T(H)1 phenotype of follicular helper T cells indicates an IFN-gamma-associated immune dysregulation in

patients with CD21low common variable immunodeficiency. J Allergy Clin Immunol 2018;141:730–40.

96. Yang R, Avery DT, Jackson KJL, et al. Human T-bet governs the generation of a distinct subset of CD11c(high)CD21(low) B cells. Sci Immunol 2022;7: eabq3277.

97. Du SW, Arkatkar T, Jacobs HM, et al. Generation of functional murine CD11c(+) age-associated B cells in the absence of B cell T-bet expression. Eur J Immunol 2019;49:170–8.

98. Rubtsova K, Rubtsov AV, Thurman JM, et al. B cells expressing the transcription factor T-bet drive lupus-like autoimmunity. J Clin Invest 2017;127:1392–404.

99. Mouat IC, Morse ZJ, Shanina I, et al. Latent gammaherpesvirus exacerbates arthritis through modification of age-associated B cells. Elife 2021;10:e67024.

100. Keller B, Strohmeier V, Harder I, et al. The expansion of human T-bet(high) CD21(low) B cells is T cell dependent. Sci Immunol 2021;6:eabh0891.

101. Pisitkun P, Deane JA, Difilippantonio MJ, et al. Autoreactive B cell responses to RNA-related antigens due to TLR7 gene duplication. Science 2006;312: 1669–72.

102. Deane JA, Pisitkun P, Barrett RS, et al. Control of toll-like receptor 7 expression is essential to restrict autoimmunity and dendritic cell proliferation. Immunity 2007; 27:801–10.

103. Brown GJ, Canete PF, Wang H, et al. TLR7 gain-of-function genetic variation causes human lupus. Nature 2022;605:349–56.

104. Christensen SR, Kashgarian M, Alexopoulou L, et al. Toll-like receptor 9 controls anti-DNA autoantibody production in murine lupus. J Exp Med 2005;202: 321–31.

105. Christensen SR, Shupe J, Nickerson K, et al. Toll-like receptor 7 and TLR9 dictate autoantibody specificity and have opposing inflammatory and regulatory roles in a murine model of lupus. Immunity 2006;25:417–28.

106. Johnson JL, Scholz JL, Marshak-Rothstein A, et al. Molecular pattern recognition in peripheral B cell tolerance: lessons from age-associated B cells. Curr Opin Immunol 2019;61:33–8.

107. Goronzy JJ, Weyand CM. Understanding immunosenescence to improve responses to vaccines. Nat Immunol 2013;14:428–36.

108. Sadighi Akha AA. Aging and the immune system: an overview. J Immunol Methods 2018;463:21–6.

109. Hayflick L, Moorhead PS. The serial cultivation of human diploid cell strains. Exp Cell Res 1961;25:585–621.

110. Frasca D, Diaz A, Romero M, et al. Age effects on B cells and humoral immunity in humans. Ageing Res Rev 2011;10:330–5.

111. Frasca D, Diaz A, Romero M, et al. B cell immunosenescence. Annu Rev Cell Dev Biol 2020;36:551–74.

112. Riley RL, Khomtchouk K, Blomberg BB. Age-associated B cells (ABC) inhibit B lymphopoiesis and alter antibody repertoires in old age. Cell Immunol 2017; 321:61–7.

113. Miller JP, Cancro MP. B cells and aging: balancing the homeostatic equation. Exp Gerontol 2007;42:396–9.

114. Swain SL, Kugler-Umana O, Kuang Y, et al. The properties of the unique age-associated B cell subset reveal a shift in strategy of immune response with age. Cell Immunol 2017;321:52–60.

Artificial Intelligence for Clinical Flow Cytometry

Robert P. Seifert, MD[a],*, David A. Gorlin, MS[b],
Andrew A. Borkowski, MD[c,d,e]

KEYWORDS

- Machine learning • Artificial intelligence • Flow cytometry • Hematopathology
- Clinical flow cytometry

KEY POINTS

- Machine learning applications in flow cytometry are no different than any other laboratory test and require rigorous scientific validation before clinical use.
- The applications of machine learning models on flow cytometry data are promising but there is a near-absence of prospective trials and few interinstitution studies.
- A barrier to clinical adoption is the opaqueness of machine learning algorithms, which can be remedied by back-gating important diagnostic features to a 2-dimensional histogram, showing the hematopathologist "how the model thinks."
- Future work requires thoughtful design and transparency of training data selection and processing.

INTRODUCTION

One of the most, if not the most, useful tool in any hematopathology workflow is flow cytometry. This high-dimensional technique measures individual cell characteristics and quantifies intensity of expression of cell antigens on cell populations by way of fluorescent antibody staining. Generally speaking, instrument data are collected in a tabular format in Flow Cytometry Standard (FCS) file format, with fluorescence intensity being logarithmic in nature. Interpretation of these data is historically limited to the pattern recognition skills of the hematopathologist and medical technologist. Accurate diagnosis is incumbent on proper analysis, which includes gating on diagnostically relevant populations and examining marker expression in 1- or 2-dimensional projections.

[a] Department of Pathology, Immunology and Laboratory Medicine, University of Florida, College of Medicine, 4800 Southwest 35th Drive, Gainesville, FL 32608, USA; [b] University of Florida, College of Medicine, 1600 Southwest Archer Road, Gainesville, FL 32610, USA; [c] National Artificial Intelligence Institute, Washington, DC, USA; [d] Artificial Intelligence Service, James A. Haley Veterans' Hospital, 13000 Bruce B Downs Boulevard, Tampa, FL 33647, USA; [e] University of South Florida Morsani School of Medicine, Tampa, FL, USA
* Corresponding author.
E-mail address: rseifert@ufl.edu

Clin Lab Med 43 (2023) 485–505
https://doi.org/10.1016/j.cll.2023.04.009
0272-2712/23/© 2023 Elsevier Inc. All rights reserved.

labmed.theclinics.com

Analysis is time-consuming and has been estimated to take between 5 and 15 minutes per sample.[1] Analysis consists of multiple manual steps:

1. Importing the FCS data file into the analysis software.
2. Defining the gating hierarchy.
3. Selecting gate boundaries.
4. Selecting sample-level features that are appropriate for classification (diagnosis, prediction, and/or prognosis).
5. Defining the thresholds for the aforementioned features for classification.
6. Documenting the classification.

Thus, analysis can lack reproducibility and can scale poorly with interrogation of several markers or samples[2]; this is burdensome for pathology departments at smaller community hospitals, considering it has been estimated that approximately 50% of flow cytometry cases lack diagnostic abnormalities.[3,4] However, thorough surveys on this subject are limited. Moreover, if an abnormality is identified, reflex "add-on" flow cytometry studies will be performed and analyzed.[3] Staff shortages compound the issue, with estimates showing a vacancy rate of 10.1% in US flow cytometry laboratories.[5]

Machine learning (ML), a component of artificial intelligence (AI), has shown promise for improving health care since the late 1970s.[6,7] For example, ML machine learning has blossomed in surgical pathology diagnosis with computer-driven algorithms reading digitized histologic images and rendering diagnoses[8,9]; this culminated in the first ever Food and Drug Administration (FDA)-cleared digital pathology product in 2021.[8] The FDA is interested in fast-tracking ML software applications under a new "Software as a Medical Device" category.[6]

ML has existed in health care and pathology for decades in the form of linear or logistic regression and decision trees. The clinical utility of such algorithms is validated on large, heterogenous patient populations, ideally using randomized, prospective clinical trials. Modern ML algorithms are no different in their design and utility.

ML algorithms have been demonstrated to have high accuracy in automated pattern recognition, particularly where pathologist-driven decision-making can falter: fatigue or analysis of a large volume of detail.[10] Whereas the human analyst relies on proper sequential gating of 2-dimensional plots, modern ML models can simultaneously interrogate FCS data in all possible dimensions. Modern ML models can be applied to the preanalytical, analytical, or postanalytical phases of hematopathology diagnosis as follows:

- Preanalytical: prescreening for high-risk cases.
- Analytical: adjunctive diagnostic input, abnormality identification.
- Postanalytical: quality assurance and improvement.

In this review, the authors aim to educate the reader on current practices in ML, highlight advancements in ML flow cytometry applications, and share a vision of the future. This is the first review article of ML application in this discipline to date. Although the Definitions section is longer than in other articles in this series, the authors hope it can serve as a quick reference when encountering ML in the wild. They also aim to "teach you to fish" by way of our evaluations of publications in this field.

HISTORY

Automated classification of blood cells has existed for almost as long as clinical flow cytometry in the form of discriminate functions such as linear or logistic regression.[11] For each feature in a data set, a linear regression function determines the relationship between numeric variables and a binary output classification (**Fig. 1**A); this allows for

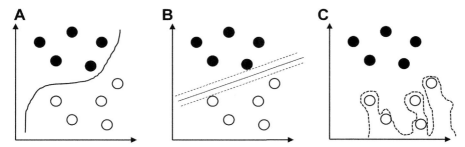

Fig. 1. (*A*) The solid line represents a logistic regression function separating the filled dots from the empty dots in a 2D histogram. (*B*) An SVM creates a decision boundary (*solid line*) based on the maximum degree of separation between the 2 clusters of data. (*C*) The model represented by the dotted line is overfitting on the empty dots.

classification of data by generalization of features and forms the basis for many complete blood count platforms. In essence, when gating on a flow cytometry scatter plot, the authors visually generate a discriminate function. Such functions can be calculated and automated by a computer for a given kind of data using a training set with known properties. In principle, this reduces the dimensionality of data to what is called a vector of observations that conveys the important features.

Other mathematical methods exist to reduce data's dimensionality, of data including principal component analysis and cluster analysis. In principal component analysis, the original variables of a data set are transformed into linear functions, computed ordinally such that the first new linear function accounts for the most variation in the data, the second for the next most, and so on.[11] The so-called principal component then is the new linear function that accounts for the largest variation in the data. Cluster analysis classifies members of a population based on measured variables and is typically hierarchical. In fact, this mathematical methodology defined the clusters of differentiation ("CD" markers).

In flow cytometry, such dimensionality reduction tools can improve visualization of data, as they allow the analyst to compare marker behavior across cell populations beyond a defined gating strategy. A variety of other clustering algorithms, including t-distributed Stochastic Neighbor Embedding, SPADE, FlowSOM, and flowMeans, have been developed over the decades.[12,13] However, the output of these algorithms mimics standard flow cytometry gating and must still be interrogated by an analyst in a 2-dimensional scatter plot; this is a subjective process, and, with some algorithms such as SPADE, the analyst must understand what is represented by each cluster, which is visualized out of the usual biological context with no differential expression of antibody fluorescence displayed.

Development in this area seems to have stalled since the Flow Cytometry Critical Assessment of Population Identification Methods, or FlowCAP, summit in 2014.[13] We hypothesize that thought leaders have focused instead on newer ML algorithms.

ML applications in health care are exciting, but daunting to the uninitiated, with discussions on the topic being either exaggerated or overly technical. The authors hope to disentangle this in the next section.

DEFINITIONS
Artificial Intelligence

Artificial intelligence is the study and development of computer algorithms that can perform tasks generally thought to require human intelligence.[14] In medicine, applications initially involved discretely programmed, rules-based classification algorithms but these have limited utility in that they struggle with classifying unique data and lack contextualization. Examples of the latter in flow cytometry are discussed in the History section. In the last decade, AI has become synonymous with using statistical tools such as ML and neural networks to perform various kinds of pattern recognition. ML is a branch of AI in which algorithms learn from a given set of data and generate a model that can be applied to new sets of data.[15] ML models are generated by evaluating different features or points of interest in the raw data available. In medicine, these features can be as simple as vital signs, medications, or smoking histories that point to a classifier such as a patient's risk for cardiovascular disease.[6]

Classically, ML models relied on expert, manual identification of important features within a set of data[15]; this was dependent on a priori knowledge of the experts and kept models blind to features that may actually be relevant for optimal function of the model. For example, a model designed to estimate the Ki-67 proliferation index by immunohistochemistry on a whole slide image could do so by counting dark brown–colored pixels. However, such a model may overestimate the proliferation index in the setting of confounders such as overstaining and hemosiderin or melanin pigment. Deep learning is a branch of ML based initially on the neuronal architecture of mammalian brains in which the algorithm can derive important features from a data set on its own, with minimal to no human input.[15] Such ML models require extensive training.

During training, an ML algorithm performs a kind of regression on the data. It assigns weighted significance to features in a training data set, which at first can be random or manually assigned. The model then attempts to classify the input data given the presence of those features and calculate the loss or error in its classification. The algorithm then attempts to minimize this error by adjusting the weights accordingly during multiple iterations of a process called gradient descent. Finally, when an appropriate threshold of accuracy is reached in the training set, the model's accuracy can be validated on a validation data set.

Model Development

Whether for flow cytometry or image recognition, ML model development follows similar steps, and understanding modern ML model development is crucial. Ultimately, an ML model should be treated no differently than any other laboratory test validation. The steps of model development are summarized in **Table 1**.[10,15]

Glossary

Following is an alphabetized glossary of technical terms related to ML development.

Classifier

A classifier is a component within an ML model performing mathematical operations on features and generating an output that becomes an element of the ultimate classification of the input sample for the model.[16]

Decision trees

A decision tree is a flowchart composed of interrogations nodes resulting in classification of a sample. A classic example in hematopathology is the Hans criteria for immunohistochemical classification of diffuse large B-cell lymphoma cell of origin wherein each node of the decision tree asks a yes/no question, approaching a classification[17] (**Fig. 2**A). Alone, decision trees are sensitive to noise in the training data set; however, they can be combined into what is termed a random forest classifier.[15,16]

Table 1	
Steps of machine learning model development	
Step	**Actions**
1	*Identify if ML is the appropriate tool for the problem.* Some problems may be solvable with a discretely programmed method instead.
2	*Obtain "big data."* ML training requires large quantities of data to produce generalizable results. If the training data set was generated by only one institution, it may not be generalizable.
3	*Prepare high-quality data.* "Garbage in, garbage out": high-quality data are free of errors, accurate, complete, consistent, and relevant to the problem. It must be in a format software can interpret. Irrelevant dimensions or variables should be removed to avoid overfitting. If performing supervised learning, the data set must be labeled consistently with a reliable ground truth.
4	*Select an optimization metric.* During each iteration of model training, a metric can be calculated to assess the degree of error. This metric is referred to as the loss function or cost function. As training progresses, the model attempts to minimize the loss function. Different model types have different options for this function so understanding how a given loss function will shape the model is critical.
5	*Train the model.* The data obtained and prepared in steps 2 and 3 are often split into 2 groups at the onset of model development: training and validation. The conventional split of the initial data set is 80% training, 20% validation. The combination of training and validation cohorts is sometimes called the discovery or development cohort. The model, in training, iterates over the training data set, making small adjustments to improve future predictions. In addition, some model types require adjustment of hyperparameters to obtain optimal results that depend greatly on the task and data format. The data set that accommodates this is sometimes called the tuning set and should be derivative of the training set, not the validation set.
6	*Validate the model.* In a given ML experiment, multiple different model types may be trained on the same data set and then their accuracy is assessed by comparative evaluation using the validation set. It is crucial that the validation set consists of data that are completely independent of the training set. Doing otherwise would be like seeing the answers to an exam, beforehand. A validation method that accommodates for smaller data volumes, as in flow cytometry, is the K-fold cross-validation, described later.
7	*Test the model.* The validated model must be tested on new data using real-world conditions to prove reproducibility and generalizability. Few published works, particularly related to flow cytometry, have done this. The test set must contain data that have not been evaluated by the model in step 5 or 6 and should preferably come from multiple institutions. Although the loss function can be used again to evaluate performance, it is an abstraction, and it is more useful to apply statistical methods commonly used in the evaluation of other diagnostic laboratory tests, including receiver operating characteristic curve (summarized with area under the curve [AUROC]), sensitivity, specificity, and positive/negative predictive value. It is imperative at this step to investigate for patterns of misclassification errors made by the model, and if significant to the application, correct them by repeating steps 2–7.
8	*Deploy the model.* Best practices are still being debated for deployment. Any deployment would require conversations with key stakeholders, end users, and information technology specialists to ensure the model functions as intended, and, more importantly, its results are interpreted correctly by the hematopathologist and clinician.

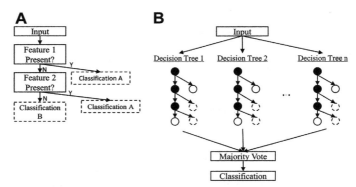

Fig. 2. (*A*) Classic decision tree. (*B*) Random Forest Classifier with n component decision trees.

F1 score
F1 score is the harmonic mean (a mathematical method for averaging ratios) of positive predictive value and sensitivity of an ML model. It is a way of representing a model's performance with a single number that captures poor values. It can be weighted based on how many of a given class are present in the data set.

Feature
Features represent the input variables of an ML model.[10,16] Features can be processed before input. For example, some flow cytometry ML models have concatenated (joined) the data from all channels of a given tube into one line of a large database.[18]

Gradient boosting
During training, the ML model, as well as individual classifiers within the model in some algorithms, attempt to optimize the loss function by iteratively adjusting weights, resulting in a decrease (descent) of the loss function over time. A powerful mathematical technique called boosting enhances this process, particularly for weak classifiers, by forcing them to concentrate on training set features that were missed in previous iterations. These techniques tend to minimize bias but are prone to overfitting.[15,16] XGBoost is a popular example of a gradient boosting algorithm.

Hyperparameter
Various ML model types contain so-called hyperparameters that are variables that influence the model's learning and performance, allowing for fine tuning.[16] These hyperparameters should only be adjusted during a model's training and tuning with their performance on the validation data set. Caution must be taken in overtuning a model's hyperparameters, as, in theory, doing so could achieve 100% accuracy on the training set but poor generalizability to other data sets due to overfitting. The model type XGBoost, for example, has several adjustable hyperparameters that allow it to adapt to different tasks.[10,18]

K-fold cross-validation
Ideally, after model training, sufficient untested samples remain for adequate validation, and the samples within the validation data set are as randomly distributed as those in the training set; this is a problem for small data sets. To mitigate this, the full data set is divided randomly into *k* folds, typically 10, with a combination of folds being used for training and a separate combination for validation over *k* iterations, resulting in an average estimate of error.[16] For example, a 5-fold cross-validation on

100 flow cytometry cases would result in 5 groups of 20 (**Fig. 3**). The first iteration would train the model on groups 1 to 4 and validate on group 5. The second iteration trains on groups 2 to 5 with validation using group 1 and so on. The average error (or accuracy) for all 5 iterations would then be reported for the validation. Mathematically, this tends to overestimate error, which is desirable[16]; this is ideal for testing different ML algorithms on smaller data sets; however, candidate models for clinical use should still undergo validation on an independent data set.[10] See also Leave-One-Out Cross-Validation.

Label
The label, or annotation, identifies for the ML model the proper classification of a given sample.[16] For example, in a supervised learning model, a tube from a positive chronic lymphocytic leukemia case could be labeled "CLL," whereas a tube from a normal blood case could be labeled "Normal."

Leave-one-out cross-validation
Similar to k-fold cross-validation, leave-one-out cross-validation can be helpful to evaluate for error when only small data sets are available. In this process, N-1 cases are used for training and the single "left out" case is used for validation, with the entire process repeated N times and the average error reported. See also k-Fold Cross-Validation.

Loss (or cost) function
Loss function is the metric by which an ML model's accuracy is evaluated during training that guides subsequent corrections.[10,15,16]

Neural networks/deep learning
More classic ML models, such as random forest classifiers, can fail when there is a high degree of variation/complexity in the input, such as with analysis of an image.[15] More effective models learn abstractions from the input, by way of dimensionality reduction. This kind of model is termed deep learning.

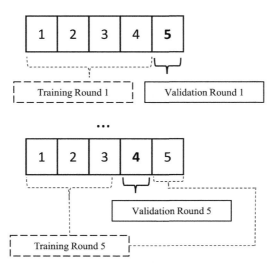

Fig. 3. Example of k-fold cross-validation with 5 folds showing the first round of validation and then later the fifth iteration. The results of all 5 rounds would be averaged and reported.

A neural network is a deep learning construct consisting of layers of interconnected nodes (**Fig. 4**). Between the input and output layers are multiple, so-called, hidden layers. Multiple input and output connections exist between each node in a layer with nodes in adjacent layers. Within a given node, mathematical operations are performed with the goal of abstracting features from the original input data.[15] The connections between nodes have weights that are adjusted during model training to avoid errors in classification, and there are different mathematical approaches to refining the weights. Different neural network constructs exist for a variety of applications.

Convolutional neural networks. Convolutional neural networks (CNNs) have been effective at interpreting images.[15] CNNs are termed such because they are composed of so-called convolution layers. These layers attempt to learn motifs from local data points, such as nearby pixels in an image and are combined with pooling layers, which attempt to generalize the higher-level features, such as a structure within an image. CNNs have been shown to be less prone to overfitting, which is discussed earlier.[15]

Overfitting
An ML model can be trained too well on its training set. Substantial amounts of suboptimally curated data tend to produce models inclusive of irrelevant features beyond those needed to create an accurate classification (**Fig. 1**C); this impairs a model's generalizability in classifying data other than that which it was originally trained. Various mitigation techniques have been used to avoid this problem of overfitting, including regularization or early stopping. Regularization smooths the fit of a model to minimize overfitting. Early stopping halts model training before overfitting can occur.[10,16]

Parameter
Parameters are the internal values of an ML model derived from the training data set to achieve correct classification of an input.[16]

Python, RStudio
Python, RStudio is a commonly used free, open-source software tool for curating data and training ML models. A popular software package for ML within Python is scikit-learn.[19]

Random forest classifier
A random forest classifier (RFC) is an ML model design algorithm wherein each component decision tree is composed of a random selection of features and each is trained on a random sample of training data, with the output of the model being

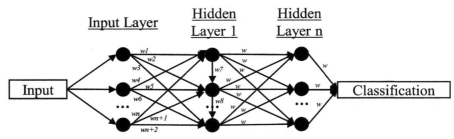

Fig. 4. A neural network with n hidden layers and n nodes. Each connection contains an individual weight, *wn*, that is adjusted throughout the training period.

decided by majority vote of the component decision trees[15] (**Fig. 2**B). Such algorithms minimize overfitting but can be less accurate if the input data are highly complex.

Supervised versus unsupervised

ML models can be trained in a supervised or unsupervised manner. Consider this analogy: a hematopathology fellow analyzes a flow cytometry panel and dictates a draft interpretation into the electronic health record. This draft is reviewed by the hematopathology attending, with feedback given to the fellow on what was correct and incorrect. The more cases the fellow sees, the more proficient he or she gets at interpreting flow cytometry data. The hematopathology attending provided supervision for the fellow. Conversely, the fellow, while on call, is required to analyze flow cytometry and communicate results directly to clinicians without direct oversight by the attending. The fellow is unsupervised (in ACGME terms, "indirectly supervised") in this example. ML models can be developed using essentially the same approach that is termed supervised, unsupervised, or semisupervised learning, the latter being a combination.[15]

In supervised learning, the ground truth is established by labeling or annotating a training data set to develop the model. In the aforementioned analogy, this was the instructive feedback of the hematopathology attending. During training, the model compares its prediction with the ground truth and adjusts itself to improve the likelihood of a correct prediction in future iterations.[15]

In unsupervised learning, no ground truth labels are present in the training data set, and the model is left to discover features in the data, unaided; this is akin to the hematopathology fellow working on-call, without direct input from the attending.[15] ML models that have undergone unsupervised training have shown humanlike diagnostic ability, although this is still a relatively new field.[10]

There are pros and cons to both concepts. Supervised learning requires tedious manual labeling of data, and generally requires subject matter expertise, the latter potentially incorporating bias, skewing the model. Unsupervised learning requires much larger data sets than supervised learning, which may not be available.[10]

Support vector machines

Support vector machine (SVM) is an ML algorithm that separates 2 classifications by maximizing the space between the decision boundary and the training set sample closest to it (**Fig. 1**B). New samples are classified based on where they land with respect to the decision boundary. This algorithm is robust to outliers but computationally heavy, performing poorly when classifications have overlap.[15,16]

Transfer learning

Transfer learning leverages a previously trained ML model for a new purpose by partially retraining the model on a new task.[15] For example, a model capable of differentiating CLL from normal could be applied to detect other B-cell lymphomas.

Uniform manifold approximation and projection

Dimensionality reduction algorithms such as t-distributed stochastic neighbor embedding can underperform with large data sets and show poor generalizability to new data. Uniform Manifold Approximation and Projection (UMAP) for dimension reduction is a newer algorithm that may be more scalable and robust to new samples.[20]

BACKGROUND

Herein the authors summarize 11 recently published endeavors to develop modern ML models for clinical flow cytometric analysis (**Table 2**).

Table 2
Summary of published machine learning applications for clinical flow cytometry sorted by ascending publication date

First Author, Year	N Cases (Specimen Types)	Instrumentation (Events/Tube)	Tubes (Colors)	Trained Classifications (N)	FCS Data Pretreatment	Algorithm Trained	Validation Method	Validation Results	Testing/Notes
Ng et al,[21] 2015	144 (tissue)	BD LSRII (500,000)	1 (9)	CHL (57), negative (47), other neoplastic (40, classified with negative)	Transformed, normalized	RFC, SVM, SVM with ad hoc dimensionality reduction. All inputs vectorized to 2D histogram.	20 excluded from training combined with 6-fold cross-validation on training	ACC RFC 85%, SVM 90%, SVM with ad hoc 95%	Single-channel "knock-out" and artificial noise had no impact on performance.
Ko et al,[22] 2018	5333 (bone marrow), split 4:1 for validation	BD FACSCalibur, BD FACSCanto II (100,000)	13 (4)	AML (1320), MDS (363), negative (3650)	Normalized, vectorized	SVM (unsupervised) after vectorization	1007, independent validation set with 5-fold cross-validation	ACC 84.6% for normal vs abnormal	Tested against separate cohort 287 cases with "abnormal" calls having worse OS, PFS
Zhao et al,[23] 2020	18,274 (blood, bone marrow) split 9:1 for validation	Beckman Coulter Navios (50,000)	3 (9)	CLL (4035), MBL (1554), MCL (275), PL (552), LPL (642), MZL (990), FL (222), HCL (201), negative (9803)	None	CNN after SOM dimensionality reduction	1827, independent validation set	F1 0.7	2348 independent cases tested, F1 0.98 for B NHL vs negative, weighted F1 0.94 for individual lymphoma classification
Gaidano et al,[24] 2020	1547 (blood, bone marrow, tissue, fluid), split 3:1 for validation.	BD FACSCalibur, Beckman Coulter FC500, Dako CyAn, Beckman Coulter Navios (various)	Various	CLL (670), FL (199), MZL (174), DLBCL (220), LPL (60), MCL (83), BL (14). Normal not included.	Removal or imputation of missing data and rare classifications.	Decision tree	386, independent validation set	ACC 89.3%	—
Ng & Zuromski,[3] 2021	3417 blood	Beckman Coulter NaviosEX (26,000)	1 (10)	Any abnormal B cell population (674), negative (2026)	Filtration of platelets, debris, then transformation. Nonnormal case representation tripled.	RFC after UMAP dimensionality reduction	10-fold time series using 80:20 split of overlapping cases from training set.	ACC 77.98% for classifying normal	569 independent, prospective test set showed ACC 93.51 %, F1 0.96 for classifying normal
Kang et al,[18] 2021	116 (blood), split 80:20 training and test set	BD FacsCanto II (769)	4 (10)	CLL (44), MBL (19), negative (53)	Filtration of early events	XGBoost decision trees (neural network, RFC, CNN also tested)	10-fold cross-validation with 80:20 split of training set	F1 0.796	24 independent test cases showed ACC 83.33% to classify malignant, F1 0.807

Study	Cases	Instrument	Institutions (panels)	Diagnoses	Preprocessing	Method	Validation	Results	Notes
Simonson et al,[25] 2021	1222 (tissue), split 80:20 into training and test set	BD LSRII (500,000)	1 (9)	CHL (321), negative (901)	Normalization, transformation. Positive cases duplicated for class balance.	CNNs individually trained on single given histogram, then combined for ensemble RFC.	5-fold cross-validation of entire data set	Similar results	244 independent test cases showed ACC 88.2%, F1 0.743
Mallesh et al,[26] 2021	10,079, 525, 2733 and 1626 cases from 4 institutions	Beckman Coulter Navios (50,000)	Various	CLL, MBL, MCL, PL, LPL, MZL, FL, HCL, negative (cohort-sized varied)	Tubes merged to single file using nearest neighbor	CNN after SOM dimensionality reduction	10-fold cross-validation on each data set comparing transfer learning vs original model	Weighted F1 scores for transfer learning ranged from 0.8 to 0.93 among institutions	Nontransfer learning model showed worse performance
Clichet et al,[27] 2022	267, split 70:30 into training and validation set	Beckman Coulter Navios (not available)	1 (10)	PCN (170), MGUS (97)	Not available	Manually selected features trained on classical gradient-boosted decision tree	Not available, separate validation cohort	ACC 95%	Independent cohort of 128 samples reportedly showed "success rate" 91%.
Simonson et al,[28] 2022	9635	BD LSRII (not available)	1 (8)	Reflex panel needed (887), no reflex panel needed (8748)	Normalization, transformation. Positive cases duplicated for class balance.	CNNs individually trained on single given histogram, then combined for ensemble RFC.	5-fold cross-validation with 80:20 splitting of training set.	ACC 94%, F1 0.63	Prospective independent cohort of 376 cases over 3 mo showed ACC 94%, F1 0.62.
Monaghan et al,[29] 2022	531	BD FACSCanto II (30,000)	5 (8)	APL(32), AML not APL(200), ALL(131), non-neoplastic cytopenia (168)	Normalized, vectorized	SVM (unsupervised) after vectorization	5-fold cross-validation with 80:20 splitting of training set.	Overall ACC 94.2%	N/A

Abbreviations: ACC, accuracy; AML, acute myeloid leukemia; CHL, classic Hodgkin lymphoma; FL, follicular lymphoma; HCL, hairy cell leukemia; MBL, monoclonal B lymphocytosis; MCL, mantle cell lymphoma; MDS, myelodysplastic syndrome; MZL, marginal zone lymphoma; OS, overall survival; PFS, progression-free survival; PL, prolymphocytic leukemia; SOM, self-organizing map.

Ng, et al, 2015

Although not widely adopted, some investigators have shown that classic Hodgkin lymphoma can be detected by flow cytometric analysis. [21] These investigators aimed to develop an ML model capable of detecting classic Hodgkin lymphoma in flow cytometric data from tissue samples by comparative validation of SVM and gradient-boosted RFC-derived models. One hundred forty-four samples from a single-tube, 9-color flow cytometry panel, previously validated for use in the detection of classic Hodgkin lymphoma, was used for training and validation. A BD LSRII flow cytometer was used. The training set consisted of 80% of these cases. FCS data were log-transformed, then normalized, and each of the 78 possible 2-dimensional histograms was plotted and vectorized into one long vector per case. Additional transformations were tested before ML training.

The validation cohort consisted of 20% of cases excluded from training and an additional 20 cases. Six-fold cross-validation was performed on the validation cohort, showing an accuracy of 85%, 90%, and 95% for RFC, SVM, and SVM with ad hoc dimensionality reduction, respectively. In addition, leave-one-out cross-validation was performed and identified a subset of cases that were consistently misclassified. Cytometer noise was artificially introduced to the data set and the process repeated showing similar results. Removal of single flow cytometry parameters did not seem to significantly alter the accuracy. Back-gating identified a population of CD5(+), CD71(+), and CD30(+) T cells with increased CD45 as well as a population of debris that the models defined as most useful features for classification.

Ko, et al, 2018

These investigators attempted to create an SVM-based ML model that could differentiate between acute myeloid leukemia (AML), myelodysplastic syndrome (MDS), and normal in preinduction and postinduction bone marrow flow cytometry specimens. [22] All cases had a 4-color, 13-tube myeloid panel performed, with more than 100,000 events per tube, using either a BD FacsCalibur or BD FacsCanto II with the fluorescence intensities of Calibur-performed cases normalized to Canto II levels. Data from 5333 cases were split 80:20 into the training and validation sets. All FCS data were normalized, then cell attributes from each tube were vectorized and those vectors combined into a case-level vector for input into an SVM. The SVM consisted of a multivariate Gaussian mixture model that was trained unsupervised.

Five-fold cross-validation on the independent validation cohort demonstrated an accuracy of 84.6% (95% confidence interval [CI] 82.9%–86.3%) for classifying normal versus abnormal (AML or MDS) across both instrument types.

The model was then tested against a separate cohort of 287 cases, and survival analysis (overall survival, progression-free survival) by Kaplan-Meier statistics was plotted against the model output (normal or abnormal). Cases categorized as normal by the algorithm showed significantly longer overall and progression-free survival versus abnormal.

Zhao, et al, 2020

These investigators attempted to develop an ML model for classifying B-cell non-Hodgkin lymphomas in blood or bone marrow by first applying an unsupervised dimensionality reduction technique to individual tubes in a case. [23] Diagnostic classes included CLL, monoclonal B lymphocytosis, prolymphocytic leukemia, mantle cell lymphoma, lymphoplasmacytic lymphoma, marginal zone lymphoma, follicular lymphoma, hairy cell leukemia, and normal. Instrumentation included a Beckman Coulter

Navios with more than 50,000 events collected per tube as part of a 3-tube, 9-color B-cell panel. The development set consisted of 18,274 cases, which were split 90:10 into training and validation cohorts. These cases included 4035 CLL cases and 9803 normal cases. An independent data set for testing was collected using only cases dated after the development set to mirror a production environment. This test set consisted of 2348 cases with slightly more normal cases (66.56% vs 53.64% in the development set). No ad hoc relinearization or transformation of the FCS data was performed. Each tube for a given case underwent unsupervised self-organizing map dimensionality reduction, similar to UMAP. The model for this step was trained using one random sample from each class within the development set. The output was then fed into a CNN model for training.

At validation, the final model demonstrated an F1 score of 0.7.

At testing, the final model demonstrated an F1 score of 0.98 in classifying B-cell non-Hodgkin lymphoma versus normal and an F1 score of 0.94 for individual lymphoma classifications after weighing for representation in the test set. Misclassifications demonstrated immunophenotypic similarity (ie, marginal zone lymphoma vs lymphoplasmacytic lymphoma), and there were no false-negative CLL cases.

Gaidano, et al, 2020

These investigators aimed to compare classical decision tree models for B-cell non-Hodgkin diagnosis trained from flow cytometry data collected on blood, bone marrow, tissue, and fluid cases over a nearly 2-decade time period.[24] Instrumentation included BD FACSCalbur, Beckman Coulter FC500, Dako CyAn, and Beckman Coulter Navios. Diagnostic classes included CLL, follicular lymphoma, marginal zone lymphoma, diffuse large B-cell lymphoma, lymphoplasmacytic lymphoma, mantle cell lymphoma, splenic lymphoma, hairy cell lymphoma, and Burkitt lymphoma, with the latter 3 being the least well represented. Normal was not included. CLL was the most common diagnostic class (670/1547 cases). As panel constituents varied, the investigators removed data if fewer than 50% of cases contained a given antibody and mathematically calculated missing values in other cases based on the mean value for a given diagnostic class. One thousand five hundred forty-seven samples were randomly split 75:25 into training and independent validation cohorts. The decision trees were trained using grid search analysis and Gini impurity split criterion. Four models were developed; however, only the model that excluded MiB1 and Bcl2 (due to poor adoption of these markers in practice) as well as cases of hairy cell leukemia and splenic lymphoma (due to paucity of cases) are discussed.

At validation, this model showed an overall accuracy of 89.3% (no 95% CI given) for B-cell non-Hodgkin lymphoma subclassification. As this was a classic decision tree, marker importance to accurate classification could be directly scored, and this identified CD5, CD10, and CD200 as the top 3 most important markers.

Ng, et al, 2021

In pursuit of a model capable of autoverifying normal cases, these investigators attempted to create a model that could differentiate normal blood from blood containing an abnormal B-cell population (including B-cell non-Hodgkin lymphomas and B-acute lymphoblastic leukemia) by reducing event dimensionality with the UMAP algorithm and then training an RFC.[3] Data were collected from 3417 blood flow cytometry cases wherein each case consisted of a single 10-color B-cell panel obtained from NaviosEX cytometers, although some individual cases included repeat runs. Cases were filtered to excluded pegged events, platelets, and doublets and cases had approximately 26,000 events. The data underwent hyperbolic arcsine transformation; then cases were chronologically split 80:20 into training and validation groups. The proportion of normal in the training and validation groups was 74.13% and 76.11%, respectively. Differential down-sampling was performed on the training group to triple the representation of nonnormal cases. The UMAP algorithm was applied to both groups reducing the dimensionality of each event in a case into a 2-dimensional histogram. Training was performed using an RFC. Validation was performed using overlapping groups of 1000 cases from the training set in order to simulate a production environment using a 10-fold fixed-window time-series cross-validation instead of a traditional 10-fold cross-validation, as the former may better simulate training on retrospective data and testing on new "future" data that would be subject to different degrees of instrument variation than in the retrospective training cohort.

At validation, the model's ability to classify normal (for autoverification applications) showed an accuracy of 77.98% (95% CI 75.9%–80%) and area under the ROC curve (AUROC) 0.8472 (95% CI 0.83–0.864).

In examining the model's ability to classify B-cell malignancies, false-negative cases included monoclonal B-cell lymphocytosis and B-cell non-Hodgkin lymphomas of unusual phenotype not present in the training set. The model's ability to classify B-cell non-Hodgkin lymphomas was also evaluated and showed an accuracy of 96.02%.

A separate cohort of 569 cases selected from dates after the training set was used to test the model; this showed classification of normal cases to have an accuracy of 93.51%, sensitivity 99.23%, negative predictive value 96.69%, positive predictive value 92.82%, AUROC 0.9653, and F1 score 0.96.

Kang, et al, 2021

These investigators attempted to compare the following ML algorithms in their ability to distinguish CLL from normal blood: neural network, CNN, random forest classifier, and gradient-boosted decision trees (XGBoost). [18] One hundred sixteen cases were used in this study, including 53 normal samples and 63 cases of CLL. The CLL cases included 19 that met criteria for the diagnosis of monoclonal B-cell lymphocytosis. These data were randomly split 80:20 for training and a separate test set. FCS data were obtained from BD FacsCanto II instruments wherein each patient case consisted of a 4-tube, 10-color B-cell panel. Early events from each tube were excluded, and 769 events per tube remained, which were then concatenated, including all channels, such that each row represented one patient sample. A 10-fold cross-validation was performed with 80:20 splitting of the original data set.

At validation, the XGBoost model showed an F1 score of 0.796 with less than 10% standard deviation in accuracy.

The separate test set showed XGBoost to have the best performance (sensitivity 67.67%, specificity 100%, accuracy 83.33%, F1 score 0.807). The RFC achieved an accuracy of 79.16% with the neural network and CNN performing poorly (accuracy of 51.09% and 45.65%, respectively). Of the 24 test cases, 4 were incorrectly identified as a false negative during validation, and all 4 met the criteria for monoclonal B lymphocytosis. Further model testing is pending.

Simonson, et al, 2021

Continuing the work described in Ng and colleagues, 2015, these investigators tested an ensemble CNN classic Hodgkin lymphoma classifier constructed in a way that is more analogous to a flow cytometry analysts' approach to histogram interpretation. [25] Individual CNNs were trained on single flow cytometry plot interpretations and then used, in ensemble, to train an RFC. One thousand two hundred twenty-two samples (321 positive, 901 negative) were randomly split 80:20 into training and validation sets. The training set was further subdivided approximately 2:1 into training sets 1 and 2. During training, positive cases were duplicated for class balance. FCS data, which generally contained greater than 0.5 million cells, was normalized and then converted into 78 two-dimensional histograms representing all possible pairwise combinations of a 9-color panel. Each of the 78 histograms was fed into one given CNN classifier. The CNN classifiers were then validated for overfitting on training set 2 (data not available). The trained CNN classifiers then used training set 2 as input for the training of the RFC.

The final RFC model, using the independent validation set, showed accuracy 88.6%, precision 82.7%, sensitivity of 69.4%, and AUROC of 0.93.

Because of the structure of this ML model, features important for classification could be visualized, and the investigators proposed that evaluation of nonviable cells along with lymphocyte ratios, and not detection of Hodgkin cells, may play a role in accurate classification.

Mallesh, et al, 2021

These investigators aimed to extend the work initially published by Zhao and colleagues[23] by attempting transfer learning using their previously developed B-cell non-Hodgkin lymphoma classifier on new flow cytometry data, including data from 3 other institutions. [26] One test group was a 5-color B-cell panel from the same institution, whereas the remaining 3 groups consisted of 8-, 9-, and 10-color panels from 3 separate institutions (10,079, 525, 2733, and 1626 cases, respectively, with disparate ratios of normal to abnormal). All used Beckman Coulter Navios cytometers with an average of 50,000 events collected per tube. To accommodate for differences in the number of tubes, all tubes for a given case were merged into a single file using a nearest-neighbor technique that assumes an event in one tube is similar to an event in another tube in terms of shared marker expression, allowing for the imputation of missing values. Application of nearest-neighbor merging was first tested on the original model that showed no difference in F1 scores. The model processed the merged FCS data as previously described.[23] Evaluation of transfer learning was performed using a 10-fold cross-validation for each new data source and compared with a similar cross-validation without transfer learning (original model).

Validation of the transfer learning model demonstrated a class-weighted F1 score (95% CI) of 0.93 (0.92–0.93) for the 5-color panel and 0.93 (0.91–0.95), 0.85 (0.91–0.95), and 0.8 (0.73–0.87) for each of the outside institutions. The nontransfer learning model showed 0.92 (0.91–0.93) for the 5-color panel and 0.92 (0.9–0.93), 0.76 (0.69–0.83), and 0.69 (0.63–0.74) for each of the outside institutions.

Clichet, et al, 2022

These investigators attempted to develop a model capable of differentiating plasma cell myeloma from monoclonal gammopathy of undetermined significance (MGUS) using flow cytometry data with a more classical ML approach wherein relevant features were manually selected ad hoc rather than as a component of model training. [27] Features selected were percentage of pathologic plasma cells, percentage of total plasma cells, the ratio of plasma cells to CD117(+) precursors, degree of CD27 expression on pathologic plasma cells, and the pathologic plasma cell to normal plasma cell ratio. The cohort used for training and validation consisted of 170 plasma cell neoplasm and 97 MGUS cases and was split 70:30. Flow cytometry was performed on a Navios flow cytometer. A stochastic gradient boosting algorithm was applied to generate a decision tree model.

At validation, this model reportedly showed an accuracy of 95% for classifying MGUS versus plasma cell myeloma.

A separate cohort of 128 samples from 2 outside institutions with different instrumentation reportedly showed a "success rate" of 91%; however, details for this experiment are not provided.

Simonson, et al, 2022

Continuing their previous work, these investigators aimed to investigate prospective, real-time deployment of an ML model for triaging additional flow cytometry panels in the setting of clonal B cells. [28] They developed a model to classify if a screening flow panel would require a reflex B-cell lymphoma panel. The training cohort consisted of 9635 eight-color flow cytometry screening cases, of which 887 (9.2%) had the reflex panel ordered. This cohort was split (67:33) into training sets #1 and #2 for training of the individual CNNs and RCF as described previously with normalization and transformation of the FCS data before training.[25] For class balance, positive cases were copied up to 10-fold during training. A 5-fold cross-validation of the model was performed with 80:20 splitting of the training set.

At validation, the model showed an accuracy of 94% and F1 score of 0.63. In addition, the investigators investigated whether enriching the FCS files for CD19(+) events would improve performance, and it did not.

Using python scripts, the investigators prospectively monitored 376 new screening panels performed over the course of 3 months, with the trained model being applied automatically. The model's decision to perform the reflex panel was compared with the laboratory's decision to perform the reflex panel; this showed an accuracy of 94% and F1 score of 0.62. Inaccurate classifications consisted of cases in which the reflex panel was not feasible (ie, low cell count) or not justified for clinical reasons. Interestingly, the model's probability distribution for the "reflex" classification is much wider versus "no-reflex," to which the investigators suggested implementing a very low threshold for "reflex."

Monaghan, et al, 2022

These investigators attempted to extend the work presented by Ko and colleagues[22] by training and validating an ML model for the discrimination of acute promyelocytic leukemia (APL), AML not APL, acute lymphocytic leukemia (ALL), and nonneoplastic cytopenias in bone marrow specimens. [29] All cases were collected on BD FACSCanto II instruments using an 8-color myeloid panel with approximately 30,000 events per tube. The development set consisted of 531 cases (31.6% non-neoplastic cytopenias) with evaluation performed using a 5-fold cross-validation splitting the development set 80:20 into training and validation cohorts. FCS data were normalized, and then a Gaussian mixture model was applied for vectorization and fed into an SVM as described earlier.[22]

Validation showed an overall accuracy of 94.2% and 99.5% AUROC with accuracies ranging from 87.5% to 97.6% among classes. The largest group of misclassifications was acute leukemia misclassified as nonneoplastic cytopenias (16 cases). This group had a significantly lower blast percentage and higher lymphocyte percentage. No differences in data acquisition were identified. Although no cases were misclassified as APL, 2 had low blast percentage and were misclassified as nonneoplastic cytopenia, whereas another 2 were misclassified as AML not APL for undetermined reasons. There was no difference in model performance in classifying monocytic differentiated AML.

DISCUSSION

The authors reviewed 11 recent publications in which ML classification models were applied to flow cytometry data. In general, ML models showed what could be considered near "expert level" accuracy and F1 score at validation and testing, regardless of data pretreatment or algorithm used. Also impressive was the diversity of diagnostic categories in which ML models were effective, covering almost the breadth of hematopoietic malignancies. Regardless, the authors would hesitate to describe any one algorithm as a clear winner at this time. Most misclassifications could be attributed to plausible phenotypic similarities or case types missed by human analysts such as low-level monoclonal B lymphocytosis. Although these results are promising, the environment in which they were tested is limited, with only one study testing their model in a truly prospective manner.[28]

Conceptually, bigger data sets are usually better for model training. The disparity in the number of training cases in the review is impressive, with some models being effective having only been trained on a few hundred cases; this is, perhaps, due to the volume of discrete tabular data points within an FCS file robustly representing the data's more global features. However, the number of events per tube varied widely in the reviewed studies, ranging from 769 to 500,000 with similar performance at validation. It is interesting that most investigators performed class balancing wherein the positive diagnostic category was oversampled at training to be equal in proportion to normal. Yet, roughly 50% of flow cytometry cases are negative in practice, raising the question of what realistic class balance would show if tested in this discipline.

One of the most appealing applications of this data-augmented decision-making is to support diagnostic pathology laboratories in smaller community health care systems that lack a large workforce of hematopathologists. Flow cytometry data collected at large academic institutions where these models are developed may perform differently in hospital systems with different flow cytometry procedures. Few studies have expanded their work beyond initial model validation. Mallesh and colleagues demonstrated that although transfer learning could yield acceptable results, performance still deteriorated when applying one institution's model on another's data. The paucity of data beyond this study is a major barrier to demonstrating generalizability.[30]

One solution is so-called federated model development.[31] Pooling data for model development and testing is challenging due to privacy and security concerns regarding the raw data. However, in federated development, the model, which contains only decision weights and no protected health information, is circulated among institutions instead and enhanced collaboratively.

A challenge to federated model development is the lack of standardization among flow cytometry panels between institutions. To address the nonuniformity, some investigators either discarded missing antibody data or imputed it based on average fluorescence intensity for a given diagnosis. Both options are problematic, as they can bias model performance against a particular cohort. More work is needed in this area.

The concept of "expert level" accuracy should also be scrutinized as a goal for model development, although the performance to date is an impressive demonstration of this technology. No models discussed took clinical information into account, as would a hematopathologist. Instead, the authors suggest focusing on fit-for-purpose design with an emphasis on model deployment in terms of preanalytical, analytical, and postanalytical phases of clinical laboratory testing. For example, Simonson and colleagues showed that a model trained to triage specimens for reflex B-cell non-Hodgkin lymphoma testing was plausible in the preanalytical phase.[28]

The nomenclature and design of studies is inconsistent in the current literature; however, many groups such as TRIPOD-AI aim to standardize design and minimize bias.[32] Such initiatives can improve the readability of such literature and allow for more 1:1 model comparison. Although training set demographics were consistently reported, it would be of value to the field for future publications to include supplementary examples of deidentified data after every step of ad hoc processing (such as normalization) such that readers could judge the effects such change may have on model training. Descriptive statistics were not consistently presented, and there are few standards in the general literature. The authors suggest the inclusion of the 95% confidence interval of the accuracy and the F1 score, although the model's application may warrant discussion of other parameters. In addition, the ground truth in model evaluation can range from triage of a specimen to definitive World Health Organization classification/International Consensus Classification. How these ground truths are established should be clearly explained in a study and should be fit-for-purpose to the model's application. More methodology details should be disclosed in future work so reproducibility studies can be attempted.

As a discipline, flow cytometry is behind surgical pathology in ML implementation; however, catching up can be expedited. Flow cytometry data already has a tabular representation, which holds an advantage over models analyzing hematoxylin and eosin photomicrographs that require more hard drive space and RAM as well as complicated ML algorithms to process. Interestingly, some studies performed numerous mathematical transformations to FCS data, whereas others fed the raw data directly into their model in training. A standard strategy may emerge as this field advances.

Another limitation clinical ML models have demonstrated is the propensity to amplify biases is our diagnostic process.[33] These have particularly been worrisome for historically underrepresented social demographics in clinical trials. In January of 2021, the FDA revised a 5-point plan to standardize ML practices that reduce the risk of these biases and create transparency for patients about the use of their data.[34]

ML algorithms can be confusing to clinicians who are often uncomfortable using a product they do not understand. If the users do not trust the prediction, they will not use the model. There is interesting work regarding model trustworthiness in the broader field that can be adapted to study design post-hoc, adding another layer of performance evaluation.[35] These investigators propose what is essentially "backgating" in flow cytometry. Backgating a flow cytometry ML model can illustrate what features were important for classification and build trust in the end user if the feature makes biological sense. If done well, these findings could lead to marker or ultimately drug discovery. Some of the aforementioned investigators have explored "backgating" models, but the features extrapolated as important, in some cases, were inexplicable; this could suggest a model may be overfitting. Moreover, many pathologists feel as though some level of experience coding ML models is required to understand its practical uses in the clinic. At large institutions, there is often a data scientist available to help design tools for a study; however, such data scientists may be unavailable in smaller community hospitals. Eventually, packaged software applications and plug-ins with user-friendly interfaces will help alleviate this barrier.

SUMMARY

In this review, the authors discussed the history of automation in flow cytometry as well as the fundamental principles of ML. They explored some of the recent studies and approaches in implementing ML into flow cytometry workflows to both diagnose and survey treatment response in hematologic malignancies. These applications are promising but not without their shortcomings. Explainability of an ML model used in flow cytometry may be the biggest barrier to adoption, as they contain "black boxes," in which a complex network of mathematical processes learns features of data that are not translatable into real language. The authors discussed the current limitations of ML models and the possibility that without a multiinstitutional development process, these applications could have poor generalizability to larger populations. They also discussed ways that particular biases can be reduced in these models and what widespread deployment of augmented decision-making could look like.

CLINICS CARE POINTS

- ML applications in flow cytometry are no different than any other laboratory test and require rigorous scientific validation before clinical use.
- The applications of ML models on flow cytometry data are promising but there is a near absence of prospective trials and few interinstitution studies.
- A barrier to clinical adoption is the opaqueness of ML algorithms, which can be remedied by backgating important diagnostic features to a 2D histogram, showing the hematopathologist "how the model thinks."
- Future work requires thoughtful design and transparency of training data selection and processing.

DISCLOSURE

The authors have nothing to disclose.

REFERENCES

1. Rahim A, Meskas J, Drissler S, et al. High throughput automated analysis of big flow cytometry data. Methods 2018;134:164–76.
2. Ji D, Putzel P, Qian Y, et al. Machine learning of discriminative gate locations for clinical diagnosis. Cytometry 2020;97(3):296–307.
3. Ng DP, Zuromski LM. Augmented human intelligence and automated diagnosis in flow cytometry for hematologic malignancies. Am J Clin Pathol 2021;155(4): 597–605.
4. Oberley MJ, Fitzgerald S, Yang DT, et al. Value-based flow testing of chronic lymphoproliferative disorders: a quality improvement project to develop an algorithm to streamline testing and reduce costs. Am J Clin Pathol 2014;142(3):411–8.
5. Garcia E, Kundu I, Kelly M, et al. The American Society for clinical pathology 2020 vacancy survey of medical Laboratories in the United States. Am J Clin Pathol 2021;157(6):874–89.
6. Thomas LB, Mastorides SM, Viswanadhan NA, et al. Artificial intelligence: review of current and future applications in medicine. Fed Pract 2021;38(11):527.
7. Yu K-H, Beam AL, Kohane IS. Artificial intelligence in healthcare. Nature biomedical engineering 2018;2(10):719–31.
8. Stephens K. FDA authorizes prostate AI software. AXIS Imaging News 2021.
9. Raciti P, Sue J, Ceballos R, et al. Novel artificial intelligence system increases the detection of prostate cancer in whole slide images of core needle biopsies. Mod Pathol 2020;33(10):2058–66.
10. Liu Y, Chen P-HC, Krause J, et al. How to read articles that use machine learning: users' guides to the medical literature. JAMA 2019;322(18):1806–16.
11. Shapiro HM. Practical flow cytometry. Hoboken, NJ: John Wiley & Sons; 2005.

12. Van Gassen S, Callebaut B, Van Helden MJ, et al. FlowSOM: using self-organizing maps for visualization and interpretation of cytometry data. Cytometry 2015;87(7):636–45.

13. Aghaeepour N, Finak G, Hoos H, et al. Critical assessment of automated flow cytometry data analysis techniques. Nat Methods 2013;10(3):228–38.

14. McCarthy J, Minsky ML, Rochester N, et al. A proposal for the dartmouth summer research project on artificial intelligence, august 31, 1955. AI Mag 2006;27(4):12.

15. Lee MD, Elsayed M, Chopra S, Lui YW. A No-Math Primer on the Principles of Machine Learning for Radiologists. Seminars in Ultrasound, CT and MRI 2022;43(2): 133–41.

16. Hastie T, Tibshirani R, Friedman J. The elements of statistical learning: data mining, inference, and prediction. Springer series in statistics. New York: Springer; 2009.

17. Hans CP, Weisenburger DD, Greiner TC, et al. Confirmation of the molecular classification of diffuse large B-cell lymphoma by immunohistochemistry using a tissue microarray. Blood 2004;103(1):275–82.

18. Kang, A.S., Kang, L.C., Mastorides, S.M., et al., Machine Learning Approaches to Automated Flow Cytometry Diagnosis of Chronic Lymphocytic Leukemia. arXiv preprint arXiv:2107.09728. 2021.

19. Pedregosa F, Varoquaux G, Gramfort A, et al. Scikit-learn: machine learning in python. arXiv. arXiv preprint arXiv:1201.0490. 2012.

20. McInnes L, Healy J, Melville J. Umap: Uniform manifold approximation and projection for dimension reduction. arXiv preprint arXiv:1802.03426. 2018.

21. Ng DP, Wu D, Wood BL, et al. Computer-aided detection of rare tumor populations in flow cytometry: an example with classic Hodgkin lymphoma. Am J Clin Pathol 2015;144(3):517–24.

22. Ko BS, Wang YF, Li JL, et al. Clinically validated machine learning algorithm for detecting residual diseases with multicolor flow cytometry analysis in acute myeloid leukemia and myelodysplastic syndrome. EBioMedicine 2018;37: 91–100.

23. Zhao M, Mallesh N, Höllein A, et al. Hematologist-level classification of mature B-cell neoplasm using deep learning on multiparameter flow cytometry data. Cytometry 2020;97(10):1073–80.

24. Gaidano V, Tenace V, Santoro N, et al. A clinically applicable approach to the classification of B-cell non-Hodgkin lymphomas with flow cytometry and machine learning. Cancers 2020;12(6):1684.

25. Simonson PD, Wu Y, Wu D, et al. De novo identification and visualization of important cell populations for classic Hodgkin lymphoma using flow cytometry and machine learning. Am J Clin Pathol 2021;156(6):1092–102.

26. Mallesh N, Zhao M, Meintker L, et al. Knowledge transfer to enhance the performance of deep learning models for automated classification of B cell neoplasms. Patterns 2021;2(10):100351.

27. Clichet V, Harrivel V, Delette C, et al. Accurate classification of plasma cell dyscrasias is achieved by combining artificial intelligence and flow cytometry. Br J Haematol 2022;196(5):1175–83.

28. Simonson PD, Lee AY, Wu D. Potential for process improvement of clinical flow cytometry by incorporating real-time automated screening of data to expedite addition of antibody panels: a single laboratory analysis. Am J Clin Pathol 2022;157(3):443–50.

29. Monaghan SA, Li J-L, Liu Y-C, et al. A machine learning approach to the classification of acute leukemias and distinction from nonneoplastic cytopenias using flow cytometry data. Am J Clin Pathol 2022;157(4):546–53.
30. Radakovich N, Nagy M, Nazha A. Artificial intelligence in hematology: current challenges and opportunities. Curr Hematol Malig Rep 2020;15(3):203–10.
31. Rieke N, Hancox J, Li W, et al. The future of digital health with federated learning. NPJ digital medicine 2020;3(1):1–7.
32. Collins GS, Dhiman P, Navarro CLA, et al. Protocol for development of a reporting guideline (TRIPOD-AI) and risk of bias tool (PROBAST-AI) for diagnostic and prognostic prediction model studies based on artificial intelligence. BMJ Open 2021;11(7):e048008.
33. Gianfrancesco MA, Tamang S, Yazdany J, et al. Potential biases in machine learning algorithms using electronic health Record data. JAMA Intern Med 2018;178(11):1544–7.
34. Artificial Intelligence/Machine Learning (AI/ML)-Based Software as a Medical Device (SaMD) Action Plan. 2021.
35. Ribeiro MT, Singh S, Guestrin C. " Why should i trust you?" Explaining the predictions of any classifier. Paper presented at: Proceedings of the 22nd ACM SIGKDD international conference on knowledge discovery and data mining2016.

Advances in Clinical Mass Cytometry

Abhishek Koladiya, PhD[a], Kara L. Davis, DO[a,b,*]

KEYWORDS

- Mass cytometry • High-dimensional • Cytometry • Protein • Signaling
- Infectious disease • Neuroscience • Clinical research

KEY POINTS

- Mass cytometry enables system-level monitoring of immune cells to study cellular mechanisms driving disease conditions.
- Reproducibility, high sensitivity, and robustness of mass cytometry assays make mass cytometer a suitable tool for clinical sample analysis.
- Clinical applications of mass cytometry allow therapeutic decision making and patient stratification.

INTRODUCTION

As patient-tailored therapies are becoming routine, improved methods for comprehensive profiling of responses at the single-cell level are required. Flow cytometry (FCM) is a commonly used tool for this task in clinical research applications including cancer, infectious diseases, cardiovascular disease, and immune monitoring. Development of novel fluorophores, laser technology, and data analysis methods have allowed an increase in the number of parameters able to be measured per cell, doubling each year (Roederer Law for FCM), which has led in development of novel functional and phenotypic assays detecting up to 30 markers per cells.[1–6] Moreover, arrival of spectral FCM that captures the entire emission spectrum of every fluorophore has pushed this limit to 40 to 43 markers per cell.[7,8] However, spectral overlap of fluorescent dyes remains a key limitation for FCM, and although it can resolved mathematically using compensation, with increases in parameters, the spectral overlap remains challenging to remove.[9–14] Additionally, application of FCM for clinical samples remains challenging, because larger sample volumes are required to test several combinations of antigen fluorochromes and to account for spillover correction; additionally, robust standardization of instrumentation is needed to achieve

The authors have no conflict of interest to disclose.
[a] Department of Pediatrics, Stanford University School of Medicine, Stanford, CA, USA;
[b] Center for Cancer Cell Therapy, Stanford University, Stanford, CA, USA
* Corresponding author. 265 Campus Drive, Lorry Lokey Stem Cell Building, Stanford, CA 94305.
E-mail address: kardavis@stanford.edu

0272-2712/23/© 2023 Elsevier Inc. All rights reserved.

reproducibility and comparable results between cytometry experiments.[15,16] Despite this, clinical laboratories rely heavily on FCM for many cellular phenotyping assays.

Mass cytometry or cytometry by time of flight (CyTOF) addresses many limitations of fluorescence and spectral FCM as it utilizes rare earth metal-tagged antibodies and inductively coupled plasma ionization to detect up to 50 parameters per cell.[17,18] Because of the elimination of fluorescent dyes, compensation is usually not required, and even with a limited volume of sample, the maximum number of markers per cell can be measured. However, CyTOF does not eliminate spillover. A minor spillover between CyTOF channels occurs because of metal impurity, oxidation, and mass overlap.[1] With proper experimental design, these limitations can be addressed.[19,20] Compared with FCM panel design, CyTOF panels are relatively easy to design and do not require extensive domain knowledge. Additionally, sample multiplexing of samples eliminates batch effects and leads to comparable results between CyTOF runs. All these features make CyTOF an ideal tool for clinical research.

Here is discussed development of CyTOF assays that enable single-cell detection of surface and intracellular proteins, thus enabling evaluation of cytokine production, signaling pathways, codetection of proteins and ribonucleic acid (RNA), cellular metabolism and epigenetic marks. Then the authors discuss the application of these assays in clinical research across domains including cancer, infectious disease, autoimmune disease, and neuroscience. Finally, how CyTOF could be incorporated in more routine clinical monitoring will be discussed.

CYTOMETRY BY TIME OF FLIGHT-BASED FUNCTIONAL ASSAYS

Since the advent of mass cytometry over a decade ago, assays to profile different cellular features have been developed. Here is an overview of each of these assays. A graphical representation is shown in **Fig. 1**.

Cellular Phenotyping

The human immune system consists of various cell types possessing distinct antigen specificities. Over the years, advancement in bulk transcriptomics, sc-RNA seq, and FCM has revealed novel markers (genes and proteins) defining cell types. Thus, inclusion of more markers can improve resolution into cellular identity. Theoretically, CyTOF can measure up to 100 parameters per cell. Current studies have measured up to 47 markers per cell.[21] That CyTOF can evaluate single cells in high parameters allows detection of novel and rare cell types as shown in studies of gastrointestinal disorders including innate lymphoid and T regulatory cells.[22,23]

Intracellular Signaling

Cell signaling pathways are vital for cell-cell communication and coordinate cellular proliferation and differentiation.[24,25] Signaling events are often mediated by kinases and phosphatases to regulate phosphorylation events. Deregulation of signaling leads to abnormal cell physiology and disease. The multiparameter, multiplexed nature of CyTOF makes it a natural choice for studying signaling pathways. CyTOF has been applied to study signaling networks and cell-cell communication following drug stimulation, to examine the relationship between pairs of phosphorylation sites to infer signaling networks, and to track signaling dynamics during phenotypic transitions.[26,27] Over the years, researchers have utilized this approach to study cancers including leukemia, glioblastoma, and ovarian cancers[28-30] CyTOF-based signaling analysis has been coupled with transient protein overexpression such as green fluorescent protein (GFP) and red fluorescent protein (RFP) to identify novel signaling mechanisms

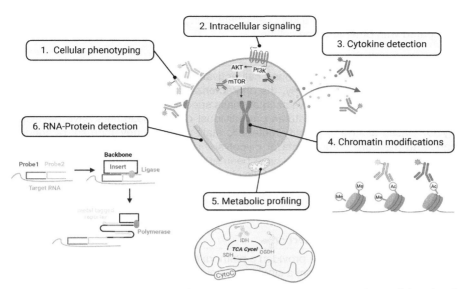

Fig. 1. Cellular view of CyTOF-based functional assays. CyTOF assays require a validated antibody to detect a target of interest. These antibodies can be used to identify molecules across various assays. Broadly, these assays can be divided into 6 subgroups: (1) phenotyping, (2) signaling pathways; (3) cytokine detection assay, (4) chromatin modification, (5) metabolic profiling, (6) RNA-protein detection.

associated with cancer progression and drug response.[31,32] Tape and collogues developed a thiol-reactive organoid barcoding in situ (TOBis) method to use CyTOF to study signaling networks between healthy and cancerous organoid cultures.[33]

Cytokine Detection

Cytokines are intracellular proteins, and their production is often regarded as a marker of immune cell function. Decades of research suggest that nearly all diseases are directly or indirectly linked with cytokine-mediated immune system activation.[34–36] Evaluating cytokine production in single immune cells from a cell mixture like PBMCs can reveal a wide range of effector functions. Such heterogeneity is better understood utilizing single-cell technologies. Microengraving-based and FLUOROSpot assays allow profiling of cytokines but are limited to 4 parameters because of spectral overlap.[37,38] FCM with proper compensation and CyTOF allows measurement of 5 to 14 cytokines per panel.[39,40]

Chromatin Modifications

Histone protein modifications including acetylation, methylation, and ubiquitination regulate chromatin structure.[41] Chromatin regulation is tightly linked with gene expression, which in turn influences cellular phenotype and function. Deregulation of histone modifications are linked with various disease conditions. Traditional methods (chromatin immunoprecipitation, Western blot) to evaluate histone modifications are performed on the bulk population. Immunohistochemistry and immunofluorescence quantify chromatin modifications in single cells but are low throughput and labor-intensive. These challenges can be addressed using epigenetic landscape profiling using cytometry by time of flight (EpiTOF), which utilizes CyTOF to detect a broad range of histone modifications using metal-tagged antibodies.[42] Applied to healthy peripheral blood mononuclear cells, EpiTOF has detected cell-type specific chromatin profiles. For instance, natural killer cells were found to fewer chromatin modifications compared with other immune cell types.

Metabolic Profiling

Cellular metabolism drives immune cell activation, proliferation, differentiation, and effector functions.[43,44] Typically, the characterization of metabolites within immune cells is done using bulk assays such as mass spectrometry or extracellular flux analysis.[45] To evaluate these features on individual cells, researchers have developed CyTOF-based assays to identify metabolic states through development of antibody panels to measure components of glycolysis, mitochondrial respiration, metabolic transporters or enzymes. These have been applied to the study of immune cells in the setting of normal activation or following chimeric antigen receptor (CAR) T cell treatment.[46,47] The application of these assays to a broad range of diseases will enable identification of metabolic alterations associated with disease that can serve as biomarkers or targets for personalized therapy.

Ribonucleic Acid-Protein Detection

Single-omics methods have provided a plethora of evidence regarding the benefits of profiling RNA and protein from a single cell. Application of these methods is shedding light on mechanisms driving treatment failure. Although these methods are sequencing based, CyTOF can also be utilized for per cell codetection of RNA and proteins. In 2016, Frei and colleagues proposed the proximity ligation assay for RNA (PLAYR) method to quantify more than 40 transcripts and proteins.[48] Briefly, cells are permeabilized, and 2 DNA oligonucleotide probes are added that are designed to hybridize at 2 adjacent regions of a target transcript. Each of these probes contains 1 region for selective hybridization to its cognate target RNA sequence and another region that acts as a template to bind and circularize 2 additional oligonucleotides called insert and backbone. When insert and backbone hybridized to the probe pair, they are amplified to produce concatenated complementary copies. Finally, the amplified products are detected using a metal-labeled oligonucleotide. This detection of transcripts can be multiplexed with traditional protein targeted antibodies to enable codetection of mRNA and protein from individual cells.

CYTOMETRY BY TIME OF FLIGHT IN COMBINATION WITH MULTI-OMICS

A primary goal of clinical studies is to extract the maximum amount of information from limited cellular material. The advent of single-cell transcriptomics (sc-RNA seq), epigenomics single-cell sequencing assay for transposase-accessible chromatin sequencing (scATAC seq), and multi-omics such as cellular indexing of transcriptomes and epitopes by sequencing (CITE seq), has enabled researchers to detect single or multiple omics layers. These methods provide a comprehensive view of heterogeneous clinical samples. Yet these methods are relatively low-throughput, subject to cell type loss, and expensive.[49] To tackle these challenges, researchers often utilize CyTOF to first phenotype cell populations, then FACS sort populations of interest for multi-omics assays[50] or integrate CyTOF data with data from other single-cell modalities.[51,52]

CLINICAL APPLICATIONS OF CYTOMETRY BY TIME OF FLIGHT
Cancer

Initial applications of CyTOF were focused on profiling cell signaling networks, phenotypic identification of tumor cells, and decoding the tumor-immune microenvironment.[28,53,54] These studies identified novel cellular features within patient groups considered to be distinct as per clinico-pathological schemes. The advent of machine learning algorithms and novel data analysis approaches have enabled the identification of features predicting disease outcomes or correlating with prognosis. Davis and colleagues performed CyTOF analysis on 60 primary diagnostic B-cell precursor acute lymphoblastic leukemia (BCP-ALL) samples to identify cells predictive of relapse in a diagnosis sample.[55] The authors developed a machine learning model to identify cells predictive of future relapse and identified the features of these cells for further study. Similarly, Leelatian and colleagues introduced a machine learning algorithm, Risk Assessment Population IDentification (RAPID), to identify phenotypically distinct cell-types correlating with patient survival in glioblastoma, a deadly brain tumor.[29] RAPID detected 4 glioblastoma-negative prognostic (GNP) populations enriched for S100 B, SOX2, p-STAT3, and p-STAT5 expression whose abundance was predictive of poor patient outcomes and 5 glioblastoma positive prognostic (GPP) populations enriched with EGFR and CD44 expression whose abundance was associated with improved overall survival.

Besides predicting cell types and disease features, CyTOF has been used to study cancer immunotherapies such as CAR T-cell therapy. CAR T treatment has shown remarkable improvement for patients with B-cell malignancies.[56,57] June and colleagues performed functional and molecular characterization of CAR T cells from 2 chronic lymphocytic leukemia patients over the period of 10 years.[58] The data suggested 2 major phases of CAR T therapy response: an initial phase dominated by CD8 CAR T cells or CD4-CD8-Helios^{high} γδ CAR T and a long-term second phase represented by Ki67+ and CD38+HLA-DR + CD95+ cytolytic CD4 T cells. In the second study, Good and colleagues focused on biomarkers associated with successful CAR T treatment in large B-cell lymphoma (LBCL).[59] The authors detected populations associated with progressive disease (PD) and complete remission (CR) at day 7 after infusion. Responding patients demonstrated a T follicular helper (T_{FH}) cell-like population (PD1+CD57+CD4 CAR T cells) and CD57+ Blimp-1+T-bet + CD8 CAR T cells, while patients with PD demonstrated an immunosuppressive T-regulatory cell-like population.

More recently, CyTOF, together with bulk and single-cell transcriptomics, imaging mass cytometry, pharmacoscopy, and 4i drug response profiling (4i DRP), has been utilized in an observation clinical trial called the Tumor Profiler (TuPro) Study for in-depth tumor analysis in order to support clinical decision making.[60] Two-hundred forty tumor samples from acute myeloid leukemia, ovarian cancer, and melanoma patients over 3 years were collected and analyzed. Preliminary results of this study demonstrated the potential of these technologies to support clinical decision making.

Infectious Disease

Infections induce broad immune responses involving the innate and adaptive arms of a healthy immune system. Mass cytometry has been widely used to study immune response to infection with human immune virus,[61–63] Ebola virus,[64] hepatitis B virus,[65] gamma herpes virus,[66] dengue virus,[67,68] and Zika virus.[69] More recently CyTOF has been employed to compare malaria-[70] and helminth-[71] induced immune response between ethnic cohorts from European, African, and Indonesian cohorts. The authors found distinct immune signatures of T-helper and innate lymphoid cells correlating with each ethnic cohort. In general, application of CyTOF to study cell types contributing to viral and pathogen responses have deepened understanding of the immune response to infection and will ultimately aid in the development of treatments and vaccines.

Mass cytometry has been utilized to study the immunopathology of severe acute respiratory distress syndrome coronavirus 2 (SARS-CoV-2). These studies were broadly focused on 2 aspects: identifying markers associated with dysfunctional immune systems[21,72] and stratifying patients with early and delayed immune responses.[73,74] Based on severity of disease, patients with SARS-CoV-2 can be classified clinically into: moderate, severe, and critical cases.[75] Studies suggested that compared with healthy donors, patients infected with SARS-CoV-2 in all clinical severity categories have increased frequencies of B cells, naïve CD4 T, and CD4+CD8+ T cells, while frequencies of naïve, memory and effector CD8 T cells were decreased. Activated CD8 T cells, dendritic cells, and macrophages were observed in moderate cases, and these cells were seen in severe and critical cases but with an exhausted phenotype. Additionally, researchers have also applied CyTOF to study immune responses following the administration of mRNA-based vaccines developed by Moderna (mRNA-1273) and Pfizer/BioNTech (BNT162b2).[76,77]

Autoimmune Disease

Inflammatory cells play a vital role in autoimmune disease progression and severity. Various research groups have exploited the multidimensional capability of CyTOF to understand immune regulation for rheumatoid arthritis (RA),[78,79] systemic lupus erythematosus (SLE),[80,81] spondyloarthritis,[82] multiple sclerosis (MS),[83,84] inflammatory bowel disease (IBD),[85] and celiac disease.[86] Some of these studies performed by independent groups identified distinct cell types associated with disease risk. Two independent studies of RA patients identified CD4 T cell-mediated pathogenesis associated with disease outcomes.[78,87] To understand the role of T cells in autoimmune conditions such as CeD, SLE, and systemic sclerosis, Davis and colleagues employed metal conjugated HLA-DQ tetramers and CyTOF. Their analysis revealed that the antigen-specific T-cell phenotype was similar to that published in RA by Rao and colleagues.[78,88] This phenotype was enriched in multiple conditions including CeD, SLE, and systemic sclerosis. Together, these studies show the power of high-parameter phenotyping to identify complex cellular features correlating with disease pathogenesis that can be used for diagnostic purposes or can serve as potential targets for therapeutic interventions.

Neuroimmune Disorders

Applications of CyTOF are not limited to the peripheral immune system. A growing body of literature highlights the unique immune environment of the central nervous system (CNS) where immune cells have varied roles in immune defense, tissue homeostasis, and neurologic conditions such as Alzheimer disease (AD) and multiple sclerosis (MS).[89–93] A CyTOF study revealed that CNS resident immune cells can be distinguished from peripheral immune cells by expression of CD44.[94] The brain parenchyma is enriched with immune cells, mainly microglia, a specialized macrophage accounting for up to approximately 10% CNS cells. Studying murine microglia using CyTOF, Mrdjen and colleagues and Ajami and colleagues reported that microglia undergo dramatic changes with respect to functional and phenotypic markers in amyotrophic lateral sclerosis and encephalomyelitis.[95,96] To better understand the role of microglia in MS, Böttcher and colleagues profiled microglia from 5 brain regions and found that in disease conditions, microglia demonstrate an activation phenotype with upregulation of CD68, CD86, CD45, and CX3CR1.[83] These studies demonstrate the utility to use CyTOF to monitor immune composition within the CNS.

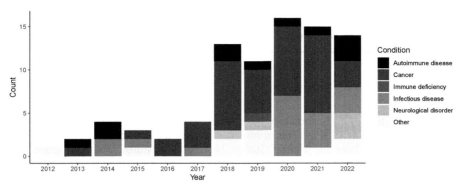

Fig. 2. CyTOF use in clinical trials. Bar graph depicting increasing number of clinical trials reported since 2012 utilizing CyTOF for correlative analyses. The data were collected from https://clinicaltrials.gov/ using "CyTOF" as a keyword.

FUTURE DIRECTIONS

CyTOF has significantly increased the ability to profile cellular populations at the single-cell level. This is beneficial particularly when the samples have low cell numbers such as in clinical biopsies. As of 2022, more than 80 clinical trials were reportedly using CyTOF (**Fig. 2**) to perform correlative assays.

Further, standardized protocols proposed by multicenter and multicohort studies suggested lower inter- and intrainstrument variability, reproducibility, sensitivity, and robustness of CyTOF-based analyses.[97,98] These facilitated researchers to include CyTOF within their state-of-the-art analytical platforms to acquire samples from clinical trials and collaborate across institutions and laboratories. The Cancer Immune Monitoring and Analysis Centers-Cancer Immunologic Data Commons (CIMAC-CIDC) network (https://cimac-network.org/) established by National Cancer Institute aims to identify biomarkers of cancer immunotherapies across clinical trials and uses CyTOF as a core assay in the context of these trials.[99] The Immunophenotyping Assessment in a coronavirus disease 2019 (COVID-19) Cohort (IMPACC) launched by National Institutes of Health (NIH) utilized CyTOF and other proteomic and transcriptomics technologies to identify biomarkers associated with effective COVID therapeutics.[100] As genomic and exome sequencing are routine tests for genetic disorders, the infrastructure proposed by these networks can be utilized as a part of clinical decision making and patient stratification.

SUMMARY

CyTOF offers system-level monitoring of the immune system in conjunction with novel biological assays to decode immune mechanisms driving disease conditions. In the past decade, researchers have exploited the high-dimensional capabilities of CyTOF to discover disease associated cell-types and cellular features that are linked to outcomes and identified biomarkers for future treatment.

CLINICS CARE POINTS

- Clinical mass cytometry overcomes challenges faced by traditional flow cytometers such as fluorescent spillover and requirement of larger sample volumes and reproducibility.

- With improved standardized operating protocols, mass cytometry can be utilized to aid routine clinical decision making.

FUNDING

K.L. Davis is the Anne T. and Robert M. Bass Endowed Faculty Scholar in Pediatric Cancer and Blood Diseases. This work is supported by Stanford Maternal and Child Health Research Institute, United States, NCI, United States U54 CA232568, NCI R01 CA251858, NCI R21 CA234529, NCI R01 CA251858-01A1S1, Mark Foundation Aspire Award, The Andrew McDonough B Positive Foundation, W81XWH-19-PRCRP-CDA Department of Defense Young Investigator Award.

STATEMENTS AND DECLARATIONS

The authors declared no competing financial interest.

ACKNOWLEDGMENTS

The authors thank all members of the Davis Laboratory for helpful discussions.

REFERENCES

1. Bendall SC, Nolan GP, Roederer M, et al. A deep profiler's guide to cytometry. Trends Immunol 2012;33(7):323–32.
2. O'Gorman MR. Clinically relevant functional flow cytometry assays. Clin Lab Med 2001;21(4):779–94.
3. Krutzik PO, Nolan GP. Fluorescent cell barcoding in flow cytometry allows high-throughput drug screening and signaling profiling. Nat Methods 2006;3(5): 361–8.
4. Maciorowski Z, Chattopadhyay PK, Jain P. Basic multicolor flow cytometry. Curr Protoc Immunol 2017;117. 5.4.1-5.4.38.
5. Mair F, Prlic M. OMIP-044: 28-color immunophenotyping of the human dendritic cell compartment. Cytom Part J Int Soc Anal Cytol 2018;93(4):402–5.
6. Vanikova S, Koladiya A, Musil J. OMIP-080: 29-Color flow cytometry panel for comprehensive evaluation of NK and T cells reconstitution after hematopoietic stem cells transplantation. Cytom Part J Int Soc Anal Cytol 2022;101(1):21–6.
7. Park LM, Lannigan J, Jaimes MC. OMIP-069: forty-color full spectrum flow cytometry panel for deep immunophenotyping of major cell subsets in human peripheral blood. Cytometry 2020;97(10):1044–51.
8. Sahir F, Mateo JM, Steinhoff M, et al. Development of a 43 color panel for the characterization of conventional and unconventional T-cell subsets, B cells, NK cells, monocytes, dendritic cells, and innate lymphoid cells using spectral flow cytometry. Cytom Part J Int Soc Anal Cytol 2020. https://doi.org/10.1002/cyto.a.24288.
9. Roederer M. Spectral compensation for flow cytometry: visualization artifacts, limitations, and caveats. Cytometry 2001;45(3):194–205.
10. Mahnke YD, Roederer M. Optimizing a multicolor immunophenotyping assay. Clin Lab Med 2007;27(3):469–85, v.
11. Bagwell CB, Adams EG. Fluorescence spectral overlap compensation for any number of flow cytometry parameters. Ann N Y Acad Sci 1993;677:167–84.

12. Ferrer-Font L, Pellefigues C, Mayer JU, et al. Panel design and optimization for high-dimensional immunophenotyping assays using spectral flow cytometry. Curr Protoc Cytom 2020;92(1):e70.

13. Roederer M. Compensation in flow cytometry. Curr Protoc Cytom 2002. https://doi.org/10.1002/0471142956.cy0114s22. Chapter 1:Unit 1.14.

14. Brummelman J, Haftmann C, Núñez NG, et al. Development, application and computational analysis of high-dimensional fluorescent antibody panels for single-cell flow cytometry. Nat Protoc 2019;14(7):1946–69.

15. Maecker HT, Rinfret A, D'Souza P, et al. Standardization of cytokine flow cytometry assays. BMC Immunol 2005;6:13.

16. Finak G, Langweiler M, Jaimes M, et al. Standardizing flow cytometry immunophenotyping analysis from the human ImmunoPhenotyping Consortium. Sci Rep 2016;6:20686.

17. Bandura DR, Baranov VI, Ornatsky OI, et al. Mass cytometry: technique for real time single cell multitarget immunoassay based on inductively coupled plasma time-of-flight mass spectrometry. Anal Chem 2009;81(16):6813–22.

18. Spitzer MH, Nolan GP. Mass cytometry: single cells, many features. Cell 2016; 165(4):780–91.

19. Chevrier S, Crowell HL, Zanotelli VRT, et al. Compensation of signal spillover in suspension and imaging mass cytometry. Cell Syst 2018;6(5):612–20.e5.

20. Miao Q, Wang F, Dou J, et al. Ab initio spillover compensation in mass cytometry data. Cytom Part J Int Soc Anal Cytol 2021;99(9):899–909.

21. Rodriguez L, Pekkarinen PT, Lakshmikanth T, et al. Systems-level immunomonitoring from acute to recovery phase of severe COVID-19. Cell Rep Med 2020; 1(5):100078.

22. van Unen V, Höllt T, Pezzotti N, et al. Visual analysis of mass cytometry data by hierarchical stochastic neighbour embedding reveals rare cell types. Nat Commun 2017;8(1):1740.

23. Kunicki MA, Amaya Hernandez LC, Davis KL, et al. Identity and diversity of human peripheral Th and T regulatory cells defined by single-cell mass cytometry. J Immunol 2018;200(1):336–46.

24. Groves JT, Kuriyan J. Molecular mechanisms in signal transduction at the membrane. Nat Struct Mol Biol 2010;17(6):659–65.

25. Yu FX, Zhao B, Guan KL. Hippo pathway in organ size control, tissue homeostasis, and cancer. Cell 2015;163(4):811–28.

26. Bodenmiller B, Zunder ER, Finck R, et al. Multiplexed mass cytometry profiling of cellular states perturbed by small-molecule regulators. Nat Biotechnol 2012; 30(9):858–67.

27. Krishnaswamy S, Spitzer MH, Mingueneau M, et al. Systems biology. Conditional density-based analysis of T cell signaling in single-cell data. Science 2014;346(6213):1250689.

28. Levine JH, Simonds EF, Bendall SC, et al. Data-driven phenotypic dissection of AML reveals progenitor-like cells that correlate with prognosis. Cell 2015;162(1): 184–97.

29. N L, J S, Am M, et al. Unsupervised machine learning reveals risk stratifying glioblastoma tumor cells. Elife 2020;9. https://doi.org/10.7554/eLife.56879.

30. Gonzalez VD, Samusik N, Chen TJ, et al. Commonly occurring cell subsets in high-Grade serous ovarian tumors identified by single-cell mass cytometry. Cell Rep 2018;22(7):1875–88.

31. Lun XK, Zanotelli VRT, Wade JD, et al. Influence of node abundance on signaling network state and dynamics analyzed by mass cytometry. Nat Biotechnol 2017;35(2):164–72.

32. Lun XK, Szklarczyk D, Gábor A, et al. Analysis of the human Kinome and phosphatome by mass cytometry reveals overexpression-induced effects on cancer-related signaling. Mol Cell 2019;74(5):1086–102.e5.

33. Qin X, Sufi J, Vlckova P, et al. Cell-type specific signaling networks in heterocellular organoids. Nat Methods 2020;17(3):335–42.

34. Brüünsgaard H, Pedersen BK. Age-related inflammatory cytokines and disease. Immunol Allergy Clin North Am 2003;23(1):15–39.

35. Schett G, Elewaut D, McInnes IB, et al. How cytokine networks fuel inflammation: toward a cytokine-based disease taxonomy. Nat Med 2013;19(7):822–4.

36. Barrat FJ, Crow MK, Ivashkiv LB. Interferon target-gene expression and epigenomic signatures in health and disease. Nat Immunol 2019;20(12):1574–83.

37. Bradshaw EM, Kent SC, Tripuraneni V, et al. Concurrent detection of secreted products from human lymphocytes by microengraving: cytokines and antigen-reactive antibodies. Clin Immunol Orlando Fla 2008;129(1):10–8.

38. Ahlborg N, Axelsson B. Dual- and triple-color fluorospot. Methods Mol Biol Clifton NJ 2012;792:77–85.

39. De Rosa SC, Herzenberg LA, Herzenberg LA, et al. 11-color, 13-parameter flow cytometry: identification of human naive T cells by phenotype, function, and T-cell receptor diversity. Nat Med 2001;7(2):245–8.

40. Bendall SC, Simonds EF, Qiu P, et al. Single-cell mass cytometry of differential immune and drug responses across a human hematopoietic continuum. Science 2011;332(6030):687–96.

41. Kouzarides T. Chromatin modifications and their function. Cell 2007;128(4):693–705.

42. Cheung P, Vallania F, Dvorak M, et al. Single-cell epigenetics - chromatin modification atlas unveiled by mass cytometry. Clin Immunol Orlando Fla 2018;196:40–8.

43. Olenchock BA, Rathmell JC, Vander Heiden MG. Biochemical underpinnings of immune cell metabolic phenotypes. Immunity 2017;46(5):703–13.

44. Klein Geltink RI, Kyle RL, Pearce EL. Unraveling the complex interplay between T cell metabolism and function. Annu Rev Immunol 2018;36:461–88.

45. Dettmer K, Aronov PA, Hammock BD. Mass spectrometry-based metabolomics. Mass Spectrom Rev 2007;26(1):51–78.

46. Hartmann FJ, Mrdjen D, McCaffrey E, et al. Single-cell metabolic profiling of human cytotoxic T cells. Nat Biotechnol 2021;39(2):186–97.

47. Levine LS, Hiam-Galvez KJ, Marquez DM, et al. Single-cell analysis by mass cytometry reveals metabolic states of early-activated CD8+ T cells during the primary immune response. Immunity 2021;54(4):829–44.e5.

48. Frei AP, Bava FA, Zunder ER, et al. Highly multiplexed simultaneous detection of RNAs and proteins in single cells. Nat Methods 2016;13(3):269–75.

49. Kashima Y, Sakamoto Y, Kaneko K, et al. Single-cell sequencing techniques from individual to multiomics analyses. Exp Mol Med 2020;52(9):1419–27.

50. Lavin Y, Kobayashi S, Leader A, et al. Innate immune landscape in early lung adenocarcinoma by paired single-cell analyses. Cell 2017;169(4):750–65.e17.

51. Dou J, Liang S, Mohanty V, et al. Bi-order multimodal integration of single-cell data. Genome Biol 2022;23(1):112.

52. Zhu B, Chen S, Bai Y, et al. Robust single-cell matching and multi-modal analysis using shared and distinct features reveals orchestrated immune responses. Nat Methods 2023;20(2):304–15.

53. Amir E ad D, Davis KL, Tadmor MD, et al. viSNE enables visualization of high dimensional single-cell data and reveals phenotypic heterogeneity of leukemia. Nat Biotechnol 2013;31(6):545–52.

54. Chevrier S, Levine JH, Zanotelli VRT, et al. An immune atlas of clear cell renal cell carcinoma. Cell 2017;169(4):736–49.e18.

55. Good Z, Sarno J, Jager A, et al. Single-cell developmental classification of B cell precursor acute lymphoblastic leukemia at diagnosis reveals predictors of relapse. Nat Med 2018;24(4):474–83.

56. Mueller KT, Maude SL, Porter DL, et al. Cellular kinetics of CTL019 in relapsed/refractory B-cell acute lymphoblastic leukemia and chronic lymphocytic leukemia. Blood 2017;130(21):2317–25.

57. June CH, Sadelain M. Chimeric antigen receptor therapy. N Engl J Med 2018;379(1):64–73.

58. Melenhorst JJ, Chen GM, Wang M, et al. Decade-long leukaemia remissions with persistence of CD4+ CAR T cells. Nature 2022;602(7897):503–9.

59. Good Z, Spiegel JY, Sahaf B, et al. Post-infusion CAR TReg cells identify patients resistant to CD19-CAR therapy. Nat Med 2022;28(9):1860–71.

60. Irmisch A, Bonilla X, Chevrier S, et al. The Tumor Profiler Study: integrated, multiomic, functional tumor profiling for clinical decision support. Cancer Cell 2021;39(3):288–93.

61. Cavrois M, Banerjee T, Mukherjee G, et al. Mass cytometric analysis of HIV entry, replication, and remodeling in tissue CD4+ T cells. Cell Rep 2017;20(4):984–98.

62. Manganaro L, Hong P, Hernandez MM, et al. IL-15 regulates susceptibility of CD4+ T cells to HIV infection. Proc Natl Acad Sci U S A 2018;115(41):E9659–67.

63. Bekele Y, Lakshmikanth T, Chen Y, et al. Mass cytometry identifies distinct CD4+ T cell clusters distinguishing HIV-1-infected patients according to antiretroviral therapy initiation. JCI Insight 2019;4(3):e125442.

64. McElroy AK, Akondy RS, McIlwain DR, et al. Immunologic timeline of Ebola virus disease and recovery in humans. JCI Insight 2020;5(10):e137260, 137260.

65. Le Bert N, Gill US, Hong M, et al. Effects of hepatitis B surface antigen on virus-specific and global T cells in patients with chronic hepatitis B virus infection. Gastroenterology 2020;159(2):652–64.

66. Kimball AK, Oko LM, Kaspar RE, et al. High-dimensional characterization of IL-10 production and IL-10-dependent regulation during primary gammaherpesvirus infection. ImmunoHorizons 2019;3(3):94–109.

67. Chng MHY, Lim MQ, Rouers A, et al. Large-scale HLA tetramer tracking of T cells during dengue infection reveals broad acute activation and differentiation into two memory cell fates. Immunity 2019;51(6):1119–35.e5.

68. Tian Y, Babor M, Lane J, et al. Dengue-specific CD8+ T cell subsets display specialized transcriptomic and TCR profiles. J Clin Invest 2019;129(4):1727–41.

69. Michlmayr D, Kim EY, Rahman AH, et al. Comprehensive immunoprofiling of pediatric zika reveals key role for monocytes in the acute phase and No effect of prior dengue virus infection. Cell Rep 2020;31(4):107569.

70. de Jong SE, van Unen V, Manurung MD, et al. Systems analysis and controlled malaria infection in Europeans and Africans elucidate naturally acquired immunity. Nat Immunol 2021;22(5):654–65.

71. de Ruiter K, Jochems SP, Tahapary DL, et al. Helminth infections drive hetero-geneity in human type 2 and regulatory cells. Sci Transl Med 2020;12(524): eaaw3703.

72. Wang W, Su B, Pang L, et al. High-dimensional immune profiling by mass cy-tometry revealed immunosuppression and dysfunction of immunity in COVID-19 patients. Cell Mol Immunol 2020;17(6):650–2.

73. Chevrier S, Zurbuchen Y, Cervia C, et al. A distinct innate immune signature marks progression from mild to severe COVID-19. Cell Rep Med 2021;2(1): 100166.

74. Burnett CE, Okholm TLH, Tenvooren I, et al. Mass cytometry reveals a conserved immune trajectory of recovery in hospitalized COVID-19 patients. Im-munity 2022;55(7):1284–98.e3.

75. Yang X, Yu Y, Xu J, et al. Clinical course and outcomes of critically ill patients with SARS-CoV-2 pneumonia in Wuhan, China: a single-centered, retrospective, observational study. Lancet Respir Med 2020;8(5):475–81.

76. Neidleman J, Luo X, McGregor M, et al. mRNA vaccine-induced T cells respond identically to SARS-CoV-2 variants of concern but differ in longevity and homing properties depending on prior infection status. Elife 2021;10:e72619.

77. Kramer KJ, Wilfong EM, Voss K, et al. Single-cell profiling of the antigen-specific response to BNT162b2 SARS-CoV-2 RNA vaccine. Nat Commun 2022;13(1): 3466.

78. Rao DA, Gurish MF, Marshall JL, et al. Pathologically expanded peripheral T helper cell subset drives B cells in rheumatoid arthritis. Nature 2017; 542(7639):110–4.

79. Zhang F, Wei K, Slowikowski K, et al. Defining inflammatory cell states in rheu-matoid arthritis joint synovial tissues by integrating single-cell transcriptomics and mass cytometry. Nat Immunol 2019;20(7):928–42.

80. O'Gorman WE, Kong DS, Balboni IM, et al. Mass cytometry identifies a distinct monocyte cytokine signature shared by clinically heterogeneous pediatric SLE patients. J Autoimmun 2017. https://doi.org/10.1016/j.jaut.2017.03.010. S0896-8411(16)30412-7.

81. van der Kroef M, van den Hoogen LL, Mertens JS, et al. Cytometry by time of flight identifies distinct signatures in patients with systemic sclerosis, systemic lupus erythematosus and Sjögrens syndrome. Eur J Immunol 2020;50(1): 119–29.

82. Al-Mossawi MH, Chen L, Fang H, et al. Unique transcriptome signatures and GM-CSF expression in lymphocytes from patients with spondyloarthritis. Nat Commun 2017;8:1510.

83. Böttcher C, Fernández-Zapata C, Schlickeiser S, et al. Multi-parameter immune profiling of peripheral blood mononuclear cells by multiplexed single-cell mass cytometry in patients with early multiple sclerosis. Sci Rep 2019;9(1):19471.

84. Ingelfinger F, Gerdes LA, Kavaka V, et al. Twin study reveals non-heritable im-mune perturbations in multiple sclerosis. Nature 2022;603(7899):152–8.

85. Rubin SJS, Bai L, Haileselassie Y, et al. Mass cytometry reveals systemic and local immune signatures that distinguish inflammatory bowel diseases. Nat Commun 2019;10(1):2686.

86. van Unen V, Li N, Molendijk I, et al. Mass cytometry of the human mucosal im-mune system identifies tissue- and disease-associated immune subsets. Immu-nity 2016;44(5):1227–39.

87. Fonseka CY, Rao DA, Teslovich NC, et al. Mixed-effects association of single cells identifies an expanded effector CD4+ T cell subset in rheumatoid arthritis. Sci Transl Med 2018;10(463):eaaq0305.
88. Christophersen A, Lund EG, Snir O, et al. Distinct phenotype of CD4+ T cells driving celiac disease identified in multiple autoimmune conditions. Nat Med 2019;25(5):734–7.
89. Greter M, Heppner FL, Lemos MP, et al. Dendritic cells permit immune invasion of the CNS in an animal model of multiple sclerosis. Nat Med 2005;11(3): 328–34.
90. Prinz M, Priller J. Microglia and brain macrophages in the molecular age: from origin to neuropsychiatric disease. Nat Rev Neurosci 2014;15(5):300–12.
91. Ginhoux F, Greter M, Leboeuf M, et al. Fate mapping analysis reveals that adult microglia derive from primitive macrophages. Science 2010;330(6005):841–5.
92. Schreiner B, Heppner FL, Becher B. Modeling multiple sclerosis in laboratory animals. Semin Immunopathol 2009;31(4):479–95.
93. Prokop S, Miller KR, Drost N, et al. Impact of peripheral myeloid cells on amy-loid-β pathology in Alzheimer's disease-like mice. J Exp Med 2015;212(11): 1811–8.
94. Korin B, Ben-Shaanan TL, Schiller M, et al. High-dimensional, single-cell charac-terization of the brain's immune compartment. Nat Neurosci 2017;20(9):1300–9.
95. Mrdjen D, Pavlovic A, Hartmann FJ, et al. High-dimensional single-cell mapping of central nervous system immune cells reveals distinct myeloid subsets in health, aging, and disease. Immunity 2018;48(2):380–95.e6.
96. Ajami B, Samusik N, Wieghofer P, et al. Single-cell mass cytometry reveals distinct populations of brain myeloid cells in mouse neuroinflammation and neu-rodegeneration models. Nat Neurosci 2018;21(4):541–51.
97. Leipold MD, Obermoser G, Fenwick C, et al. Comparison of CyTOF assays across sites: results of a six-center pilot study. J Immunol Methods 2018;453: 37–43.
98. Blazkova J, Gupta S, Liu Y, et al. Multicenter systems analysis of human blood reveals immature neutrophils in males and during pregnancy. J Immunol 2017; 198(6):2479–88.
99. Sahaf B, Pichavant M, Lee BH, et al. Immune profiling mass cytometry assay harmonization: multi-center experience from CIMAC-CIDC. Clin Cancer Res Off J Am Assoc Cancer Res 2021;27(18):5062–71.
100. IMPACC Manuscript Writing Team, IMPACC Network Steering Committee. Im-munophenotyping assessment in a COVID-19 cohort (IMPACC): a prospective longitudinal study. Sci Immunol 2021;6(62):eabf3733.

Moving?

Make sure your subscription moves with you!

To notify us of your new address, find your **Clinics Account Number** (located on your mailing label above your name), and contact customer service at:

Email: **journalscustomerservice-usa@elsevier.com**

800-654-2452 (subscribers in the U.S. & Canada)
314-447-8871 (subscribers outside of the U.S. & Canada)

Fax number: **314-447-8029**

Elsevier Health Sciences Division
Subscription Customer Service
3251 Riverport Lane
Maryland Heights, MO 63043

*To ensure uninterrupted delivery of your subscription, please notify us at least 4 weeks in advance of move.

9780443182846